S0-EIY-455

COMPETITION IN THE HEALTH CARE SECTOR

Past, Present, and Future

Proceedings of a Conference Sponsored
by the Bureau of Economics,
Federal Trade Commission
March 1978

Edited by
Warren Greenberg, Ph.D.
Bureau of Economics
Federal Trade Commission

Aspen Systems Corporation
Germantown, Maryland
1978

Library of Congress Cataloging in Publication Data

Main entry under title:
Competition in the health care sector: past, present, and future.

Includes bibliographies and index.
1. Medical economics—United States—Congresses.
2. Competition—United States—Congresses.
I. Greenberg, Warren. II. United States.
Federal Trade Commission. Bureau of Economics.
RA410.53.C652 338.4′7′36210973 78-24573
ISBN 0-89443-081-5

Library of Congress Catalog Card Number: 78-24573
ISBN 0-89443-081-5

Printed in the United States of America

1 2 3 4 5

Table of Contents

Acknowledgments

I would like to thank former Director of the Bureau of Economics, Darius Gaskins, Jr., Commissioner of the Federal Trade Commission, Calvin Collier, and Chairman of the Federal Trade Commission, Michael Pertschuk, for their support given to me in conducting the conference and editing these proceedings. Michael Klass, Assistant Director, Economic Evidence, Bureau of Economics, also provided encouragement and allowed me time to complete these extra-curricular tasks. Finally, my secretary, Diane Hammond, went way beyond her secretarial duties and provided excellent administrative assistance.

I would also like to thank Bess Townsend of the Federal Trade Commission for her diligent editorial pen and Betsy Zichterman and Ron Lewis, Supervisor, of the Word Processing Center of the FTC's Bureau of Economics for their important contribution in typing the most difficult sections of this manuscript.

Summary

These Proceedings stem from a conference conducted by the Bureau of Economics, Federal Trade Commission (FTC), on June 1 and 2, 1977, in Washington, D.C. Attended by more than 600 people, the conference was an effort by the Bureau to explore and evaluate, with solicited papers from economists and social scientists, the role of competition in the health care sector.

The views expressed at the conference do not necessarily reflect the views of the Bureau of Economics or the FTC but, instead, consistent with the complexity of the subject, represent the diversity of viewpoints of the participants from the FTC, from HEW, academic institutions, labor, the private sector, and nonprofit institutions.

Furthermore, the papers differ in their use of technical jargon and mathematical exposition common to most economists, and language suitable for non-economists and public policy-makers. This schizophrenia is, in part, due to my instructions to the economist-authors to remain true to our profession while respecting the nontechnical background of most of the audience.

As with most gatherings of economists and social scientists, no unanimity was reached with respect to public policy toward health care. Indeed, the conference highlighted how much we do not know about the proper doses of competition which might be injected into this industry, although there were examples in many of the papers suggesting how competition—both price and nonprice—might be expanded.

The Proceedings are divided into four sections: (1) opening remarks and introduction, (2) competition in selected sectors, (3) insurance and alternative delivery systems, and (4) competition and regulation. In each section the main papers are followed by one, two, or three shorter comments. Although a broad range of topics is covered, the limits of conference time prevented the inclusion of several areas of wide interest such as the pharmaceutical, dental services, and para-physician services markets.

OPENING REMARKS AND INTRODUCTION

In his opening remarks FTC Chairman Michael Pertschuk stresses the importance of the health care industry, but acknowledges that the costs of health care are constraints of which we should be cognizant. Pertschuk suggests that health care can be classified as a business, but, nevertheless, the "concept" of competition in health care must be "responsibly explore[d]" by the FTC.

Theodore Cooper, former Assistant Secretary for Health, and current Dean of the Medical College and Provost for Medical Affairs, Cornell University, agrees that "economic factors" are important in health policy deliberations. Cooper does note, however, that the FTC emphasis on competition in the medical marketplace is at variance with that of Congress and the current Administration. Cooper also asserts that competition does exist in the health care sector—such as the competition for patient referrals—but differs from price competition usually envisioned by economists.

A central tenet of economic theory is that resources which produce goods and services will flow to the lines of endeavor in which the highest returns can be captured. All things held constant, an increase or decrease in the supply of goods or services will decrease or increase the price of the goods or services. In contrast, all things held constant, an increase or decrease in the demand for goods or services will increase or decrease the price of goods or services. These basic laws of supply and demand have such powerful predictive power that many economists believe their theoretical framework can be applied to any industry in the economy. Is the medical care industry or health care sector different? Are there market imperfections which inhibit the laws of supply and demand from operating and which make impossible the economists' goal of an optimal use of resources? If there are such restrictions, antitrust public policy, which has a pro-competitive bias, may be inappropriate for segments of the medical sector.

Mark Pauly answers yes, no, and maybe to the query "Is Medical Care Different?" depending on the extent of consumer experience with an illness or unexpected illness and the type and scope of medical care contacts with physicians. It is the absence of information of the appropriate price-quality level that is the most important "potential" difference between medical care and other goods. Burton Weisbrod, commenting on Pauly's paper, suggests that the usual efficiency criteria employed by economists are not necessarily adequate for the health industry; in his view health and medical care may be different because of the public's concern with distributional access (not usually considered by economists) rather than allocative efficiency. Further, Weisbrod contends that the difficulties consumers have in evaluating medical services should caution public policymakers that any goal of stimulating competition through more information should include both price *and* quality information to consumers.

COMPETITION IN SELECTED SECTORS

The imperfections of information are stressed again in "Competition among Physicians" by Frank Sloan and Roger Feldman. The authors devote a considerable portion of the paper to analyzing the extent to which physicians can create their own demand. Although any alleged ability of physicians to create their own demand must take into account a reduced net price that patients pay in the presence of insurance coverage, surely some of this alleged creation in noncovered physician services must be due, in part, to consumer ignorance. Sloan and Feldman use standard economic analysis—termed the neoclassical framework of economists—to evaluate previous economics literature on the ability of physicians to create their own demand. Although they conclude there is some empirical evidence to suggest that physicians can create their own demand, it is not clear that all explanatory variables are accounted for in order to make a definitive judgment.

Sloan and Feldman point to elements in the market for physicians' services that, in their opinion, might be deemed monopolistic. Advertising prohibitions have made "comparison shopping" difficult and may contribute to a wide dispersion of physician fees and consequent monopoly power. The role of the medical society's relationship with Blue Shield is suspect, whereas physician-promulgated relative value scale pricing techniques are found to be relatively innocuous. Finally, Sloan and Feldman remark on restrictions and licensing requirements of nonphysician providers, suggesting that they "often appear to serve the financial interest of physicians."

Uwe Reinhardt devotes most of his comment to the methodology, assumptions, and conclusions of the Sloan-Feldman exposition of the physician-induced demand controversy. Reinhardt perceives a bias toward the neoclassical or traditional school in the Sloan-Feldman paper as opposed to the Parkinsonian school which allow for increases in demand from factors other than changes in price. Demonstrating that econometric research will reach equivocal results in most cases, even a well-fitted equation (a significant positive partial correlation coefficient between physician fees and the physician-population ratio indicating a physician's ability to induce demand) will be clouded by the physician's ability to order ancillary services and diagnostic tests. Furthermore, even if econometric research could demonstrate that there is some market-determined limit to the physician's price-output policy (as there must be) one would not know whether or not the treatments delivered at that limit include useless services. Reinhardt concludes that "tracer analysis," which evaluates the *entire* treatment of various conditions under various alternatives, may be the best solution to understanding the physician-induced demand controversy.

Donald Yett, like Uwe Reinhardt, focuses on the Sloan-Feldman treatment of the physician's ability to create his own demand. Yett believes that complex socioeconomic variables associated with physician conduct make it difficult to isolate monopoly power even if significant partial correlations can be found between physician-population ratios and per capita utilization. Indeed, Yett is inclined to question all of Sloan and Feldman's empirical evidence which assumes monopoly power by the physician.

David Salkever concludes that competition does exist in the hospital services market but is "based primarily upon the availability and sophistication of services and facilities rather than price." Since this type of competition tends to raise rather than lower price, modifications in insurance arrangements, the financing mechanism that accounts for more than 90 percent of expenditures on hospital services, must be made in order to move toward a semblance of price competition. Salkever does caution, however, that even with a change in the amount and type of insurance, the role of the physician in admitting patients and the high degree of hospital concentration found in many local markets can impede competition.

John Rafferty endorses Salkever's view that a focus on insurance mechanisms for hospital reimbursement is the most important issue for competition among hospitals. Rafferty warns, however, that a stress on price-oriented competition may pose problems for maintaining a given level of quality care.

INSURANCE AND ALTERNATIVE DELIVERY SYSTEMS

When examining the performance of firms in an industry, most economists focus on the rates of return and output of the leading firms. Typically, the firms that are studied are those which have profit-maximizing incentives. In their paper, H. E. Frech and Paul Ginsburg analyze the not-for-profit firms. Frech and Ginsburg find that Blue Cross, because of its exemption from property and premium taxes in some States and its exemptions from required reserves and other regulatory requirements, have developed "administrative slack" in the operation of their Plans. Furthermore, Frech and Ginsburg maintain that because Blue Cross and Blue Shield are beholden to hospital and physician providers there are incentives for them to sell a more complete version of insurance than the commercial carriers. The effect of Blue Cross in the health insurance market is to raise hospital prices rather than control costs. Rising prices of hospital services are of serious concern and public policy, according to Frech and Ginsburg, should consider a removal of the advantages Blue Cross enjoys vis-a-vis the commercial insurers.

Not surprisingly, David Robbins of the Health Insurance Association of America commends the Frech-Ginsburg analysis since their policy prescriptions are generally to put Blue Cross on an equal footing with the commercial insurers. Robbins does suggest, however, that the Frech-Ginsburg paper leaves out a significant explanation of the market power of Blue Cross; *viz.*, the lower prices, compared to commercial insurers, that Blue Cross negotiates with hospitals for hospital services.

Administrative slack or inefficiency, allegedly shown by Frech-Ginsburg, is disputed by Blue Cross Association's Howard Berman. Berman cites a 1975 Government Accounting Office analysis which shows that commercial insurers are less efficient than Blue Cross, and a March 1976 *Social Security Bulletin* study which suggests that Blue Cross has the lowest ratio of operating expense as a portion of premium income of all insurers.

Insurance reduces the net price of services to the consumer; assuming the usual downward sloping demand curve, more services will be demanded in the presence of insurance than without insurance (although, of course, the consumer must bear the cost of increased premium rates in the long run). In addition, more services will be demanded at each of many possible prices which shifts the entire demand curve and raises prices of services. Joseph Newhouse concentrates on another effect of insurance, that of induced technological change, which tends to "increase the rate of medical care price and expenditure increases relative to the competitive market." Newhouse's model would predict a faster rate of price increase in services covered, in most part, by insurance compared to medical services less heavily covered by insurance. Newhouse claims that his results are consistent with the view that a competitive model has been eroded for hospital services (heavily covered by insurance) compared to physician, dental, and drug services less heavily covered by insurance. Therefore, Newhouse expects that hospital prices and expenditures could continue to increase at "above average" rates for a long period of time.

In their paper Lawrence Goldberg and Warren Greenberg examine competition that once existed in the 1930's among for-profit insurers before a physician-sponsored health insurance plan entered the market. This form of competition was based on cost control efforts that Goldberg and Greenberg relate in their description of insurance firms questioning the procedures and methods of physicians. They suggest that the emergence of a physician-sponsored health insurance plan, Oregon Physicians' Service, put an end to competitive cost control efforts by the private for-profit insurers.

A final paper in the session on Insurance, Competition, and Alternative Delivery Systems provides examples of how HMO's might compete and illustrations of competition among alternative delivery systems. Alain

Enthoven suggests that imperfections in the health industry are such that "simple generalizations" about the competitive impact of HMO's are "almost impossible to sustain." Enthoven does suggest that HMO's be put on an equal footing with fee-for-service and "the subsidy of more costly systems of care through Medicare, Medicaid, and the tax laws" be eliminated. In general, Enthoven believes that the government must take positive action to create a fair market test between the fee-for-service sector and alternative delivery systems.

Stuart Schweitzer, in reviewing the Goldberg-Greenberg and the Enthoven papers, citing a theory of economics known as the "Theory of the Second Best," cautions that injecting doses of competition in only sections of the complex health care industry might not lead to more efficiency in the entire industry. In addition, Schweitzer asserts that the Goldberg-Greenberg paper, which examines competition among for-profit insurers, and the Enthoven paper, which examines competition between health maintenance organizations and the fee-for-service sector, although both "thoughtful" and "carefully drawn," suffer from an absence of empirical evidence which would shed light on their plausibility.

COMPETITION AND REGULATION

The final section of the volume addresses the policy alternatives of competition and regulation in the health care sector. To what extent might these policies complement or conflict with each other in achieving quality care at reasonable cost? Economists have a predisposition toward competition; yet, if enough imperfections exist in the market, regulation can conceivably be a preferable "second-best" alternative. To achieve a broad spectrum of discussion, this section consists of a varied set of papers from scholars and practitioners of different perspectives and persuasions.

Clark Havighurst espouses the view that more competition and less restrictive regulation would be the desired remedy to control health care costs and deliver the health care mix desired by consumers. He contends that the existence of laws which exempt health care premiums paid by employers from taxation acts as an incentive to employers to provide more health care benefits than are desired by consumers. Furthermore, Havighurst advocates strict enforcement of antitrust laws and the use of trade regulation rules by the FTC to discourage boycotts by medical societies and physicians of those insurance companies monitoring physician procedures. According to Havighurst, one of the most important endeavors that the antitrust authorities can undertake is to strengthen the market mechanism to enable the for-profit insurers to control costs.

In contrast to Havighurst's relatively sanguine view of the role of competition in the health sector, Stuart Altman and Sanfrod Weiner embrace a more skeptical approach. They claim that existing incentives and laws make a return to market forces in health impossible; hence, public regulation must be the inevitable "second best" alternative. But, claim the authors, regulation which controls output rather than encouraging changes in physician and hospital incentives will not be fruitful. The most important way that incentives should be changed is an explicit organizational strategy that concentrates on behavior within the hospitals.

The final paper deals with the similarities of the 17th century guilds and present-day licensure and restrictive practices of the medical profession. Lee Benham believes that the guild philosophy is "still accepted in our attitude toward the role of competition, production and dissemination of information, and consumer choice." Benham is not hopeful about changing the effects of the guild system; rather, he believes that the benefits of the system will go to those most able to muster political support.

The comments in the session on competition and regulation seem to be as varied as the institutions represented by the participants. John Pisarkiewicz, Jr., a member of the Federal Trade Commission staff, strongly endorses Havighurst's call for market forces and vigorous competition in this industry. But he adds a cautionary note when he suggests that the theoretical underpinnings of a free market for health care may be difficult to achieve in practice. Jesse Steinfeld, Dean of the School of Medicine, Medical College of Virginia, reiterated the view of many of the participants, suggesting that if our goal is improved health, emphasis should be on health education, exercise, avoidance of tobacco, and other preventive techniques. In addressing the issue of competition, Steinfeld claims that competition exists in a form not considered by others at this Conference. There is, for instance, competition among students to be admitted to professional schools and competition among researchers to discover the causes of various diseases. Competition as a policy option of the Federal Government should only be pursued as part of an overall national health policy.

Richard Shoemaker, Assistant Director, Department of Social Security, AFL-CIO, comments on the Havighurst paper by denying the "semblance of a market at all in the health industry." For example, the medical profession is a monopoly in the medical marketplace which prevents a free play of competitive forces. Shoemaker believes that the antitrust laws should be applied to this monopoly—one of the most important endeavors, in his opinion, that the FTC could undertake.

Harold Cohen, Director, Health Services Cost Review Commission, State of Maryland, agrees with Altman and Weiner's paper that the effectiveness of regulation depends on changing the incentives of hospitals, physicians, and—Cohen adds—local regulators. Cohen concludes by suggesting that Altman and Weiner's case for regulation as a "second best" is not made. In fact, he says the potential physician dominance of regulation may make it the "first worst."

Although endorsing competition as the most desirable method of resource allocation, Anne Somers, Professor, Department of Community Medicine, Rutgers Medical School, suggests two characteristics of the health care industry which might make this industry respond differently to doses of competition. First, for the most of the medical care sector, the economist's assumption of the sovereign consumer is, in reality, a myth. Second, the government is "inextricably involved in virtually every aspect of the decisionmaking." Like Steinfeld, Somers believes the answer to quality care at lowest possible cost lies in a large-scale cooperative public-private effort and not necessarily in competition or regulation.

A FINAL STATEMENT

Are there themes common to the 10 papers and 12 comments on the state—past, present, and future—of competition in the health care sector? Can some tentative conclusions be reached? Although strict unanimity is absent, I suggest the following as possible findings:

(1) Competition does exist in the health care sector, but it is not necessarily the type of competition that exists in other industries or is helpful in restraining monopoly power. For example, competition may take the form of new, and perhaps better, equipment and technical apparatus, without regard to cost considerations. Competition which tends to control the cost of medical care is not as apparent but it did exist once in the State of Oregon and might exist between HMO's and the fee-for-service sector.

(2) There are several reasons for atypical competition in the health care industry. Among them are the pervasive influence of government, the special role of the physician, and other peculiar characteristics of the industry. These latter characteristics include the lack of information from providers and the existence of insurance which reduces prices to consumers of health care services. Finally, the uncertainty surrounding medical care is so great that physicians themselves are unsure of many outcomes.

(3) Although the health care industry may not conform to the economist's ideal of competitive behavior, there were no obvious answers as to what form appropriate public policy might take. However, most observers believe that, even in view of the health industry's special characteristics, antitrust has, at least, some place in public policy. At the same time most authors believe that current public policy, with its

emphasis on regulation, is not working optimally and the desired amount of government intervention has not yet been found.

(4) Finally, there was a strong consensus that more research is needed on competition in the health care industry. Most papers reflect the lack of empirical work on this industry and are only strong beginning steps toward a better understanding of competition in the health care sector.

* * *

This is a staff report, prepared by the Commission's Bureau of Economics. The Commission has not adopted the report in whole or in part. Hence, all statements, conclusions, and recommendations contained herein are solely those of the staff responsible for its preparation.

* * *

Part One

Opening Remarks and Introduction

Remarks

Michael Pertschuk
Chairman, Federal Trade Commission

As everyone must know, it's not easy to get a handle on the economics of health care, much less focus on the specific issue of competition. While there are examples of more flexibility in the field of physician training and practice—doctors' unions, prepaid group practices, community health cooperatives, free clinics, and so on—we have to admit that the practice of medicine remains one of the last strongholds of private entrepreneurship. Despite the large infusion of Federal, State, and local tax money into medical care, the physician population still operates with rather remarkable independence.

But physicians ought not to be singled out either for special honor or opprobrium. The entire health community—the *health industry,* if you will—has become the object of careful scrutiny by the public guardians of the country's trust and treasure. We all need the health industry so very much; it's not an overstatement to say that our lives depend on a strong, vigorous, responsive health industry. But not at any price. *Not at any price.*

That is our issue today and tomorrow. Accessible and affordable quality health care is something every American has come to expect. How many times in the past several years have consumers spoken of the "right" to quality health care, as if it were the same as the right to education or to police and fire protection? Yet, those other essential public services are supported out of a general tax base and are administered by officials subject to the rule of the ballot box.

No such controls are the rule in the health sector. Quite the contrary. The money is generated in a variety of ways: third-party payments, Government subsidies, reinsurance guarantees, private fund-raising, complex tax incentives, and old-fashioned cash fees for service.

The providers of care are generally not public officials. They are answerable primarily to their colleagues—and there is great suspicion that such accountability is more apparent than real. We know we need them—but we also know that, thus far, we have failed to control the escalating costs of the health care they provide.

The Federal Trade Commission is not a health or medical agency. To paraphrase a President who was hardly our patron saint, Calvin Coolidge, "the business of the FTC is business." And we recognize, along with most Americans, that the delivery of health care is business, an industry of vast proportions and vital effect. Health care has become our business. I have no apologies for that; in fact, one might ask, "What took the FTC this long?"

An answer to that is embarrassingly simple: The Commission—like most other agencies of Government—was slow to admit that one possible way to control the seemingly uncontrollable health sector could be to treat it as a business and make it respond to the same marketplace influences as other American businesses and industries.

> Is it possible, for example, to give enough information to patients so that they may shop for the best care at the lowest price they can afford?
>
> Is it possible to promote prevention and wise self-care as an alternative to costly reparative medicine and high-priced prescription drugs and devices?
>
> Can health care be marketed under all the requirements for full disclosure and non-deception that other marketed services must fulfill?
>
> Would Gresham's Law dominate a health marketplace in which providers compete on terms both of price and quality?

We don't know the answers. No one—whether American or foreign-born—has experienced such a marketplace. Yet, of all the societies on earth today, ours would seem to be the only one that could still inject competition into the provisions of health care, allow prices to respond to consumer demand, and maintain standards of quality care that reduce or even eliminate the risk of death or disability.

The FTC is now in the process of receiving documents subpoenaed from the American Medical Association and certain State and local medical societies. Our intention is to learn how self-regulation—professional control over voluntary and State agencies—really works. There is reasonable doubt that the medical profession, by itself or through friendly State governments, is completely open to innovation, competition, quality control, or consumer choice. We are also beginning the same process with the American Dental Association and several of the ADA's State and local affiliates.

We may conclude, one day in the future, that self-regulation—however inadequate—is better than strong Government regulation. There is serious doubt that the Civil Aeronautics Board has been a boon to passengers. And after nearly 10 years of piled-on law and regulation, the Medicare and Medicaid programs have benefited the providers of health care as much—and in some cases more—than they have benefited patients. Certainly Secretary Joseph Califano has indicated as much in the recent HEW reorganization which produced a new Health Care Financing Administration with a specific mission: to control the costs of Medicare and Medicaid before they completely control the rest of *us*.

But it is far too early to draw any rigid conclusions. Those of us who sit on the Commission know that competition in the health sector is a concept we must responsibly explore. Our minds are open to the ideas that will come from such ground-breaking conferences as this one. I want to thank the many people who are coming together with us today and tomorrow to give of their time, their ideas, and their good will. I was delighted to learn from Warren that the fees charged by the lawyers and economists on our program are still lower than the fees charged by the physicians we are all talking about. Maybe the reason lies in the fact that there is still no "competition industry" that sets its own high fees. But it would be dreadful if, several years from now, the FTC has to run another conference on "competition in the health care *competition* industry." We would have only ourselves to blame.

Remarks

Theodore Cooper, M.D.
Dean, Medical College and Provost for Medical Affairs, Cornell University

I have often dreamed of being turned loose in a field of economists, particularly health economists. Forget what I would have done were I turned loose—I suppose it would have depended on the time. Nevertheless, over a period of time, I have come to be a fan of many economists and I have developed an admiration for the discipline. I suppose I agree with the famous statement of John M. Keynes (p. 383) that "the ideas of economists and political philosophers both when they are right and when they are wrong are more powerful than is commonly understood. Indeed the world is ruled by little else. Practical men who believe themselves to be quite exempt from any intellectual influences, are usually the slaves of some defunct economist."

Grudgingly, I have to admit that one can no longer discuss health policy without an appreciation of the importance of economic factors. It is my fervent hope that economists who aspire to be health policymakers will come to appreciate the importance of the medical factors. Therefore, I am delighted to appear on this program—certainly not as a spokesman for medicine (and certainly not as a spokesman for the Administration) and not as a spokesman for the consumer—but at least as a token, a symbol, a recognition—that important discussions on health matters should include the direct participation of the profession—preferably the practicing profession (in contradiction to myself).

We in medicine have learned that the public can understand a great deal, even about technical matters, when decisions have to be made, and that even if the patient does not wish to choose himself or herself, he or she wants to know what is being chosen and wants to be consulted. In a like manner, you in other fields of expertise who are diagnosing the ills of the medical profession need to be sure that your key consultations include the consumers and health professionals, for your remedies need to be "doable" even if not emotionally or philosophically acceptable to the profession. How many times have I seen proposals containing "neat" ideas, some of which become law or regulations that prove to be impractical monstrosities and, though generated from the highest motives, become ineffective and inefficient programs. And to be "doable," you must seek the evaluation and participation of those who actually do the service. Theoreticians are needed to help formulate strategies, but practitioners are needed to see the limits and deficiencies and practitioners are needed to put the plan in action.

The political and technical discussions about health policy will contine to expand (and, since they will be in larger and larger spaces, will follow the gas laws). The concern is largely how much money is being spent; it used to be that the discussions were tempered by statements of progress and concerns for quality and perhaps how much service. Now even that rhetoric is largely gone or, if present, largely distorted. It is now only the amount of money that is of concern, and the drive comes from the fact that 40 percent of the money comes from *public* sources.

Speeches are made about the fact that nine cents of every Federal dollar goes for care in the field of health. Apparently that is too much. What is satisfactory and why? I am not sure I understand the criteria. What are the criteria by which we determine the proper Federal role?

It certainly seems that the Federal Trade Commission has views on this fundamental question which differ by about 180 degrees from those of Congress and the present Administration. Whereas the FTC appears to seek to have market forces direct the performance of the health professions, the governmental forces seek to control the professions; for example, by stipulating the mix of specialties, by limiting payments, by directing the allocation of capital improvements. That is not free trade—that is restraint of trade. The reason for mentioning it in this setting is that we will hear about "competition" (a free enterprise term) and that should include the meaning of "competition" for the public dollar. When I used to point out solemnly that our national expenditures in health were exceeding 8 percent of GNP, the public audiences, the consumers, if you will, yawned.

On the other hand, I have been told more than once by well-informed, educated persons that he or she went to the doctor and got an examination, tests, X-rays for about $150-$200 and, to their apparent chagrin, nothing was wrong. Hence, the fee was outrageous. I suppose if something bad was found, the fee would appear reasonable.

I have heard very often that the relief of pain in the chest or restoring the ability to swallow, or the relief of indigestion was "worth a million dollars." That turns out to be a figure of speech. Rarely does such a feeling remain when it is time to pay the bill or part of the bill. Of course, the altered response is greater if the net result proves not to meet the patient's expectation. But these are predictable human responses. It is why lawyers who take criminal cases often want the fee ahead of time.

Comments such as these are usually brushed aside in "serious" conferences like this one, yet an appreciation of the facts is fundamental to the personal participation of providers and of the consumer of services in the health field. And if you want competition to work you have to understand the reasons why people use the services. Relatively few people (in my opinion) seek services to stay well. Most seek services to remove a real or perceived complaint—an abnormality. It is a bit much for experts (usually well) to contend that 75 percent of visits to physicians are "not needed." It is also interesting, but often not cogent, to assert that there are too many unnessary hospitalizations. What is meant by "unnecessary" in the theoretical land of "if" is that when one reviews the longitudinal history of an encounter, one concludes (from the vantage point of the reviewers) that the issue could have or should have been dealt with in some other way. We cannot continue to make the citizenry health conscious, disease concerned, symptom aware and expect them not to seek some attention. We cannot continue to tell workers and beneficiaries that they are entitled to more health benefits (in lieu of income), to sell them multiple insurance policies that encourage the use of in-patient resources, and then say we didn't mean for it to cost money. We cannot continue to insist on more dignified personal care with only single or double rooms, with high density nursing, better food service, and the "best and newest" of equipment, higher wages for staff and then say we should be able to have these improvements at a standard price that is different from that of prices in the rest of the economy. And we cannot continue to enfold new social problems into the medical care system for their attention (like new programs at hospitals for compulsive gamblers) and expect service costs to go down.

By the way, if my memory serves me correctly, the escalation of costs of the programs of other nations is not really below that of the United States, even though they spend less per capita.

Where "competition" fits in the scheme of things is unclear. If this conference can clarify that issue, it will be a great success. If it can explain how competition should work for the doctor, the patient, the hospital, it will be an extraordinary achievement. If it gives new ideas, it will be a milestone.

I assume that most people will concentrate on price competition, perhaps as envisioned by HMO advocates or prepaid plan enthusiasts or those who advocate prospectively negotiated fixed fees, as a mechanism for containing cost. And in some regards I suspect patients will consider these approaches and be willing to choose between price differentials—if they can understand why one "care plan" is cheaper than another. *Nevertheless,* there is a tendency of the public to be suspicious of reduced costs and cut rates in health care. Indeed, they often equate higher prices with better quality of care.

I hope we also hear about other forms of competition in the health field because, in my view, there is some pretty intense competition in the practice of the health professions in the area of patient referrals.

There is considerable interest in retaining patients by offering quality service in locations that are more accessible. Patients are attracted to physicians and dentists and others by what they know or hear of the capability of the person or group (i.e., reputation), and the patients will choose on this basis. It is not likely that many will choose on price, particularly when a third party is paying the bills.

Obviously, (1) making more health professionals, including doctors, has not satisfied those who proposed this maneuver as a cornerstone of policy; (2) lowering financial barriers to access has not suited more critics; (3) building more facilities has been indicted as an evil; (4) allaying ignorance through research and improving service through technology now appear to some to have been a bad thing to do.

What, then, can bring this great system back into consonance with those who expect more from it—for less?

Perhaps we need more *competition,* but the competition should probably come from those sectors of the economy that hold the real key to health—those sectors that control the standard of living.

REFERENCE

J. M. Keynes, *The General Theory of Employment, Interest and Money,* New York 1936.

Is Medical Care Different?

*Mark V. Pauly**
Professor of Economics, Northwestern University

As the title suggests, this paper will address the question of whether medical care is different from other goods and services, in the sense that a different kind of analysis or different kinds of supply and demand models are appropriate for medical care. At present, in the literature the answer to this question is a definite "yes." Both Selma Mushkin and Kenneth Arrow have argued that medical care is indeed different from other goods and services. Broadly speaking, the differences they list can be grouped under three headings: (1) greater *uncertainty* on the part of demanders; (2) *risk* associated with the random occurrence of illness; and (3) *absence of profit-seeking behavior* by providers of care. Arrow goes on to assert that these intrinsic differences explain the peculiar organization of the real-world medical care industry, with its set of governmental and quasi-governmental restrictions.[1]

In what follows I will assert that reality and theory are actually much less forthright than this literature suggests. I will not even say that the appropriate answer to the question is "yes or no"; it is rather, "yes, no, and maybe." In particular, I want to argue (1) that yes, there are currently some kinds of medical care and some kinds of situations in which the economist can use the same or similar methods of analysis as he uses for other industries reasonably well; but (2) no, there are other kinds of medical care for which the usual tools are not appropriate; while (3) there may be still other kinds of medical care for which competition (or more precisely an analogue to competition), and the usual analysis of competition, might not work perfectly, but might work reasonably well.

Competition currently may not work here because of restrictions on the

* I am grateful to Uwe Reinhardt, Gerald Goldstein, Barry Friedman, and members of the student-faculty seminar at Northwestern for suggesting a number of ideas and saving me from a number of errors. Remaining errors are my own.

actions of some of the participants. I also need to sound a pessimistic note, however; because we have not yet developed the appropriate method to handle group (3), and because that group may be large, we are at present nearly powerless to make any useful normative a priori statements, or many useful positive ones, about much of the medical-care sector. I will suggest that Arrow's assertion that the special characteristics of the industry arise from attempts to achieve optimality is at least open to serious question. I will also consider the effect of insurance coverage and supplier motivation on the distinctiveness of this industry. The main emphasis, however, will be on uncertainty, both because it seems most distinctive, and because the peculiarities on the supply side may not arise from anything intrinsic to the activity of supplying medical care, but, rather, from the way the supply side has adapted to uncertainty-generated restrictions on demand.

In what follows, I will first make some important distinctions among types of medical care. Then I will indicate why the economist's use of the competitive model as a tool of analysis is useful for some kinds of care, but why neither it nor the orthodox analyses of what to do when competition is absent is appropriate for other kinds of care.

TYPES OF MEDICAL CARE

It is, I believe, a grave mistake to try to characterize all of the services we lump under the general name of "medical care" in a similar way. There are several groupings of those services which should be distinguished: One may, for example, group by the extent of consumer experience.

Group (1)—Services which are purchased relatively frequently by most households.

Group (2)—Services a typical producer produces relatively frequently but which a typical consumer can consume relatively infrequently, perhaps once in a lifetime.

Group (3)—Services which a typical producer produces and a typical consumer consumes relatively infrequently.

In group (1) I would include such services as pediatric care, normal deliveries (especially after the first child), most of routine dental cavity repair and prevention, prescription drugs for common or chronic conditions, most non-prescription drugs, and routine care for persons with chronic conditions. In group (2) I would include such procedures as appendectomies, hysterectomies, hospitalization for acute gastrointestinal distress, pneumonia and many other common reasons for hospitalization. In group (3) I would include experimental and unusual procedures, including most of those undertaken in severe medical emergencies. There are no clear dividing lines among these groups, but rather various shades of gradation; the general notion of the distinctions should be clear.

There is another kind of threefold classification that will also be relevant for the following discussion. Some kinds of medical care are what might be called "diagnostic"; the critical elements are (1) the "care" consists primarily of information but (2) this information is usually peculiar to particular individuals. What one purchases is not a statement of what kinds of symptoms or test results are generally related to what kinds of conditions, but rather an assessment of what *his* symptoms and test results suggest. Another kind of care is what may be called "prescriptive-informative." This consists of general statements on the outcome of various courses of treatment on individuals with a particular diagnosis. Information is also being purchased here, but it is of somewhat more general nature than in the first case. How general it is depends on whether the diagnosis is common or rare. The third classification of care is that which is "active-therapeutic." This involves some time-consuming action by the provider: administration of an injection, a surgical procedure, or a normal delivery. Most medical-care contacts will have elements of some or all of these three types, but, again, the conceptual distinction among them will be useful.

ECONOMIC ANALYSIS AND INDUSTRY DIFFERENCES

With these distinctions in mind, let us turn to considering the types of analysis that might be applied. An economic analysis of an industry usually involves both positive and normative discussion, although the ultimate purpose for worrying about competition is normative. In positive analysis the critical characteristic of the "typical" industry is that suppliers maximize profit, or something analogous to profit. The normative question is usually couched in terms of efficiency or Pareto optimality. The strategy is usually to inquire whether competition is feasible, and, if it is, whether a competitive equilibrium would be efficient. If efficiency could be achieved, suggested Government intervention takes the form of insuring that the competitive preconditions are (approximately) present. If competitive equilibrium is infeasible, or if production with a large number of sellers would not be efficient, suggested intervention is usually the public utility model, with Government enforced barriers to entry and price regulation.

The primary reason for departure from the competitive model is the possible existence of unexploited economies of scale or of natural monopoly. In medical care, economies of scale are generally not important. In some rural markets natural monopoly may still occur, and hospitals probably display increasing returns to scale over some small sizes. In the urban and suburban areas in which the great bulk of the population lives, economies of scale either in ambulatory or hospital care are probably not very important, except for uncommon specialized procedures. Likewise, in such areas the number of sellers of medical services is large, again, except for the rare specialized service. On these grounds, then, the competitive market, with all of its nice optimality properties, should be expected to emerge once any governmental or cartel restrictions are removed.[2]

The missing condition in the medical care industry is surely not the absence of large numbers of sellers and buyers in most markets or for most types of care. Rather, if there is a missing condition, it is the absence of *consumer information.* The problem is even more complex. What consumers buy, in their diagnostic or prescriptive-informative transactions, is primarily information itself to be used in guiding future transactions. So we have a multiproduct industry in which the quality, quantity, and characteristics or content of one of the products—information—affects the demand of other products.

Consumer ignorance would have two consequences for efficiency. First, it may prevent the emergence of competitive equilibrium, because a seller may continue to sell some output even if his price is higher or his quality lower than that of some other sellers; firm demand curves are not perfectly elastic. Second, without any information necessary to determine quality, consumers may be purchasing a quality level lower than the utility-maximizing one.

So there are two alleged differences on the demand side between medical care and a typical industry: (1) Consumers are not informed and (2) what is demanded is not a typical commodity, but is information itself. We do have an attempt to analyze the medical-care industry which does make specific and clear reference to these characteristics: Arrow's classic article. I will argue that, where it is applicable, Arrow's discussion is unhelpful and possibly misleading in answering the question of appropriate analysis. I will assert that the appropriate analysis is surely more difficult, and certainly less conclusive, than what Arrow presents. While this is a negative conclusion, it is surely desirable, at this conference, to face up to the difficulties we are likely to encounter.

CONSUMER INFORMATION ABOUT TYPES OF MEDICAL CARE

It is generally alleged that consumers of medical care are very poorly informed. Karen Davis, for example, presents a typical argument:

> The nature of health care is such that the consumer knows very little about the medical services he or she is buying—possibly less than about any other service purchased. Some choices about

> medical care are made solely by patients. But a very large part of the decision making is done by physicians — diagnosis, treatment, drugs and tests, hospitalization, frequency of return visits are all substantially under the physician's control. . . . While the consumer can participate in policing the market, that participation is much more limited than in almost any other area of private economic activity. (Karen Davis, pp. 22, 23.)

The surprising thing about this statement, considering its strength, is that no evidence is provided, nor is there any suggestion as to how large a part is "a very large part." The statement that consumers are not well-informed about medical care may seem so obvious as not to require empirical documentation. But I will argue that things are not so easy.

Some information about the price and quality of medical care is costly, but it does not necessarily follow that consumers are poorly informed about all types of care. For some types, information may be relatively cheap (and so relatively extensively obtained). For some types, individuals may generate a substantial amount of information as a by-product of other activities. We do acquire a considerable amount of information simply by random contacts as consumers or as observers. For instance, a person who uses a particular physician's services necessarily acquires some information from the experience he has with the outcomes of those services. He may well want to incur costs to obtain additional information, even to the extent of purchasing more services than he otherwise would to generate more information, but it is possible that he may "automatically" be well informed.

Most of medical care, like most services, is an experience rather than a search good, to use Philip Nelson's terminology. Still, there may be some information on price or quality obtainable by search at relatively low cost. A consumption unit can tap not only its experience, but also the experience of friends. If each household's experience provides a relatively good estimate of quality, a given household can have both an idea of the quality of provider it is currently using, and, by contacting friends at a nominal cost, a good idea of the quality and price of some other providers as well.[3] If people select the highest quality provider for a given price in the subset of providers on which they have information, each household is likely eventually to become informed about high quality providers, so that information will become fairly complete. Of course, not all persons have friends, and so not all persons will face a low price for information. But, as has been suggested by Steven Salop, and by Sanford Grossman and Joseph Stiglitz, if enough people are well-informed, the remainder can appropriately judge quality by price and so there is no need for them to become well-informed.

It is not possible in this study to provide a definite measure of the types of medical care on which consumers are reasonably well informed. No large-scale empirical work has been done on this question; "reasonably well-informed" (like workable competition) is not even easy to define. However, I believe that it is possible to offer some numerical conjectures about that portion of total national health expenditure that might, as a starting point, be suggested as impossible to disprove as being the "reasonably well-informed" portion. Roughly, these types would be ones for which individual consumption units are likely to have fairly extensive experience, or whose outcomes are easy to judge either during or soon after the performance of the service.

In another sense, these estimates may understate the extent of reasonably well-informed purchases. Referrals from a primary care physician are the primary determinant of type of provider for many of those procedures with which an individual consumer does not have extensive experience.

If the consumer does have a reasonable amount of information on the quality of referrals provided by the primary care physician, he may still be effectively informed. This point will be discussed more extensively later.

Approximately what fraction of total medical-care spending goes for the types of care described above? Of all non-hospital physician visits, approximately 10 percent were made to pediatricians in 1971. About 10 percent of all other visits were for general checkup, immunization and vaccination, or pre- or post-natal care. Half of all physician visits were made for chronic conditions. While there is surely some overlap between these categories, it seems reasonable to conclude that at least half of ambulatory care physician visits are made by persons who might be reasonably well informed. On average, physicians spend approximately one-quarter to one-third of their time at the hospital; physicians' services were about 23 percent of all health-care spending,[4] so "informed" ambulatory care physician purchases are about 8 percent of total spending (.5x.75.x.23). For hospital care, about 10 percent of all discharges are for normal delivery, and this is about 5 percent of total spending. Total expenditure on all drugs was 10 percent of total personal health-care expenditures in 1973, and a reasonable approximation of the well-informed part would be about 5 percent. Routine dental care would add perhaps another 4 percent. A final, and somewhat more questionable category, is that of nursing home care which is about 7 percent. In total, then, perhaps one-fourth or more of total personal health-care expenditures might be regarded as "reasonably informed." [5]

I do not contend that consumer information is perfect; for most final consumption goods that is rarely so. What I suggest is that information is sufficiently extensive to permit an outcome at least as close to the competitive equilibrium as might occur with other "usual" services. This is not to imply that the information could not be improved; removal of institutional barriers to information might still produce an improvement in welfare, though that improvement need not be very large.

What might one mean by a "reasonably" or "appropriately" well-informed purchaser? The consumer seeks informaton on both price and quality. There appears to be no important intrinsic difference between medical care and other industries in generating or transmitting price information. Of course, existing laws prohibiting advertising may limit actual consumer knowledge of prices, and there may be some questions of product homogeneity which need to be answered for valid comparisons. The critical uncertainty is that about *quality*—both the quality of therapeutic performance, and the quality (accuracy) of diagnostic or prescriptive information. Without such information available to consumers, sellers can perhaps continue to sell even if they raise prices above the "going" level because they can convince consumers that they provide higher quality or because the customers of the seller who raises prices would prefer paying a higher price for a more certain level of quality rather than using a lower priced service whose quality is more uncertain.

It may be so obvious that consumers are ignorant about medical care quality as not to require proof. It is important to note, however, that there are two reasons why it is not the *total* amount of perceived consumer ignorance that is relevant to a discussion of the desirability and feasibility of competition. First, not everyone agrees on how quality is to be defined or measured. In particular, the qualities that particular consumers value may not be the qualities that experts measure. So consumers may not seek information about qualities which are irrelevant to them, appear to the experts to be uninformed, and yet be appropriately informed.

The second, and more important, reason is that everyone, including the experts, is imperfectly informed on much of medical care quality. Quality could be defined as the relationship between various characteristics of the medical-care process and differences in health outcomes. Consumers do not know, for example, whether board-certified surgeons are likely to produce better outcomes than non-board-certified ones, whether tonsillectomy on average improves children's health, or whether a particular laboratory test is useful. Consumers cannot evaluate quality. *But neither can anyone else.* No one knows whether board certification, tonsillectomies, or some lab tests will improve health outcomes or not. I would argue that much of the uncertainty that the consumer has about medical care quality, even (or especially) in the narrow sense of the relationships between characteristics and expected health outcome, is of this type.

In this sense, medical care is different from many other goods: The relationship of use of the good to the outcome is much more certain for, say, sugar or baking powder, than it is for medical care. It is this *irreducible* uncertainty that we often think of, *but this kind of uncertainty may be mostly irrelevant to any notion of competition.* (It is necessarily relevant only in the sense that some form of insurance may be desirable to deal with it.) The kind of uncertainty that is relevant is that which represents information about quality which the seller has but the buyer does not. Arrow has, of course, remarked on this asymmetry of information, noting that it is information about outcome (what will happen), not process (how things work) which is relevant. One should add, however, that there may not be more *reducible* intrinsic uncertainty in this type of medical care than elsewhere. For the types of care discussed in this section, there may still be considerable ignorance (say, about whether well-baby checkups really make a difference). But this is primarily irreducible uncertainty.

Paradoxically, for irreducible uncertainty to be irrelevant, it is necessary not only that consumers know that they are ignorant, but also that they know that those from whom they purchase are ignorant as well. For example, consumer uncertainty about the indications for tonsillitis or the value of board certification will not interfere with the proper functioning of the market if and only if consumers know that physician experts are themselves ignorant on these questions. The physician must not be able to persuade the consumer that medical knowledge is greater than it actually is. The ironic conclusion is that one of the most useful types (and probably one of the least expensive types) of information that could be provided to patients is information on what is *not* known by medical science and physicians.

CONSUMER IGNORANCE AND SECOND BEST

Another type of care is that which occurs rarely for any individual, so that his own experience, or even that of his necessarily limited contacts and friends, conveys relatively little information. Without incurring costs which are large enough to matter, he cannot become very well informed. At least at present, markets in this type of care may depart considerably from the competitive one. How much of currently observed consumer ignorance is intrinsic to the service and how much is due to the present set of institutional arrangements is unknown. We do not even know how great the extent of ignorance is. It does seem clear, however, that (a) with sufficient expenditure of real resources, any purchaser could become well informed but (b) information is sufficiently costly that it would not pay to become approximately well informed. The fundamental problem is that we have no notion, or even a suspicion, of what the equilibria in markets with imperfectly informed consumers would be like, and what is more important, whether there are institutional restrictions that could be put on the market to improve matters. (We do not even know if equilibrium necessarily exists.) As it stands, we can show that almost anything could be optimal, but we cannot show that anything actually is. Some examples: Restricting consumer choice is ordinarily not desirable. As will be shown, however, if information itself is costly, barring types of outputs or types of providers that few people would choose anyway may be cheaper and more desirable than providing information. A second example: It is ordinarily desirable that potential purchasers know prices. But if it is cheap to become informed about price, but expensive to become informed about quality, it is possible that more consumers may mistakenly purchase lower priced but even inappropriately lower quality care when price information is available than would occur if provision of information on price or quality were limited, as by advertising restrictions. Some information may be worse than no information.[6] All these things could occur, and a priori reasoning cannot distinguish the real from the possible. This is equivalent to saying that we are dealing with a second best problem, with imperfect markets, imperfect consumers, and an imperfect regulator. What is the appropriate method of analysis?

Arrow has considered this problem most directly in his paper. He begins by stating the two fundamental theorems of welfare economics: (1) Competitive equilibrium is Pareto optimal, and (2) every Pareto optimum is a competitive equilibrium for some distribution of income. He then argues that medical care is different: Because of lack of consumer information and the absence of markets, principally in insurance, the present peculiar institutional arrangements have arisen to improve matters. "The special structural characteristics of the medical-care market are largely attempts to overcome the lack of optimality. . . ."

While this is surely possible, the problem is that such arrangements do not *necessarily* improve matters; we have no assurance that these characteristics really are attempts by politicians and medical trade associations to do what the welfare economist would suggest. Where the market would achieve competitive equilibrium, we know that public intervention *could not* improve matters. When it seems reasonable to suppose that the market would not satisfy the usual competitive conditions, we only know that public intervention *might* improve matters. But it is a big step from "might" to "will."

Whether lack of consumer information provides an explanation for existing institutional arrangements, with competitive restrictions as an unfortunate by-product, or whether it simply furnishes an excuse for what would otherwise be unacceptable use of Government to preserve monopoly, is impossible to say. Arrow is misleading in arguing that "the first step in the analysis of the medical-care market is a comparison between the actual market and the competitive model." The competitive model is irrelevant to an analysis of the medical-care market; the relevant comparison is between the actual market and what equilibria could be achieved under alternative institutional arrangements.[7] In such a world, welfare economics cannot furnish reasons; it can only furnish excuses. While it is surely true that the optimal equilibrium might be achieved by chance, or by a government mystically endowed with the appropriate knowledge and incentives, the relevant model is one in which information has a real cost, and all organizations face the same information production technology.

What is obviously necessary, and has not been developed, by Arrow or anyone else, is a theory which shows why and how welfare-increasing restrictions would be expected to emerge from the interaction of self-interested providers and consumers. That is, we need a theory to explain why and how a desirable "social contract" would be expected to be chosen. One can, of course, invoke the vague notion that whenever Pareto optimal moves exist, institutions will emerge to facilitate these moves, but any satisfactory explanation would surely require more. One would like to know, for example, whether the circumstances surrounding the Abraham Flexner report (or the medieval medical guilds) might reasonably be interpreted as the welfare economist's social contract. One would also want a theory to predict what specific *kinds* of restrictions would be expected to emerge from such bargaining: What are the desirable "constitutional" rules?

The second-best model is more relevant; it is also enormously more difficult. I will argue that without developing it, we are really fighting with shadows, and may cheapen what work we do perform. One of the attractive features of the competitive model is that strong welfare predictions can be derived without information on what demand and production functions look like. We shall not get off nearly so cheaply here; whether or not a rearrangement can improve matters depends on the actual magnitudes of costs and benefits. One important element in the development of such a theory is the notion that the configuration of equilibrium depends upon the empirical technology for the production of information.

Searching for Price and Quality

In this section I first provide some discussion of a possible positive model of equilibrium. Then I consider the normative analysis of ways to produce welfare improvements on this equilibrium.

It is clear that in part this model will be similar to existing search models, and in part it will be a kind of monopolistic competition model, except that neither free entry nor economies of scale are necessarily assumed. Unfortunately the monopolistic competition theory for even the simple model in which only price is uncertain is far from complete, and the multiplicity of monopolistic competition models, equilibria, and welfare evaluations of outcomes is an embarrassment of riches. While the theory of a consumer searching from a distribution of prices is fairly well settled, how that distribution comes into existence has not been fully explained (Michael Rothschild).

One way of sorting out the problem is to consider alternative reasons for departures from optimality and alternative corrective policies. There are two sorts of corrective policies I will discuss: (1) policies to correct prices or entry, given information; and (2) policies to correct information or compensate for incorrect information, given prices and entry.

In this section I wish to assume that information is given to be less than full, and ask how the market might be expected to perform. If consumers are not fully aware of the quality of all providers, providers may be able to raise prices above the competitive level. To the extent that this power differs in different submarkets, providers may move in response to income differentials. The sort of result one can get is presented in a particularly striking way by M. Satterthwaite. He develops a model in which the information a consumer has on any individual physician's price or quality depends upon the experience that the consumer and his friends have had with that physician. In a town with, say, two doctors, there will be relatively extensive experience, and each consumer will have a reasonably good idea of the quality level provided by each doctor. Now let the number of physicians increase. On the average, the number of experiences (his own and friends') per physician will decrease, and so the consumer will be less well-informed about any physician. This can cause individual physician demand curves to become less elastic, and price to increase when the number of physicians increases. No recourse to a non-maximizing or target income model is necessary.

From the welfare viewpoint, this model suggests possible gains from regulating prices or from limiting mobility, because free entry may lead to higher prices. A. M. Spence makes the argument that price limitation is likely to be infeasible in general in monopolistic competition, but even the notion of maximizing welfare subject to a profit constraint may suggest that some restriction on entry may be desirable.

But again "maybe" is not "will be"; the power of a priori reasoning is limited to posing questions, not answering them. This type of result seems to be what one gets out of most of the "new" monopolistic competition literature; the extent of monopoly is something that needs to be known before one can judge empirically whether the monopolistic competition equilibrium is or is not subject to improvement.

Knowing About Knowledge: Implications for Licensing

The previous section asked the question of possible welfare improvements, given some level of less-than-perfect information. In this section I want to concentrate on information itself. I want, first, to suggest a somewhat different way of evaluating the performance of an industry in which much of the output is information. Consider the three classifications or stages of care: diagnosis, prescription, and therapy. (Ordinarily they will follow in this order.) From the consumer's viewpoint, the three are obviously related, in the sense that his demand for therapy depends upon the quantity and the content of the other types of care purchased for an episode of illness. But suppose that each seller at a prior stage thinks that he cannot affect demand *from him* by the content of the advice he provides. Finally, and this is critical, assume that the consumer can perfectly evaluate the *quality* of each kind of care. By quality here I mean the usefulness of outcome from each stage. For example, for diagnosis, quality would mean the accuracy of diagnosis. For prescription it would mean the accuracy of advice about the outcomes to expect from various courses of therapy, given some diagnosis. For therapy, quality refers to the outcomes expected from performance of given therapeutic procedures on patients with given diagnoses.[8] Outcomes here means all the outcomes or characteristics that the consumer values, and is not limited to morbidity or mortality.

If the consumer was fully informed about these qualities, then the outcome would, I conjecture, be Pareto optimal. This differs from the usual notion of consumer information in that knowledge of "quality" applies not to the advice, but to the advisor, not the performance, but to the performer. The consumer is still ignorant about specifics, but he can judge which provider sells the high quality advice; he knows the provider's reputation.

There are some implications here for the notion of agency. If the consumer is well informed about primary-care physicians' general performance as agents, the referring physician will be a perfect agent. It is not necessary that the consumer be informed about the evidence concerning a particular referral, any more than a buyer of a pocket calculator needs to second-guess the manufacturer's choice of input suppliers.

In the real world, neither the assumption of independence of demands nor that of full consumer information about quality may hold. More to the point, there appear to be real resource costs of making demands independent and consumers fully informed. These resource costs are of three types. First, resources must be used to evaluate the quality of different providers. Second, the information must be made available to potential consumers. And third, consumers must expend real resources (primarily time) to "process" the information provided. All of these observations suggest that in equilibrium consumers are not likely to be fully informed. Given that information will not be complete, is this industry then different in the sense that public intervention in information provision may be required?

One kind of efficiency-improving public intervention can occur when provision of information itself is not cost effective.[9] If the cost of providing information to all consumers is sufficiently high, it may be cheaper to ban the good or service than to provide information which indicates that it is of lower quality. Some consumers lose when (low) quality levels are banned, but the gain to the rest may be substantial.

If there are costs of getting information to consumers, or if consumers incur a cost in processing it, then it is possible that either producer liability for lower than expected levels of quality or prohibition of certain qualities or quality proxies may be appropriate (C. Colantoni et al.). In medical care, both approaches are used. Providers are liable for negligent behavior which results in adverse outcomes under malpractice law. "Unqualified persons" (usually everyone except a physician) are legally forbidden to render certain medical-care services. The malpractice question does not appear to differ from that of products liability generally, and so I will emphasize the second (prohibition or exclusive licensing) approach.

There is a tradeoff among denying their ideal choice to relatively more knowledgeable persons, saving ignorant ones from their mistakes, and saving on information costs for all. It is surely *possible* that at least some consumers will be made better off if some low quality products are banned, and that the gain to them will exceed the loss to others. Consumer ignorance alone is not sufficient, of course; one needs to show that ignorant consumers are more likely to misestimate the chance of injury from a "low-quality" provider. We are prohibited from saying more by the old problem—second best. While such rules may improve aggregate welfare, it is not necessary that they do so, and one cannot tell a priori.

One way to settle the question is by a cost-benefit type of study. But perhaps some crude beginnings can be made first. While it is true that one does not wish simply to count heads, but rather willingness to pay (Walter Oi), as a rough approximation it does seem reasonable to assert that a good case can be made for banning quality levels which would be almost no one's choice if fully informed, but which would be regarded as decidely inferior by many.

Perhaps surprisingly, there appears to be almost no empirical work designed to answer this question: How heterogeneous are demands or tastes for types of medical care? Nor has there been any investigation, other than Bunker and Brown's study of physicians' families, to indicate what a fully informed consumer would do.

EXCLUSIVE LICENSURE AND POLITICAL CHOICE

In practice, laws typically govern the provider and not (within broad limits) his performance. These laws do more than just certify competence. They restrict the performance of certain actions to people with certain qualifications. One rationale for this policy would involve a kind of regress. Consumers do not have sufficient information to choose medical care on their own, so they hire an expert, the physician, to guide their choices. They do not have sufficient information to choose a physician, so, in effect, they can gain from having the Government hire experts to guide their choices of physicians. If people prefer to have their choices of quality guided or restricted, that is a service which the market can also surely provide. The critical question is whether there is any reason to suppose that public provision, via Government, of this choice of expert, and the restriction on individual choices it implies, is likely to be different from and superior to market alternatives. There are two possible reasons. First, the choice itself may in some sense be "better." Second, limiting choice to a small set of options, even if it is arbitrarily chosen, may improve matters.

To answer the question of whether choice is "better," the following non-transformation theorem on the usefulness of public intention will be useful. *The mere transfer of the locus of choice from the market to the political process does not transform consumers into better judges of quality, nor does it necessarily improve the decisions made.*

Since in a democratic policy the ultimate political choice of experts must rest with the voters, it is not clear how "government" (i.e., political regulation) can improve matters. Second-best reasoning suggests that a set of governmental (or other) experts *could* choose restrictions on quality or information which might make consumers better off than they would have been with no limits on quality or information. But the non-transformation theorem says that if these experts could be chosen by the polity, in the political choice of advice, it is approximately true that they could also be chosen in the market. If consumers in the advice markets would not choose the best experts, it is hard to see why they would be more likely to do so in the political market: It is not obvious why or how the transfer of the locus of choice would lead to better choices. There is, of course, a problem of public goods or non-exclusion in the production of information about qualifications, a point which will be discussed shortly.

The actual level that would be chosen would depend on the preferences of voters and the strength of lobbyists or other special interests. To take the simplest voter model: Suppose voters are to choose a minimum quality level for medical care, suppose their preferences for quality levels are absolute, and suppose that the preferences of the median voter (i.e., the voter with median quality preferences) would be decisive. In equilibrium, all quality levels below the optimal quality of the median voter would be banned.

In a more general model, the choice by any individual of his optimal level of quality obviously depends on the price he pays for different quality levels. But if the relationship of price to quality is being determined in an imperfectly informed market, should one expect a voter to take present prices as an indicator? If he does so, this would lead to possible biases in choice.

One may object that the approval of quality levels in medical care by medical examining boards or other government officials is so far removed from either the concern or the power of an average voter, and so frequently combined with other aspects of an election campaign, that voter choice is irrelevant. There are two alternative models. In one, choice is made ultimately by an elected official. Voters choose a governor, say, who appoints board members. But this just puts the process through another regress, and does not change anything fundamental. Instead of choosing the expert, voters choose a general expert agent who picks specialized experts of all sorts.

The second model is one in which voter preferences do not affect the outcome, but those of special interests do. This is a regulatory capture theory; the analytical problem, in a profession such as health where there are lots of special interests, is to explain why some special interests have captured more than others. Whatever the outcome, there is no reason to expect the choice to be "right" in any welfare sense; quality could be too high or too low, but it would only be an accident for it to be appropriate.

Even if the choice is not necessarily better, there are other important differences between market and political choice. One of the most important ones is the uniform and exclusive characteristic of political choice, compared to the pluralistic nature of market choice. This characteristic represents a mixed blessing. The advantage of political choice, as suggested above, is not that the choice is better, but, rather, that reduction in diversity of sellers, even if it is fairly arbitrary, can save buyers the cost of determining quality. For some this is a gain; for others, it is not.

For example, a person who knew he was ignorant about choosing the type of practitioner to treat an illness might well select an expert whose advice would be: You should always seek treatment from someone with a Doctor of Medicine degree. But a person who is more knowledgeable might sometimes wish to seek treatment from someone with less training. In market choice, both of these individuals could have their preferences satisfied, but in an exclusive licensure political arrangement they could not. If the first person is the one with median preferences, exclusive licensure might well be enacted into law, because it would save the decisive individual the cost of finding out what training a given provider of care had received, even if (as is likely to be true) this cost is small. As usual, majority rule equilibrium could be optimal, but it need not be.

There is indeed a kind of external cost imposed on an individual by the existence of quality levels he would not choose if fully informed. If the quality level exists, he would have to determine, at some cost, whether any given provider was of that quality level or not. If he bans quality levels he would not choose anyway, he suffers no loss in utility and he saves himself the cost of finding out whether a provider is or is not of that quality level.

Can it be desirable to ban once certification is provided? Given that certification occurs, it is hard to believe that the cost of examining a label is more than trivial. There is, however, an incentive for the decisive individual to support exclusive licensure rather than certification. With certification he would have to bear some of the cost, whereas banning a set of non-preferred quality levels is costless to him.

A third kind of difference between market and political choice is that political choice may be able to deal with the public good nature of the information production process in a superior way. Resources are consumed to measure quality levels. Once the information on quality has been produced, the amount of it available to any one individual is not diminished by the use of it by another individual. So exclusion of anyone by a positive price is inefficient, and yet the market cannot supply the information unless a positive price is charged.

The logic of this argument is impeccable, and it perhaps applies more strongly to medical care than to some other goods, since the cost per capita of providing information on a physician may be higher than that of providing information on, say, a dishwasher, both because of the difficulty of evaluation and because dishwashers are branded while physicians are not. Even so, the argument seems of limited relevance because (1) much of the cost of providing information is the private good, distribution of the information, rather than the public good, production of the information, and (2) the market price of information is still likely to be sufficiently low that those to whom information is more than trivially useful will still be willing to buy it. Those who would be excluded would be those for whom the information would not have been of much value anyway; while they could be worse off, the loss in per capita welfare would be small. Finally, there is no reason to suppose that actual governments would choose the ideal amount or type of this public good (information) anyway.

There is a fourth difference which is of importance. The consumer has little experience of his own on the outcomes of services provided by a particular seller. He wishes to obtain such information. Clearly, the lowest cost source of the information is the seller himself; for instance, the physician or hospital would be in the best position to know how many adverse outcomes there were among their patients. The same information could be obtained by an independent survey of their patients, but this would obviously be more costly. Those sellers whose quality is high, relative to their price, would obviously be eager to furnish information, but those whose quality was low relative to price would be unenthusiastic about having that fact made known. One solution in a market arrangement would be to list the fact of refusal to provide information, and that alone might be some testimony, even if mute, to the quality actually provided.[10] The Government does, however, have the legal power or the financial leverage to extract this information from all providers. The legal protection it gives to a physician's records it alone can take away. In this sense, it possesses an advantage over voluntary market arrangements in providing accurate information at low cost.[11]

There are, of course, some private organizations that possess the data needed to generate useful information at low cost. Third-party payers of various types could in principle profile that part of the activity of various providers which is covered by insurance. It is of some interest to speculate why, for example, insurers who are concerned with overuse have not informed their insureds about which physicians or hospitals have unusually high claim rates. Of course, the offended parties might retaliate by refusing to accept assignment, but if that is all the threat that is needed, the value of the information could not have been very great.

To summarize: It is easy to exaggerate the ability of government to deal with imperfect information in a way which is superior to the market. The main advantage it possesses arises from its ability to remove, with sufficient reason, a guarantee of property rights in information that it itself provided at an earlier stage. It also can avoid free rider problems, but this at most would give it a role in certification. The principles involved here appear to be general, and not specific to medical care. With regard to the type of care we are considering, one cannot rule out the possibility that it could be desirable to have more information than there currently is. If this information were made available, then this part of the sector might be further analyzed with the usual tools of economic analysis.

INFORMATION AND INTERRELATED DEMANDS

The preceding discussion looked at the possibility of obtaining information from "outside" sources. I remarked that, for the individually-infrequent types of care, there seems to be little such purchase of information from non-physician sources, although information in the form of referrals is very common. Much of the information we buy about the need for procedures we buy from physicians who may provide us with both the information about a procedure and the procedure itself. Since there clearly *can* be an incentive in such an arrangement to distort information, especially if there is excess capacity in the therapeutic service at the going price, why do consumers buy advice *and* treatment from the same seller?

The reason, as suggested by Michael Darby and Edi Karni, is that it is often cheaper to purchase all types of services from the same provider than from different providers. Once I have purchased diagnosis from a given physician, I can purchase therapy or prescriptive advice from him more cheaply than from another physician who would have to repeat at least some of the diagnostic workup.

In this sense, the diagnosing physician can influence the demand for his or others' services at later stages, and may do so in ways intended to enhance his income. In addition, if a diagnosis is required in order to obtain additional services, he can in principle extract all of the consumer's surplus in his charge for diagnosis. The way in which demands for information and care are related is not yet known, although some work has been done (Mark Pauly (1977), (1975), Dennis Smallwood and K. Smith).

The extent to which this power can be exploited by the physician may, however, be severely limited. The expected loss imposed on the consumer cannot exceed the expected cost advantage of single over multiple providers. In concrete terms, this cost advantage appears to be relatively slight. For example, Eugene McCarthy was able to offer second opinions on surgical procedures at a cost of about $40. This is less than 5 percent of the typical cost for an in-hospital surgical procedure. The expected utility loss, measured in dollars, of unnecessary surgery cannot exceed $40. The perhaps surprising result is that, when the second opinion program was voluntary, and covered by insurance, relatively few persons took advantage of it. Clearly, they expect the loss from unnecessary surgery to be small; whether this belief is true or erroneous is not yet clear. Here again, consumers may be so ignorant that they do not even conceive that their physician's advice is not the most accurate he could give.[12] This could also explain why they do not buy second opinions, although it would surely be relatively cheap just to inform consumers that a second opinion would be useful.

INSURANCE

The incidence of illness is random. This leads to a demand for insurance against medical bills on the part of risk-adverse individuals. There are other goods subject to such randomness in demand; for example, all classes of repair service, for which there also tend to be forms of insurance, either explicit policies or as service contracts. What is truly distinctive about medical care is not the risk or consequent insurance as such, but, rather, the way in which insurance benefits are determined.

The great bulk of health insurance is purchased by reasonably well-informed group purchasers, and premiums are reasonably well equated to risk, the two conditions necessary for an efficient competitive market (tax considerations aside). There are some problems raised by insurer ignorance about the probability of loss, but these adverse selection difficulties do not seem of much quantitative importance. Indeed, most of the concern in public policy with respect to selection is not that health insurers sell insurance (at low rates) to bad risks they cannot identify, but that they refuse to sell insurance (at low rates) to bad risks they *can* identify. The market works, but it leaves a residue of persons unable or unwilling to buy insurance. The only real puzzle here is why longer term health insurance against the possibility of becoming a bad risk—guaranteed renewability without strings attached—is not more common. There is potentially a more serious problem if individual insurers cannot measure the *total* amount of health insurance an individual has bought. Since his losses will be functions of his coverage (moral hazard), premiums cannot be appropriately tailored to risks (Pauly (1974)).

The absence of markets for some risks, much emphasized by Arrow as a reason for inefficiency, is now generally viewed as caused by irreducible moral hazard or transactions-information costs. On a priori grounds, one cannot show that it is amenable to improvement (with the possible exception of the relatively small market for individual insurance).

As noted above, the primary distinguishing characteristic of health insurance is the way in which benefits are paid. Much of medical care is covered by an insurance which does have a unique characteristic; the insurance payment depends, not on the amount of loss, but on the expenditure made to repair the loss. This insurance distorts demand curves, reduces the incentive for search, and reduces the extent of competition. But with suitable translations from gross to net price, these alterations, however much they affect welfare, do not affect the extent of competition more than any other similar price reduction, as long as the differences among insurances are limited to paying different fractions of unlimited total expenditures. Problems do arise when insurance covers full cost or full price (perhaps up to a limit), because then there can be no price competition among sellers at prices below the limit.

If insurance plans can place restrictions on use, then there can be a kind of competition based on the appropriateness of these restrictions and the extent to which they are enforced. In a sense, the argument here about market-generated restrictions on quantity is analogous to the earlier argument about market-generated restrictions on quality. It is the consumer's interest to have his use of care restricted in situations where there is moral hazard, as long as he recoups the savings in lower insurance premiums. Health maintenance organizations are a way of restricting quantity to deal with moral hazard. The consumer gets more than just quantity restriction in an HMO; he also gets group practice (possibly, though not demonstrably, more efficient) and restriction on his choice of providers. The more puzzling question is why other third-party payers have not only been unsuccessful but even uninterested in ways of controlling moral hazard. Does this indicate a failure of competition or an inefficient consequence of competition?

There are some possible reasons why typical third-party insurers have in general been unwilling to control use directly. An insurer who wishes to control use by some form of utilization review or denial of benefits can generally expect to be able to offer his insurance package at lower premiums.

Of course, there is a cost; some benefits will not be provided and some bills will not be paid. The essence of the moral hazard-welfare loss argument is that the reduction in premiums from controlling use exceeds the value to the individual of the care that would otherwise have been received. Such a gain can be realized, however, only if insureds of this carrier are able to recoup in lower premiums the full reduction in expenditure that restriction on their behavior implies.

There are two reasons why the insureds may not be able to capture all of these benefits. First, it may be that restrictions imposed on, say, physician or hospital behavior with respect to one set of insureds changes the use, in a quantitative sense, of other insureds. An insurer-sponsored second-opinion program for unnecessary hospitalization may reduce the total cost of hospital care not only to its insureds, who bear the time and inconvenience cost, but also for other insureds, if physicians behave in approximately the same way toward all patients. Certain kinds of reduction in use, such as in routine nursing care, would not even be under the control of the insurer, since such services are not itemized, nor would any reduction in use of such services reduce premiums proportionately.

The second reason is the tax treatment of insurance premiums, especially employer-paid premiums. The implicit costs of reduced use are fully borne by the insureds, but the benefit of premium reductions are shared with the Treasury because offsetting increases in money income are taxed. This implies, not only that the fraction of expense covered by insurance will be too large, as has been pointed out by Martin Feldstein (1973a) and others, but also that efforts to reduce use via regulations or controls will not be carried far enough.

Where these conjectures are true is not currently known, or even investigated. It can hardly be alleged that they represent failures of the competitive system as such. Rather, they arise in large part from tax distortion or from average-cost pricing schemes often followed by non-profit hospitals. The solution might be changes in tax treatment or pricing policies. Another option would be to subsidize those cost control activities which generate external benefits.

DIFFERENCES ON THE SUPPLY SIDE

Most of Arrow's discussion of suppliers is hypothetical in nature: Since it would be desirable that physicians or hospitals not take advantage of the imperfect knowledge of consumers, physicians are "supposed" to follow a higher ethical code, and non-profit hospitals are "supposed" to behave in a less mercenary fashion. Unfortunately, he does not provide any suggestions of ways to tell whether providers are doing what they are supposed to do, or indeed, any explanation of why one should have supposed that they would behave this way in the first place. Here again, but in a more qualified way, he seems to be arguing that since these institutions should, in an (first-bet) optimal state, behave this way, they must be doing so.

In this section I consider briefly the theory that might be constructed to explain the behavior of suppliers of medical care. The behavior of this industry seems different enough to suggest that models different from those of the conventional firm should at least be tried. In line with the normative focus of this paper, however, it is important to note that non-wealth-maximizing behavior of suppliers does not necessarily, or even probably, cause outcomes which are non-optimal.

So in what follows I will present some aspects of possible "different" models of medical-care provider behavior, not only to show why, in a positive sense, behavior might be expected to be different, but also to show that these differences do not necessarily imply inefficiency. I will not provide a full treatment of such models because that will be done by other papers at this conference.[13]

It is widely suggested that physicians are not wealth maximizers. It is plausible to argue that physicians may place lower values than other suppliers on money income relative to leisure and relative to their own evaluations of the quality or accuracy of output they provide.

There are two possible reasons. First, it is likely that these nonpecuniary aspects of work are normal goods. Since physician incomes are relatively high, one might expect these income effects to predominate. Second, physicians are not selected in the same way as other entrepreneurs. A successful owner or manager is likely to be one who has worked hard for the financial rewards that success brings. He is likely to be relatively more responsive to financial incentives than a person selected without regard to his financial responsiveness. Because the limited number of medical school-places are allocated on some basis other than financial responsiveness, and because medical care can be provided only by persons who have completed medical education, it is likely that physicians will be less responsive to financial rewards than would a typical provider in another industry. If entry into medicine were not limited, a good bit of this different behavior might be expected to disappear.

The question which is still of particular interest is the following. Given the present process for selecting and training physicians, does the absence of wealth-maximizing behavior suggest inefficiency? At first, one might suppose that the answer to this question should be yes. Absence of wealth maximization implies the possible absence of cost minimization, and that is obviously inefficient. There is even fairly strong empirical evidence that physicians do choose less than the cost-minimizing amount of non-physician inputs in managing their own practices (Uwe Reinhardt). It is difficult to suppose that this arises from unplanned ignorance by physicians. The easiest explanation is based on the "utility-from inefficiency" gambit—the argument that physicians actually *choose* to be inefficient, because of the subjective cost of supervision and control. They may even choose not to obtain information on ways to perform such supervision, because of the subjective cost of both the information and the supervision.

Is this "inefficiency" inefficient? The answer is that, if the incentives faced by physicians reflect the real tradeoff between inefficiency and supervision cost, it would not be desirable either to induce or to compel physicians to reduce costs and increase their money incomes. This anomalous result is based on the notion that the payment that would have to be made to induce the physician to provide more supervision, or the payment he would be willing to make to avoid supervision, would exceed the cost reduction. Public good aspects of information may suggest a role for government in subsidizing information to physicians on how to organize their practice in more profitable or more efficient ways, but I would regard the hypothesis of government ability to reduce significantly producer ignorance as even less plausible than its ability to reduce consumer ignorance.

There is a second peculiar effect of non-maximizing behavior that comes from the interrelatedness of information content and demand for therapeutic care. It is often suggested that, because the physician can control the content of the advice he provides to patients, the physician who wants to increase his income will generate demand for his own output. It is further suggested that the empirical observation that demand is related, *ceteris paribus,* to the availability of physicians supports this view.

I have argued above that the ability of physicians permanently to shift demand may be severely constrained, and I regard the empirical evidence that demand is shifted to be very weak. Nevertheless, it is important to note that, in theory, observation of an availability effect based on information manipulation may require that physicians *not* be income or wealth maximizers. If a physician mazimizes his income, he will choose that level of informational accuracy that maximizes the price he can get for any quantity from him. If the number of physicians increases, this reduces each physician's share of total quantity demanded at any price, but the maximum price at any given total quantity is not changed. So the observed market demand curve will not shift. One way to get such shifting is to assume that physicians value accuracy, and are only willing to trade off accuracy for income as their incomes get sufficiently low or the reward for inaccuracy gets sufficiently high. The normative implication of this discussion is that control of physician stock, below the free entry level, can be welfare increasing if physicians are not wealth maximizers.[14]

With respect to hospitals, we note that one of the most striking aspects of empirical studies of hospital behavior, dominated by not-for-profit and governmental firms, is that it is almost all consistent with the assumption of profit maximization. Suppliers respond, prices rise, and incomes increase when demand increases. Although there are theories to explain these facts in terms of utility-maximization (Feldstein (1971), Joseph Newhouse), it is also possible to suggest profit-maximizing explanations for hospital behavior (Pauly and Michael Redisch). The nonprofit nature of hospitals may be a distinction that does not make much of a difference. In view of empirical evidence and the need to limit this paper, I will not discuss possible theories of hospital behavior further.

CONCLUSION

This paper has emphasized consumer ignorance as the most important potential difference between medical care and other goods. I argued, however, that for some of medical care there was possibly little actual difference even in the present case, while for another part there *could* be market-like institutions to deal with it. This still leaves a third kind of care, which is by definition rare and unusual. Here some Government regulation may help, although even here its superiority over information provision is a second-best conjecture. The most plausible case for public intervention may be, not in the regulation of quality or of information flow, but in the regulation of sheer numbers of providers, especially physicians, and especially with regard to geographical distribution.

The primary message from theory for research is that more empirical information is needed to go from conjectures to fact, that theory itself cannot take us very far. Research on how well informed consumers are, and how differently they might behave with additional information, and how markets would change in response would be of high priority.

NOTES

1. There is a fourth kind of difference, which they do not list and which will not be discussed here, but which may still be of importance. Medical care is one of those goods and services to which *social concern* attaches. People other than the direct user of care are concerned about the amount that is used. This kind of concern can generate an external effect which calls for public subsidization. It need not, however, imply any difference in the operation of the market once the subsidy has been paid.

2. One qualification: If entry restrictions are removed, it is possible that firms might shrink in size to such an extent that economies of scale would appear.

3. The empirical evidence on how people select providers is skimpy. There is a strong suggestion, however, that not only are friends and relatives used as sources of advice, but especially those friends who have had experience with the provider or type of provider contemplated, and who are regarded as more knowledgeable than the direct consumer. See A. Booth and N. Babchuk.

4. Data for 1973 are used for the percent of total expenditures figures; they have changed little over recent years.

5. It should be noted that definition of the "reasonably well informed" part of total spending should *not* be based on the distinction between physician and patient-generated care. Some patient-generated care may be quite poorly informed, while some care may be suggested by the physician but still be of a sort that the consumer is capable of evaluating.

6. Consider the following example. Suppose there are two producers of a medical service, each one producing a different level of quality. Suppose that, if quality levels and marginal costs were known, all consumers in a world of identical consumers would choose the higher level quality. In the absence of information on price or quality, consumers might be randomly distributed in approximately equal numbers across the two producers. Suppose higher quality costs more, and suppose that price advertising is permitted. Ignorant consumers might now all choose the lower quality producer because his equilibrium price is likely to be lower. Those who formerly used the low quality producer may not lose, but those who switched from the high quality producer may be worse off. It is possible, therefore, that partial information can lead to an outcome in which none are better off and some are worse off.

7. This is a restatement of one of the parts of the well-known "Coase Theorem" (Ronald Coase).

8. An alternative approach which is equivalent in some cases is to consider an entire course of treatment from presenting symptoms through therapy, and to evaluate quality as the outcome of an entire course of treatment.

9. As Victor Goldberg has noted, this makes sense only if the consumer is not fully informed. If he is fully informed, he will make appropriate choices in the market. Public intervention can then only serve to make consumers worse off, as Walter Oi has noted.

10. This also suggests that wholehearted voluntary support for PSRO's which provide useful information is *not likely* to be universal among physicians, especially low-quality ones.

11. It may not be efficient to provide information on outcomes because of its incentive effects. Physicians may select cases in such a way as to improve their outcome measures, if those outcome measures cannot be perfectly adjusted for differences in underlying conditions.

12. Another result provided by McCarthy and E. Widmer suggests that consumers are not this ignorant. They compared a mandatory and a voluntary surgical second opinion program and found that the rate at which the initial recommendation for surgery was not confirmed was much greater for the voluntary program. This implies that patients *knew,* even before the second opinion, which recommendations for surgery were likely to be questionable.

13. See also Feldstein (1973b) and Davis (1972) for surveys.

14. Of course, this ignores the direct effect of numbers of physicians on consumers' own ability to generate information, a point discussed above.

REFERENCES

K. Arrow, "Uncertainty and the Welfare Economics of Medical Care," *Amer. Econ. Rev.,* December 1963, 941-973.

A. Booth and N. Babchuk, "Seeking Health Care from New Resources," *J. Health Social Behavior,* March 1972, 90-99.

J. P. Bunker and B. Brown, "The Physician-Patient as One Informed Consumer of Surgical Services," *New England J. Medicine,* May 1974, 1051-55.

R. H. Coase, "The Problem of Social Cost," *J. Law Econ.* October 1960, 1-44.

C. Colantoni, O. A. Davis, and M. Swaminutham, "Imperfect Consumers and Welfare

Comparisons of Policies Concerning Information and Regulation," *Bell J. Econ.*, Autumn 1976, 602-15.

M. Darby and E. Karni, "Free Competition and the Optimal Amount of Fraud," *J. Law Econ.*, April 1973, 67-88.

K. Davis, "Economic Theories of Behavior in Nonprofit Private, Hospitals," *J. of Econ. and Bus.*, Winter 1972, 1-13.

——, *National Health Insurance*, Washington 1975.

M. Feldstein, "The Rising Price of Physicians' Services," *Rev. Econ. Statis.*, May 1970, 121-33.

——, "Hospital Cost Inflation: A Study of Nonprofit Price Dynamics *Amer. Econ. Rev.*, December 1971, 853-72.

——, (1973a), "The Welfare Loss of Excess Health Insurance," *J. Polit. Econ.*, March 1973, 255-80.

——, (1973b), "Econometric Studies in Health Economics," in *Frontiers of Quantitative Economics*, 1973.

A. Flexner, "Medical Education in the U.S. and Canada," *Bulletin No. 4*, Carnegie Foundation for the Advancement of Teaching (1910).

V. Goldberg, "The Economics of Product Safety and Imperfect Information," *Bell J. Econ.*, Autumn 1974, 683-88.

S. Grossman and J. Stiglitz, "Information and Competitive Price Systems," *Amer. Econ, Rev.*, May 1976, 246-253.

E. G. McCarthy, and E. Widmer, "Effect of Screening by Consultants on Recommended Elective Surgical Procedures," *New England J. Medicine*, Dec. 1974, 1331-35.

S. Mushkin, "Towards a Definition of Health Economics," *Public Health Reports*, Sept. 1958, 785-93.

P. Nelson, "Information and Consumer Behavior," *J. Polit. Econ.*, March-April 1970, 311-329.

J. Newhouse, "Toward a Theory of Non-profit Institutions: An Economic Model of a Hospital," *Amer. Econ. Rev.*, June 1970, 64-74.

W. Oi, "The Economics of Product Safety," *Bell J. Econ.*, Spring 1973, 3-28.

M. Pauly, "Over insurance and Public Provision of Insurance: Moral Hazard and Adverse Selection," *Quarterly J. Econ.*, February 1974, 44-62.

——, "The Role of Demand Creation in the Provision of Health Services," paper presented at annual meeting of American Economic Association, December 1975.

——, "Information and the Demand for Medical Care," in J. Hixson and L. Krystaniak, Eds., *Theoretical Studies in Health Economics* (forthcoming, 1977).

——, and M. Redisch, "The Not-for-Profit Hospital as a Physicians' Cooperative," *Amer. Econ. Rev.*, March 1973, 87-99.

U. Reinhardt, "A Production Function for Physicians' Services," *Rev. Econ. Statis.*, February 1972, 55-66.

M. Rothschild, "Models of Market Organization with Imperfect Information," *J. of Polit. Econ.*, November-December 1973, 1283-1308.

S. Salop, "Information and Monopolistic Competition," *Amer. Econ. Rev.*, May 1976, 240-45.

M. Satterthwait, "The Pricing of Physicians Services: A Theoretical Analysis," unpublished paper, Northwestern University, April 1977.

D. Smallwood and K. Smith, "Optical Treatment Decisions, Optimal Fee Schedules, and the Allocation of Medical Resources," Northwestern University, processed, 1976.

Comment

Burton A. Weisbrod
Professor of Economics and Fellow, Institute for Research on Poverty, University of Wisconsin

All things are different from each other. All things are the same. Both of these statements, seemingly contradictory, are true. The question that Mark Pauly's valuable paper addresses is not whether health care is a "commodity" that is unique, different in *all* respects from any other commodity, but whether it is different in ways that are relevant to the development of public policy—and particularly antitrust and Federal Trade Commission policy. Can the forces of the decentralized private market be relied upon to serve "social objectives" to essentially the same degree for health care as for most other goods and services?

To begin to answer this difficult yet vital question we must first say something about what is meant by social objectives. Unfortunately, Pauly's paper is silent on this matter. Implicitly, however, he has only the goal of allocative efficiency in mind; the paper in fact deals only with the question of the ability of the private market to bring about efficiency, in the resource-allocation sense. Not once is there mention of any other social goal, and in particular there is no recognition of the distributional-equity goal. The relevant issue is whether the effect of health care on life itself does or does not warrant a different public policy-antitrust policy than is generally regarded as desirable for other commodities. The answer is not obvious. And precisely because it is not, explicit attention to the question should be a central part of a comprehensive answer to the question, "Is Medical Care Different?" The answer is complicated by the facts that not all medical care is vital to life—indeed, most is not—and that there are other goods that, even though not necessarily involving life maintenance, are generally deemed to be sufficiently important that access to them should not be determined solely by private markets—e.g., schooling and minimum quality housing.

One of the several highly useful contributions of Pauly's paper is its attempt to disaggregate "health care." He distinguishes types of care according to the degree to which the patient-consumer is a well-informed buyer. Whether or not this is a useful, or the only useful, basis for disaggregating health care—a matter to which I return, below—Pauly's analysis does highlight the danger of too quickly generalizing about all health care. It is clear that the term, health care, encompasses a variety of resource inputs (e.g., physicians, nurses, drugs) that are provided by a variety of organizational structures (e.g., solo medical practitioners working on a fee-for-service basis, prepaid group practices, hospitals), and that operate simultaneously in the public sector, private for-profit and private nonprofit sectors.

Pauly does not define "health care," but is apparently thinking about the activities that are customarily associated with physicians and hospitals. In fact, however, such a conception of the health care "industry"—a term that Pauly does not use but that I regard as useful in this context—is too narrow as a basis for public policy determination. Pharmacists, drugs, and nursing homes, for example, are all resources that frequently are "close" substitutes for (and often are complements to) physicians and hospitals. And then, of course, there are the various paramedical workers, as well as the chiropractors, optometrists, denturists, etc. As with any industry, the boundary between what should be regarded as in the industry and not in it, is fuzzy. If the categorizing variable, however, is—as I believe it should be, in this context—the marginal rate of factor substitution among resource inputs to the "health" production function—then public policy toward the health industry should recognize the breadth of resources and institutional structures that affect health. Indeed, health "care," when defined as *treatment,* disregards the contribution of *prevention,* a use of resources that affects both the subsequent demand for treatment and the probable effectiveness of that treatment. Not only should such preventive activities as vaccinations—typically administered by "medical providers"—be considered, but also occupational and environmental factors affecting health: housing, diet, smoking, job hazards, and automobile safety, to name a few.

The picture of the health care production process that is painted by Pauly—limited to treatment—is too narrow in still another sense. It reflects a static analysis, in which the state of knowledge is given and public policy is directed at how much of the knowledge should be employed, and how it should be applied. Disregarded is the critical longrun question of biomedical research policy; yet even a casual glance at advances in knowledge in recent decades discloses that the nature of our health care choices today is very much a function of the resources devoted to research and development "yesterday." Health care policy that disregards this linkage between resources devoted in biomedical R&D and the options available for prevention and treatment will, in all likelihood, yield unfortunate and unintended results. For example, consider the effect of R&D on the variable on which Pauly concentrates, how well informed the patient-consumer is. On the one hand, through time, rising levels of education are making patients more skillful consumers of health care, better diagnosticians of health problems and more able to determine whether professional help is needed. But on the other hand, advances in the state of knowledge, resulting from R&D, have continually expanded the ability of professionals to diagnosis and treat, have provided new technology and drugs, have led to the development of new types of medical and paramedical specialties, and, in general, have made the patient-consumer increasingly uncertain as to whether some new development has made his or her knowledge obsolete. Thus, the patient-consumer is less and less able to judge when a visit to a physician or other provider of health care is likely to be salutary, and is less and less able to judge whether the treatment being dispensed is or is not "satisfactory" or "optimal."

As a result of the R&D-induced changes over time in health care capability, a patient who has repeated contacts with a particular health care provider is not necessarily obtaining much useful information for evaluating the provider. When Pauly focuses on the frequency-of-purchase variable, he is arguing that patient-consumers of frequently-purchased services become sufficiently expert buyers to warrant a conclusion, apparently, that such medical care will be provided efficiently in decentralized private competitive markets. But if scientific knowledge is also expanding through time, the patient is not necessarily becoming better informed; in his repeat "purchases" he is not obtaining a larger sample of treatment effectiveness from a given "population" of health care capability, but is sampling from a changing population—a result of scientific and engineering advances.

The issue of how well informed buyers of health care are involves more than the effects of R&D. While my judgment is that consumers are generally informed rather poorly about the quality of health care being purchased —and in this judgment I differ with Pauly—I agree with Pauly's emphasis on this issue. To the extent that consumers are well informed, the case is strengthened for a public policy toward health care that regards it as like other "ordinary" commodities in the sense that consumers can be relied upon to buy efficiently, and competition, if it is present, can be relied upon to serve the role of allocating resources efficiently. (Even so, as pointed out earlier, there may still be distributional equity considerations, involving financing and access to health care, that make health care a commodity that differs from most consumer goods.)

The key reason that I am less sanguine than Pauly about consumers of health care being well informed involves the difficulty consumers have in specifiying the "counter-factual." What a buyer wants to know is the difference between his state of well-being with and without the commodity being considered. For ordinary goods, the buyer has little difficulty in evaluating the counterfactual—that is, what the situation will be if the good is not obtained. Not so for the bulk of health care (and legal representation, to cite another example). Because the human physiological system is itself an adaptive system, it is likely to correct itself and deal effectively with an ailment, even without any medical care services. Thus, a consumer of such services who gets better after the purchase does not know whether the improvement was because of, or even in spite of, the "care" that was received. Or if no health care services are purchased and the individual's problem becomes worse, he is generally not in a strong position to determine whether the results would have been different, and better, if he had purchased certain health care. And the consumer, not being a medical expert, may learn little from experience or from friends' experience —both of which Pauly regards as important sources of information—because of the difficulty of determining whether the counterfactual to a particular type of health care today is the same as it was the previous time that the consumer, or a friend, had "similar" symptoms. The noteworthy point is not simply that it is difficult for the consumer to judge quality before the purchase (as it also is in the used car case), but that it is difficult even after the purchase.

The information issue is indeed critical to determining whether medical care is different in a sense that justifies special public policy. A great deal of public policy in the consumer area is directed to promoting price competition and to expanding the provision of price information. But the importance of information on *prices* cannot be separated from the availability of information on *quality*. Pauly is quite correct in noting that providing consumers with additional price information may not enhance efficient choice if consumers are poorly informed on quality. For most commodities the assumption that consumers are well informed is sufficiently correct that governmental efforts to elicit information and competition on price are well-founded. For health care, however, and such other commodities as legal representation and much of education, Government policy that concentrates on price information should be balanced with simultaneous efforts to assure the availability of information on quality, and in a form that is widely intelligible.

The information problem for much, but not all, of health care, has given rise to a variety of mechanisms claiming to protect the consumer. In addition to direct governmental efforts involving, for example, licensure and threats of license revocation, and a legal framework permitting malpractice suits, there are private sector actions in such forms as professional ethics codes, and nonprofit-sector efforts to operate hospitals and nursing homes. The poorly-informed patient has a demand for information, but frequently he does not know either what information is needed or how valuable the information would be if he had it. As a result, the consumer is generally dependent on some agent to evaluate quality of medical care and the appropriateness of particular forms of medical care to the health conditions and preferences of the consumer. The physician's ethics code and the nonprofit organizational form are two examples of devices ostensibly designed to ensure that the ill-informed patient can "trust" the provider to act in the patient's best interest. How well such devices function is a matter deserving analysis. Moreover, development of sound public policy toward medical care should recognize that these mechanisms exist; they differ from the devices of ordinary private markets, and they may well have useful roles to play in markets in which consumers must rely upon, and trust in, experts whose judgment and advice is frequently either costly or impossible to monitor.

When the consumer information problem is recognized, the next step is to recognize that to some extent nothing can be done—at least not until the long run, when R&D can expand knowledge. Pauly notes an important fact when he points out that ". . . *everyone,* including the experts, is imperfectly informed on much of medical care. . . ." Allocative inefficiencies and inequities can develop, however, when better information is available to some persons, generally sellers, than to others, generally buyers, for this gives rise to opportunities for those with more information to take advantage of those with less, especially if the former are in positions of trust (e.g., physicians and hospital administrators).

Is medical care different? Yes and no. Yes, it is different from most commodities in the sense that (1) there is widespread interest in the distribution of access to it; and (2) unlike most goods and services, medical care is difficult for consumers to evaluate, so that they are heavily dependent on experts in whom they must place their trust, frequently without ever knowing whether the trust was warranted.

Nevertheless, no, medical care is not different from all other commodities: (a) There are other commodities the distribution of which are of general social interest; and (b) there are other commodities that, being difficult for consumers to evaluate even after the purchase, require the consumer to rely on an expert whose advice and actions are difficult to assess.

In summary, Pauly is surely right to emphasize the fact that medical care is not a homogeneous commodity, and that some forms of medical care are more routine and easier to evaluate than others. I would emphasize, however, that consumers may learn little from experience in purchasing medical care, both because technological change causes actions that are optimal (or, at least, most effective) at one point in time not to be optimal (or most effective) at a later date, and because the ability of the human physiological system to adjust makes it very difficult for the patient-consumer to determine when an improvement (or worsening) in health is attributable to a particular medical care intervention. Thus, while price information and price competition are likely to be in the interest of consumers, a balanced public policy would deal simultaneously with price and quality, both by providing information to consumers and by stimulating competition. Finally, because of the consumer's problem of evaluating quality, careful consideration is needed of the role of such "nonmarket" mechanisms as ethics codes and nonprofit organizational forms, and the role and effectiveness of regulatory mechanisms such as are used in the public utility field. When buyers have difficult quality-evaluation problems, the theorem of economics that more information—e.g.; on price—is always preferred to less need not hold.[1]

NOTE

1. For further elaboration of this point, though not specifically in the medical care context, see Russel Settle and Burton Weisbrod.

REFERENCE

R. Settle and B. Weisbrod, "Governmentally-Imposed Standards: Some Normative and Positive Aspects," forthcoming in *Research in Labor Economics*, R. Ehrenberg, editor.

Part Two

Competition in Selected Sectors

Competition Among Physicians

Frank A. Sloan
Professor of Economics, Vanderbilt University
and
Roger Feldman
Assistant Professor of Economics, University of North Carolina at Chapel Hill

Examples of monopoly in the physicians' services market abound in microeconomic textbooks. Some texts assert that the American Medical Association and its State and local affiliates are an entry-restricting cartel. Others cite Reuben Kessel's 1958 study of price discrimination by physicians. Few, our study included, question that monopolistic elements exist in this market. Yet there is considerable room for debate about specific deviations from the competitive norm, both historically and currently.

There are two levels of inquiry. The first is at the level of the individual physician. Are individual physicians local monopolists who, although constrained by a demand curve, can set the price of their services? A number of observers have questioned whether individual physicians face a meaningful demand constraint. If the physician can *shift* the demand curve for his services, he possesses considerably more market power than the ordinary monopolist. Statements about the physician's dual role as a provider of services and a "management consultant" for the patient on medical matters give a rationale for physician-generated demand, but, without empirical evidence and the underlying theory needed to interpret the evidence, they do not provide a convincing case for rejecting the standard tools of the economist's trade.

The second level of analysis looks at physicians' professional associations. Is there a cartel limiting entry into medical schools? If so, entry restraints can create monopoly profits even though individual market behavior remains reasonably competitive. Organized medicine's success in obtaining legislation limiting the roles of non-physicians and the growth of alternative forms of medical practice are complements to entry barriers. The cartel need not stop with entry restrictions. It could also engage in price fixing.

This paper addresses all of the above issues with one important exception, barriers to entry into medical schools. Persistently high internal rates of return to training in a profession over time are an index of monopolization.

Medicine appears to fit this picture: The rate of return to training has risen from 14.7 percent, in 1959 (Frank Sloan (1968)) to 22 percent in 1970 (Roger Feldman and Richard Scheffler (mimeo)).[1] By comparison, the return to a college education for men was 11 percent in 1959, 11.5 percent in 1969, and only 8.5 percent in 1974 (Richard Freeman (1975)).

However, Cotton Lindsay (1973) has recently argued that rates of return are biased upward unless corrected for hours-worked differences. His basic contention is that investment in education increases the productivity of work relative to leisure, thereby inducing substitution toward work. In markets with free entry, everyone locates along a single lifetime income-leisure indifference curve, and all income differences are equalizing.

Lindsay presents corrected estimates which show that medical training does not yield rents. But these estimates have in turn been criticized by Sloan (1976b), who claims that the data, taken from *Medical Economics* magazine, consistently overstate physicians' hours of work. Lindsay (1976) accepts this point in his reply to Sloan. In an appendix to this paper, we contribute to the discussion in two ways: First, we present a simple, "back-of-the-envelope" method for calculating any rate of return and adjusting it for hours-worked differences; second, we apply the method to 1970 data from the American Medical Association. Our results show once again that rents to medical education persist even when the rate of return is corrected for physician's longer hours of work. Subject to the caveats that rents may reflect other sources of monopoly power as well as entry barriers and the difficulties inherent in assigning pecuniary returns to ability, we see no reason for "beating a dead horse." Although medical school barriers *per se* are not stressed in this paper, one should not neglect their potential effects on performance of practicing physicians. Some economists argue, for example, that freedom from managerial responsibilities is a normal good, and excess returns may be used to "purchase" inefficiency.

We believe that competition in the physicians' services market *should* be fostered. Organized medicine has traditionally argued that anti-competitive restrictions are necessary to insure a minimum level of quality. We shall show that monopolies do not generally produce higher-quality goods. In fact, plausible assumptions lead to the opposite result; i.e., that quality is higher under competition. If patients cannot assess the quality of medical care, a notion we find implausible, one loses the normative significance of consumer demands on which the argument concerning the desirability of competition is predicated. However, assuming consumer ignorance, it takes a leap of faith to conclude that social welfare will be served by granting physicians market power.[2]

The paper is divided into four sections. Section I, entitled "Does the Supply of Doctors Create Its Own Demand?" examines the theory and evidence of the supply-created demand controversy. Although several descriptive studies have discussed supply-created demand, there has been virtually no attempt to formalize these ideas. While a formal theory cannot settle the controversy, it provides a framework for logically analyzing supply-created demand. Our theory reveals logical inconsistencies in past work on this subject. The importance of supply-created demand, in the final analysis, is an empirical issue. We review pertinent literature and find currently-available empirical evidence insufficient to settle this question. We maintain that additional empirical research can narrow the range of uncertainty.

"Gauging Monopoly Power in a Standard Market Context," Section II, analyzes monopoly by individual physicians and physicians' professional associations. To determine whether individual physicians have local monopoly power, we examine relationships between physician concentration and earnings, econometric evidence on determinants of physician fee levels and fee dispersion within local market areas, and the relationship between local monopoly power and product quality. Although some of the evidence is inconclusive, there is sufficient information to conclude that individual physicians possess some monopoly power. Assessing monopolistic practices of physicians' associations is more complex. Associations clearly have an interest in getting higher reimbursements from third parties. Organizations, however, face problems in fixing fees of individual physicians, and there is currently no evidence of widespread price fixing. We briefly examine Blue Shield and Foundations for Medical Care to ascertain whether physicians' associations, cooperating with these organizations, could cartelize the industry. Again, except in isolated cases, it is doubtful that such cartels exist.

The third section, "Recent Developments in the Physicians' Services Market," examines health maintenance organizations (HMO's), Professional Standards Review Organizations (PSRO's), and recent health manpower legislation from the standpoint of competition in the physicians' services market. HMO's are pertinent for two reasons. First, we argue the HMO's lower observed utilization rates vis-a-vis the fee-for-service mode does not necessarily imply that fee-for-service physicians generate their own demand. Second, we review legal impediments to HMO growth. The potential of HMO's to improve the performance of the fee-for-service sector may well be limited by existing restrictive laws.

PSRO's were instituted by the 1972 Amendments to the Social Security Act to assure quality and at the same time reduce costs. Presumably, the dual objective could be achieved if curbing costs reduces "waste." However, PSRO's also have the potential of reducing competition. We show that the PSRO concept is especially weak if physicians create their own demand. The large data bases being amassed by individual PSRO's could possibly be used to improve consumer information in this market; however, there are important legal impediments to such use.

Various legal restraints affecting health manpower serve the collective financial interest of physicians. Recent developments in this area are reviewed. While medical practice acts *per se* have some merit, they may often be applied against the public interest.

Section IV, "Conclusions and Implications," summarizes, indicates areas for future research, and briefly suggests how public policy can improve the performance of the physicians services market.

DOES THE SUPPLY OF DOCTORS CREATE ITS OWN DEMAND?

The Issues

As Robert Evans (1976b) notes in a recent book review on the proceedings of the 1973 International Economics Association conference on the economics of health care held in Tokyo, the specialty of health economics currently suffers from a case of acute schizophrenia vis-a-vis the matter of consumer sovereignty in the health care marketplace. In his discussion, Evans distinguishes between two groups, the N's (for "narrow") and the B's (for "broad") economists. The N's assume that the demand curve for health care services is *not* subject to shifts induced by physicians in pursuit of their own interests. Certainly the N's agree that the demand can be shifted by advertising and quality changes, including amenities that do not directly affect health. But the B's go a lot further than this. In Evans' words, the B's "assert that the provider is a predominant force in determining utilization patterns due to his/her ability to form consumer/patient preferences and to provide information on which patient choices are made. Hence, analysis of all aspects of health care, including demand, must take account of the objectives and discretionary power of the provider" (p. 534).

The differences between the N's and B's have important theoretical, empirical, and policy implications. B's would be far less interested, *inter alia,* in the results of patient demand studies. Their arguments imply the ultimate in monopoly power—the absence of a demand constraint facing the physician firm. A number of institutional features of the physicians' services market, especially fee-for-service practice, make the B's view attractive at first glance. Restricitions on advertising and the complexity of medical care make it difficult for consumers to shop for price and quality. This explains low cross-elasticities of demand among physicians. But the physician also serves in a dual role vis-a-vis the patient: He provides services *and* information about patients' medical care "needs." By controlling information, *and* because of the lack of competition, physicians may be able to manipulate patient demand.

We find the frequent statements inferring supply-created demand on the basis of consumer ignorance quite troublesome. The standard theory does not require that *everyone* possess perfect information—only that there be a sufficient number of marginal consumers both able to assess output and willing to seek it out at its lowest price. Anecdotal comments describing isolated instances in which patients have been "duped" are not convincing. To use an example of Mark Pauly, who makes this point in a medical care context: "I know even less about the works of a movie camera than I know about my own organs; yet I feel fairly confident in purchasing a camera for a given price as long as I know that there are at least a few experts in the market who are keeping sellers reasonably honest" (p. 146).

We shall argue, however, that the theoretical and empirical evidence advanced by the B's to date does not go very far beyond these statements. Although the N's case seems to us to be stronger on balance conceptually, their empirical evidence is not fully conclusive either.

Concepts

To assess the theoretical implications of supply-created demand, we adopt and extend Evans' (1974) model of physician behavior. Evans discusses the comparative statics results of his model in qualitative terms. While noting that certain predictions from his model are ambiguous, he does not, in our view, exploit its full potential. We therefore extend his model to analyze supplier-induced demand. Let, following Evans,

$$U = U(Y,W,D) \qquad (1)$$
$$W = R \cdot f(P,D) \qquad (2)$$
$$Y = R \cdot f(P,D) \cdot P - C(W) \qquad (3)$$

where: $U(\cdot)$ = utility function of a "representative" physician;
Y = physician income with utility a positive function of income;
W = physician workload with utility a negative function of workload;
D = physician's discretionary influence on patient demand;
$f(\cdot)$ = "representatiave" patient demand function;
P = price of physician's services;
R = the *population-physician* ratio in the market area, an exogenous variable in this model;
$C(\cdot)$ = the physician's cost function.

The effects of interest are $\frac{dY}{dR}$, $\frac{dP}{dR}$, and, by substitution, $\frac{dW}{dR}$. That is, if the population-physician ratio changes, how will physician income, price, and volume be affected?

Substituting (2) and (3) into (1), the physician's decision variables are price (P) and discretionary behavior (D).

The first-order conditions (with subscripts identifying derivatives) are:

$$U_P = U_Y[Rf_P P + Rf(P, D) - C_W Rf_P] + U_W Rf_P = 0 \qquad (4)$$

$$U_D = U_Y[Rf_D P - RC_W f_D] + U_W Rf_D + U_D = 0 \qquad (5)$$

Equation (4) states that price will be set where the marginal utility of goods equals the marginal disutility of work. The precise interpretation of (5) depends on whether the physician regards his use of discretionary power as a "good" or a "bad." Evans is not explicit, but we shall give physicians the benefit of the doubt. We specify that $\frac{\partial U}{\partial D}$ is negative, which implies that physicians only shift demand if they "must." They regard the use of their discretionary power as essentially bad.[3] With $\frac{\partial U}{\partial D} < 0$, (5) implies that physicians use discretionary power up to the point where the marginal utility of income from this activity equals the marginal disutilities of an increased workload and aversion to demand curve-shifting.

Totally differentiating (4) and (5) and solving, expressions for $\frac{dP}{dR}$ and $\frac{dD}{dR}$ are readily obtained.

$$\frac{dP}{dR} = -\frac{U_{PR}U_{DD} - U_{PD}U_{DR}}{\Delta} \qquad (6)$$

and

$$\frac{dD}{dR} = -\frac{U_{PP}U_{DR} - U_{PR}U_{PD}}{\Delta} \qquad (7)$$

where Δ = the Hessian determinant of second partials involving P and D; cross-derivatives $^U PP$ and $^U DD$ are negative and the determinant Δ is positive, assuming that second order conditions are satisfied. Plausible restrictions on the functions f(·) and W(·) yield positive $^U PD$ and $^U PR$[4], but do not determine the sign of $^U DR$. We therefore examine the effects of changing the population-physician ratio (R) assuming the $^U DR$ is negative (Case 1) as well as positive (Case 2).

1. Case 1: $^U DR < 0$

The first products in both (6) and (7), divided by Δ, represent direct effects of changes in R; the second products again divided by Δ, are indirect effects.

When ^{U}DR is negative, the direct effects are positive in (6) and negative in (7). As the population-physician ratio rises, price rises and the level of discretionary behavior are offsetting. A fall in D (*cet. par.*) shifts the demand schedule inward, causing equilibrium price to fall. The indirect effect of an increase in P on D is to increase discretionary behavior.

A positive $\frac{dP}{dR}$ is consistent with standard assumptions about market behavior. However, as discussed more fully below, several empirical studies of physician pricing behavior report a negative $\frac{dP}{dR}$, and the authors have often been quick to attribute this finding to physician-generated demand. *Case 1 implies that* $\frac{dP}{dR}$ *may be negative, but it must then be negative for all variables shifting the demand curve outward.* Patient income and insurance, for example, would operate on price in the same manner as a change in R. However, estimates of patient income in physician price equations have without exception been positive.

2. Case 2: $^{U}DR > 0$

With a positive ^{U}DR both $\frac{dP}{dR}$ and $\frac{dD}{dR}$ are unambiguously positive. Case 2 leaves the negative population-physician parameter estimates unexplained.

The impacts of changes in R on physicians' workloads and earnings are easily assessed, given $\frac{dP}{dR}$ and $\frac{dD}{dR}$.

$$\frac{dW}{dR} = f(P, D) + f_P \frac{dP}{dR} + f_D \frac{dD}{dR} \tag{8}$$

$\frac{dW}{dR}$ is unambiguously positive if $\frac{dD}{dR}$ is negative, and $\frac{dD}{dR}$ is positive. A positive $\frac{dW}{dR}$ is consistent with all studies we have reviewed, including those that conclude that physicians create their own demand. Of course, a positive $\frac{dP}{dR}$ could also yield a positive $\frac{dW}{dR}$, depending on the relative strengths of the offsetting effects.

$$\frac{dY}{dR} = (P - C_W) \cdot \frac{dW}{dR} + W \frac{dP}{dR} \tag{9}$$

Since $(P-C_W)\frac{dW}{dR}$ is positive for positive $\frac{dW}{dR}$, the sign of $\frac{dY}{dR}$ depends on the sign of $\frac{dP}{dR}$. With a negative $\frac{dP}{dR}$, $\frac{dY}{dR}$ could be negative even if $\frac{dW}{dR}$ is positive. Empirical studies relating physicians' earnings to a number of variables, including R, show $\frac{dY}{dR}$ to be positive.

A simpler but conceptually unsatisfactory model assumes that physicians set their workloads and prices to achieve an income target.[6] This theory predicts that an increase in physician density (a fall in R) increases fees. However, as in Case 1, if $\frac{dP}{dR}$ is negative, consistency requires that demand shift factors such as patient income and insurance have negative effects on price. On the whole, the model is unsatisfactory because it does not say how the target is set. Uwe Reinhardt suggests that the target may be set with reference to the local income distribution or according to the model physician income in the region. Meaningful empirical tests of these suggestions have not been devised.[7]

The most important contribution of economic theory is to remind the empiricist that consistency is required across a set of parameter estimates. Conclusions based on a single parameter estimate are not valid. With this point in mind, we now review literature on physician workload and patient utilization, fees, earnings, and quality-amenities associated with physicians' services.

Empirical Evidence

Physician Workload and Utilization Per Capita Population

While the theory presented above relates to workload per physician, most evidence advanced by the advocates of supplier-induced demand relates to medical services per patient or population. Services per capita (L) is defined as

$$L=\frac{W}{R}=f(P, D). \tag{10}$$

A decline in R (i.e., an increase in the physician-population ratio) could lower workload per physician and, at the same time, increase L.[8] This will occur if the elasticity of the physician's workload (W) with respect to R is positive but less than one.[9] If this elasticity were one, a ten percent decrease in R would be offset by a ten percent decrease in W, and L would not change. If the hypothetical ten percent decrease in R led to a six percent decrease in W, L would rise.

In a standard model, a decrease in R leads to a lower price which in turn promotes utilization. In a nonstandard model which includes discretionary behavior, price could rise and discretionary activities could increase quantity per capita as well. Evidence on R and L alone do not allow one to distinguish between the standard and nonstandard models.

Proponents of the supplier-induced demand hypothesis frequently cite positive associations between the area physician-population ratio and the quantity of physicians' services rendered *per patient* to support their arguments. Such two-way comparisons are not convincing because (a) the association is consistent with standard as well as supplier-induced demand models, (b) bordercrossing, and (c) physicians may locate in areas where patient demand is high. Bordercrossing arises since patients frequently cross county and State boundaries to obtain medical care, and utilization is often attributed to the place the care was received rather than to the patient's residence. In technical terms, it is not clear that the effect of physician density on use is identified in these studies.[10]

A frequently-cited study by Victor Fuchs and Marcia Kramer concludes that the supply of physicians creates its own demand. Fuchs-Kramer (FK) estimate a simultaneous system of four equations with these dependent variables: (1) quantity of services consumed by patients per capita; (2) physicians per 100,000 population; (3) quantity of medical services produced per physician; and (4) insurance benefits for physicians' services per capita. Although the gross and net (of insurance) prices of physicians' services are endogenous explanatory variables, the structural price equations are not presented. Structural equations are estimated in logarithmic form. The authors refrain from solving for a reduced form because "of the many ambiguities complicating the interpretation of most of the (structural) equations" (p. 36). FK's result therefore cannot be compared directly to our comparative statics, but aspects of FK's results are nevertheless instructive for the analysis of physician-induced demand.[11]

FK use the physician-population ratio $\left(\frac{1}{R}\right)$ as an endogenous explanatory variable in two structural equations. In the quantity per physician regression, the ratio has a negative impact on workload with elasticities in the -0.5 to -0.67 range. FK's patient utilization regression contains per capita income, the net price of physicians' services, and the $\left(\frac{1}{R}\right)$ ratio, which has a positive impact on services per capita with an elasticity of 0.4. The price elasticity is -0.2.

As the authors note, with money price included in the utilization equation, the coefficient of the $\left(\frac{1}{R}\right)$ ratio must reflect something other than the effects of the money price on utilization. FK offer three explanations:

First, they suggest that an increase in $\left(\frac{1}{R}\right)$ probably reduces mean travel time to the physician and mean waiting time in the physician's office. But they also state, "Given a low price elasticity of demand [about −.2], however, this factor alone is insufficient to account for the magnitude of the MD [the ratio variable] coefficient" (p. 36).

The relative magnitude of the time price elasticity depends on (a) the effect of the ratio on the time price and (b) the share of the time price in the total price (the sum of the money price and the time price). FK present evidence on neither. We shall discuss this issue further later in this section and, then, present evidence from other studies.

Second, FK raise the possibility of physician-induced demand. In fact, they venture that supply-generated demand may fully explain their empirical findings. Moreover, they claim that "because physicians can and do determine the demand for their own services to a considerable extent, we should be wary of plans which assume that the cost of medical care would be reduced by increasing the supply of physicians" (p. 2).

Third, FK indicate that the ratio's partial effect on utilization may be consistent with Martin Feldstein's view (1970) that there is permanent excess demand for physicians' services. If there is excess demand, an increased supply of doctors would increase utilization and thereby reduce the excess demand gap. FK reject this possibility, and we agree. Feldstein's structural equations are probably underidentified, as Newhouse and Phelps (1974) have noted. Therefore, it is inappropriate to find evidence from Feldstein's "implausible" coefficients for his permanent excess demand hypothesis.

A more recent study by Joel May (1975) investigates the effect of supply-created demand on patient utilization.[12] May includes time prices, travel time to "regular" source of care, and waiting time for an appointment in his structural equations.[13] Unfortunately, he only presents selected regression coefficients and omits those for the time price variables. Thus, we cannot assess the impact of physician availability from his utilization regressions.

Elasticity estimates corresponding to two physician variables from May (1975) are summarized in table 1. These variables are the ratio of physicians in patient care per 1,000 population for the Primary Sampling Unit (PSU) in which the individual lives (MDPOP), and the fraction of physicians in patient care in the PSU who are general (or family) practitioners (PERCGPS). A PSU corresponds to an SMSA or a county (for nonSMSA PSU's).

May concludes that the availability of health care inputs affects utilization. Since most input coefficients are statistically significant, the null hypothesis of no effect can be rejected. But the associated elasticity estimates are low, far lower than FK's. At least three additional points should be made. First, since one expects MDPOP and PERCGPS to be negatively correlated with each other and apparently positively correlated with the dependent variables, omitting the latter variable (and the case for including it is not strong) should further reduce the MDPOP elasticity. Second, a measure of office waiting time, though available in May's survey, was not included. As seen below, there is a negative relationship between MDPOP and office waiting time and the latter should have a negative impact on use. Omitting the component of the time price would positively bias MDPOP's elasticities shown in table 1. Finally, the physician-induced demand hypothesis is particularly plausible for follow-up visits. By contrast, the first visit is most likely to be patient-oriented. If so, the lower MDPOP elasticities in regressions based on persons with one or more visits are implausible.[14]

Studies of patient demand for medical care by Newhouse and Phelps (1976) and Karen Davis and Roger Reynolds suggest an impact of physician availability on utilization, but neither contain patient travel or waiting time variables. In the first study, physician availability elasticities range as high as FK's but many are lower, depending on the sample and estimator.[15] The Davis-Reynolds (DR) elasticities from a sample of the elderly are the highest we have seen; i.e., as high as 1.0. This is particularly surprising since, for persons living outside the twenty-two largest SMSA's, the authors inserted ratios corresponding to the person's Census Area broken down by SMSA and nonSMSA residence. This is clearly a source of errors-in-variables, which biases parameter estimates toward zero. Unlike other utilization regressions we have reviewed, DR exclude money as well as time prices. If one were to interpret DR's equations as reduced form equations, one has the implication that increasing the supply of doctors has a negligible or even a zero impact on workload per physician! However, this contradicts tabular evidence on physicians' workload presented by E. F. Hughes *et al.* and others, as well as FK's finding that the elasticity between workload per physician and the physician-population ratio is about −0.6.

Evans, E. M. Parrish, and Floyd Sully (EPS) assess variations in gross billings per physician (W·P) in British Columbia for the year 1969. This research supports Evans' strong policy statements regarding supplier-induced demand elsewhere (1976a, 1976b). Since Medicare (Canadian "national" health insurance) was in effect during that year, and it reimbursed on the basis of fixed fee schedules, the EPS study is really an inquiry into sources of difference in physicians' workloads. The dependent variable is the natural log of billings. Explanatory variables are dummy variables for specialty, location (dummies for physicians located in Vancouver, Victoria, and communities of 25,000 to 100,000 and 10,000 to 25,000 population), size of group, date of graduation of practitioner, and the log of the physician-population ratio.

One of the study's major findings is the small negative estimated elasticity of the physician-population ratio variable (− 0.16 in a regression for all physicians), a result consistent with DR's work on patient utilization.

Regressions based on subsamples never yield a much more negative elasticity, and in one instance, the elasticity is zero. The authors interpret the result in the main as evidence for the supplier-induced demand hypothesis.

Table 1 Effects of Physician Availability on Physicians' Services Utilization—the May Study[1]

	MDPOP		PERCGPS	
Dependent Variable	**sig.?**	**elasticity**	**sig.?**	**elasticity**
Visits to MD office per year (all cases)	yes*	+.14	yes*	+.19
Visits to MD office per year (only those with one or more visits)	no	+.01	yes*	+.14
Total visits per year (all cases)	yes*	+.19	yes*	+.15
Total visits per year (only those with one or more visits)	yes**	+.08	yes*	+.11

[1] May (1975) *at 1% **at 5%

Unfortunately, EPS do not consider the socio-demographic and geographic character of British Columbia. According to data they present (but do not discuss), 56 percent of all physicians in the Province were located in Vancouver at the time of the study. When Vancouver is combined with nearby Victoria (across the Strait of Georgia), this rises to 68 percent. About one percent were located in areas with populations of under 10,000. The distribution of practicing specialists was more uneven, with Vancouver and Victoria accounting for 87 percent of the total.

The observational unit for the regression analysis is the individual physician, but the physician-population ratios are defined for 29 hospital districts and then merged with individual physician records prior to estimation. Two of these districts are in the Vancouver-Victoria area. Many of the others are extremely rural.[16] Thus EPS have distributed the vast majority of districts over the minority of British Columbia physicians. Although the outlying areas have different per capita income, mean distance to a physician, and racial composition, EPS include no explanatory variables for these influences. Certainly they cannot be considered to be orthogonal to physician density. With regard to patient travel time, locating a physician in many northern sections of the Province may indeed lower travel time markedly, and, correspondingly, the elasticity relating travel time to physician density would reflect this. In any case, patients outside the southern region must travel great distances for certain types of care, particularly for specialized treatment. For some types of care, the pertinent market area is nearly the entire Province. To the extent this is so, the specification of 29 district market areas is inappropriate, and border-crossing could produce substantial biases which lead the unsuspecting reader to accept EPS's conclusions.

Physicians' Fees

Articles on physicians' fees by Martin Feldstein and Joseph Newhouse, both appearing in 1970, are the first econometric studies of physician fee-setting. Using an annual time series of 19 years, Feldstein concludes that the standard market model cannot explain observed behavior of physicians' fees. This result is reached after obtaining a number of coefficients with signs inconsistent with the standard model. As noted above, Newhouse and Phelps (1974) have argued persuasively that Feldstein's structural equations are underidentified. If so, implausible signs could be explained on econometric grounds.

Newhouse's (1970) evidence on the impact of physician availability on fees is based on a bivariate regression of general practitioner office visit with per capita income. Both variables were deflated by the Consumer Price Index for each of the 18 SMSA's comprising the sample. The coefficient of per capita income is significant at the five percent level (one-tail test). With income included, the partial correlation of the physician-population ratio with the fee is .55. Although Newhouse's result implies that the reduced form derivative $\frac{dP}{dR}$ is negative, this is hardly conclusive. Certainly other variables, such as area factor prices related to space, are positively correlated with the physician-population ratio and should have been included in the regression. If so, omitted variable bias is a problem. More serious, however, are the inferences about supply-created demand and target-income setting that have been drawn from such results. The coefficient of per capita income is consistent with a standard model! At a minimum, such empirical evidence leads to a standoff between the B's and the N's.

More recently, Bruce Steinwald and Sloan (1974) and Sloan (1976a) have used American Medical Association data to assess determinants of physicians' fees. Both students represent physician density with two variables: (a) the number of physicians in the physician's own specialty per 1,000 population; and (b) the number of physicians per 1,000 population in other specialties which are not necessarily competitive with the physician.

In Steinwald-Sloan, based on microdata on individual physicians, the ratios are defined for the physician's county when possible (for general practitioners) and for the State when it is not (for physicians in internal medicine, pediatrics, general surgery, and obstetrics-gynecology). The ratios are thus best measured for general practitioners. For general practitioners and general surgeons, increases in the number of competing physicians per capita lowers fees in most of the regressions. But the opposite result is obtained for internists, pediatricians, and obstetricians-gynecologists. Even though Steinwald-Sloan's price regressions contain many more explanatory variables than the earlier price studies, the positive association between fees and physician density is not universal, but remains for a number of specialties.

The Sloan (1976) study combines individual observations on physicians from 1967 through 1970 AMA surveys into State aggregates and conducts a cross section-time series analysis for the four-year period. Results are presented for general practitioners, general surgeons, and internists. A negative association is obtained for the first two specialties, but not for internists. Both studies report signs for the demand shift variables that are fully consistent with the N's interpretation of physicians' behavior.

L. F. Huang and O. Koropecky also report that physician density has a positive impact on fees and suggest that as physician density rises, physicians gain better information about what the "market will bear." According to their model, not only does higher physician density drive prices up, but since the ratio interacts with last year's price, the positive effect of the MD-population ratio is strengthened with each successive price increase. Thus, the model offers the unfortunate prediction that the ratio's effect will grow increasingly stronger in each successive time period.

While the preceding price studies use data on individual physicians or aggregates of physicians, the aforementioned Newhouse and Phelps (1976) study (NP), based on household data, is also germane to the discussion of price. NP estimated a regression for the price of a physician's office visit. In an earlier study, which used essentially the same equation specifications (Newhouse and Phelps 1974)), the authors gave four reasons for variation in price in a patient-oriented sample.[17] Two relate to quality (differences in the marginal productivity of a given unit of service) and to amenities, such as tasteful office furniture. Third, higher priced services may involve less queuing, particularly less waiting time in the office. Fourth, prices may differ because of inter-personal variation in search costs. Persons with higher time prices may engage in less search and therefore purchase more expensive services. NP, followers of the N school (at least in their work on demand), do not attribute price variation to geographical differences in physician-generated demand.

For our discussion of price, these are most important results from the NP study. First, wage income has a positive impact on the physician office visit price while nonwage income has almost no effect. This patter *suggests* that high wage patients are willing to pay a higher price for faster service.[18] Second, the physician-population ratio raises price. We argue below that a reasonable alternative to the supplier-induced demand hypothesis is that quality, amenities, and patient time vary systematically with the ratio.

Physicians' Earnings

We have seen that the physician-population ratio consistently has a positive impact on patient utilization and often has a positive impact on prices. To our knowledge, all studies on physicians' earnings show that, *cet. par.*, physicians located in high physician density areas earn less. It is useful to distinguish between unadjusted earnings and earnings adjusted for work hours. To the extent that quality and amenities vary systematically with physician density, the behavior of effort-adjusted earnings may well differ from that of fees.

Murray Brown, Alexandra Benham, and Lee Benham (mimeo.) analyze pooled cross section-time series data on physicians' net earnings from Canada's ten Provinces for the years 1961 through 1971. The main objective of this paper is to assess the effects of instituting Medicare (universal compulsory insurance) on physicians' earnings. Determinants of earnings are provincial per capita income, the percent of population covered by medical insurance (to account for variations in the years before Medicare was introduced),[19] the number of physicians per capita, and a set of dummy variables to gauge the effect of Medicare on earnings in years after the introduction of Medicare. Some regressions also include a continuous time variable to measure secular trends, such as shifts toward salaried practice and changes in referral patterns.

For purposes of this review, the estimated elasticities of earnings on the physician-population variable are pertinent. These range from –.36 to as high as –.95 when two Provinces, Saskatchewan and Newfoundland, are excluded. The elasticities (coefficients) are all statistically significant at the one percent level.[20]

Sloan (1968) estimates a seven equation model of physician location with the State as the observational unit. Both ordinary least squares (OLS) and two stage least squares (TSLS) estimators are used. Physicians' earnings is the dependent variable in one equation, and among the explanatory variables, only the physician-population ratio is considered endogenous when TSLS is the estimator. With OLS, the ratio is significant at the one percent level with an elasticity of –.60. The corresponding TSLS parameter estimate is extremely imprecise with an elasticity of –.03. Since simultaneous equation bias should drive the ratio's coefficient toward zero, the difference between the OLS and TSLS is not due to simultaneity but rather to poor performance (inefficiency) of TSLS, which frequently occurs in cross section analysis.

The above comparative statics analysis assessed the *total* impact of an exogenously-determined ratio on physicians' earnings. The Brown-Benham-Benham and Sloan OLS results directly correspond to our comparative statics analysis. If the ratio is endogenous, it disappears from explicit consideration. The –.03 elasticity then requires a structural (as opposed to a reduced form) interpretation.

Benham, Alex Maurizi, and Melvin Reder (1968) (BMR) also assess the impact of the physician-population ratio on mean earnings by State. BMR's specification is less complete than Sloan's and the R^2s are much lower than Sloan's OLS regression. BMR's elasticities for the physician-population ratio vary from –.12 to –.70, depending on the year. In the most recent year, 1963, the elasticity is –.24 but the R^2 is only .04.

Estimates of the impact of the ratio on earnings per hour and per week are available from Sloan (1975) and Barbara Kehrer. Not surprisingly, elasticities with an effort-adjusted earnings measure are lower. Sloan's estimated elasticities, based on data on individual physicians from the 1960 and 1970 Censuses, range from –.20 to –.34. Kehrer's, using microdata on physicians from a 1973 American Medical Association Survey, are negative but about half of Sloan's.

Quality and Amenities Associated with Physicians' Services

Because of significant problems, economists have been reluctant to analyze the demand for quality. To assess adequately the notion of supplier-induced demand, it is essential to isolate qualitative aspects of physicians' services. Possibly, as physician density increases, quality-amenities increase systematically. If so, empirical relationships seemingly inconsistent with the standard model may be explained by a *very* standard model according to which patients willingly pay for quality. Patients may value, for example, time spent with an "understanding" physician, physician availability by telephone at night and on weekends for which there is no separate charge, short waiting times in the doctor's office, and short delays to an appointment.

To access the relationship between quantity (W), quality and physician density, we first turn to pertinent theory. Assume that the physician sets price on the demand function P = P(W,A;Z), where A represents quality-amenities, and Z any exogenous (to the firm) demand shift variable, including R—the population-physician ratio. Since the comparative statics are slightly simpler, we specify a profit function (Y) rather than a utility function. In this formulation, the physician's shadow wage is an element of the cost function,

$$C = C(W, A).$$

$$Y = P(W, A; Z)W - C(W, A) \tag{11}$$

The first-order conditions are:

$$Y_W = WP_W + P(\cdot) - C_W = 0$$

and

$$Y_A = WP_A - C_A = 0 \tag{12}$$

Totally differentiate (11) and (12) and use Cramer's Rule to obtain total effects associated with changes in Z.

$$\frac{dW}{dZ} = - \frac{Y_{AA}Y_{WZ} - Y_{AW}Y_{AZ}}{\Delta} \tag{13}$$

From the second-order conditions, Y_{AA} and Y_{WW} are negative and Δ is positive. Taking R as the member of the Z set, assume that Y_{WZ} is positive. That is, an increase in R shifts the individual physician's demand schedule outward. There is no reason to believe R has a *direct* effect on A; i,e.; Y_{AZ} is zero. If so, $\frac{dW}{dR}$ is positive, a result consistent with the empirical studies reviewed above.

Likewise,

$$\frac{dA}{dZ} = - \frac{Y_{WW}Y_{AZ} - Y_{WA}Y_{WZ}}{\Delta} \tag{14}$$

The sign $\frac{dA}{dZ}$ depends on the cross-partial involving the decision variables $Y_{WA}(= WP_{WA} + P_A - C_{WA})$.If the demand function is separable in W and A, Y_{WA} is negative since C_{WA} is plausibly positive. With a negative Y_{WA}, $\frac{dA}{dR}$ is negative. This means that a rise in the population-physician ratio increases W along a positively-sloped marginal cost function, which makes the production of A more costly at the margin. The marginal revenue schedule for A (WP_A) is unaffected by the rise in W, and therefore growth in R leads to a reduction in quality-amenities; e.g., more hurried visits, physician unavailability by telephone, etc. If the marginal revenue schedule for A shifts downward with increases in W, a negative $\frac{dA}{dR}$ is also obtained. It is worth emphasizing that high volume practices, often found in rural areas, can be understood with reference to this model. There is no need to invoke *ad hoc* assumptions, such as "physicians respond to community need."

Studies by Sloan and John Lorant, and Sloan (1977) investigate components of A, in particular, waiting time in the physician's office and the mean length of physician visit. The Sloan and Lorant studies are based on a 1973 American Medical Association survey of physicians' practice (the data base also used by Kehrer). They found statistically significant relationships between physician density and office waiting time and between density and visit length, and both imply a negative $\frac{dA}{dR}$. The vast majority of other parameter estimates are also consistent with a negative Y_{WA}. However, although the signs of the estimated coefficients imply a negative $\frac{dA}{dR}$, the associated elasticities are all under 0.11 in abosolute value.

Sloan (1977) analyzes patient travel time and office waiting time with data grouped into 60 "communities." The data source is the 1969 Health Interview Survey, conducted by the National Center for Health Statistics. Simple correlations show that increased physician density $\left(\frac{1}{R}\right)$ is associated with decreased travel and waiting time. The correlations never exceed 0.32 (in absolute value), implying that R explains less than 10 percent of the variance in patient time. Regressions were not estimated, and thus elasticity estimates are unavailable.

Econometric research on quality-amenity variables is still in its infancy. This work suggests that prices are higher, at least in part, in physician dense areas because A is also higher there. The implied quality-amenity elasticities, as yet, are too small to explain fully the magnitude of the elasticities associating R with patient utilization.

To see this, we consider the role of one type of amenity, the time patients spend obtaining physicians' services. The method is generalizable to other dimensions of quality. Specify a demand function for visits,

$$Q = (P_N + T)^{\beta} \tag{15}$$

where: Q = quantity of visits demanded per capita;
P_N = money price net of insurance;
T = time price.

Furthermore, let

$$T = wt \tag{16}$$

and

$$T = R^{\alpha} \tag{17}$$

where: w = patient's shadow wage;
t = patient's time input;
R = population-physician ratio.

Then,

$$Q = (P_N + wR^{\alpha})^{\beta} \tag{18}$$

From (18), one can derive money (ϵ) and time price (η) elasticities:

$$\epsilon = \beta\left[\frac{P_N}{P_N + wR^{\alpha}}\right] \tag{19}$$

and

$$\eta = \alpha\beta\left[\frac{wR^{\alpha}}{P_N + wR^{\alpha}}\right] \tag{20}$$

From (19) and (20), it is evident that the patient money and time price elasticities depend on the elasticities and and the relative share of time price in total price. For consumers well insured against money prices, this share could be quite significant. Let s be the time price share and, using Fuchs-Kramer elasticities for illustrative purposes, let

$$\beta(1 - s) = -.2$$

$$\alpha\beta s = -.4$$

Using market wage for workers in private industry and follow-up office visit fee estimates for 1969 from Sloan (1977), estimates of t from Sloan and Lorant (1976) and Sloan (1977), and assuming a coinsurance rate of .8 (proportion of the charge paid by the patient)[21] and \$1.50 for out-of-pocket transport costs, added to the time price, the total price to the patient in 1969 dollars is \$12.59, and the time price share (s) is .53. With s - .53, β is $-.43$ and α is 1.7. To date, *individual* time elasticities (waiting time, etc.) less than one-tenth the *composite* elasticity have been obtained. Many features of "A" in addition to travel and waiting time are undoubtedly reflected in FK's physician-population ratio elasticity.

To date, only very few quality-amenity variables have been analyzed. The method developed here can be generalized to include other kinds of "A" variables. Further research is necessary because one appropriately attributes the "residual" elasticity associated with R to supplier-induced demand. Hopefully, this section has provided a technical basis for analysis of this important issue.

The reader lacking a vested interest in econometric applications may (perhaps, legitimately) question whether economic theory and applied econometrics will ever settle this matter. Some have attempted to make inferences about supplier-induced demand from comparisons between fee-for-service and prepaid group practice. As indicated in a later section, such comparisons at best yield ambiguous evidence on this issue.

GAUGING MONOPOLY POWER IN A STANDARD MARKET CONTEXT

As Section I indicated, the supplier-induced demand argument contains numerous weaknesses. Yet, current evidence cannot rule it out completely. Since it may be years before enough evidence is in, it is useful to pose a second question. Assuming that the standard market model holds, can we say whether the market for physicians' services is monopolistic or competitive? If not, what kinds of tests should be conducted to decide the question? We accepted the notion at the outset that physicians earn rents because of entry barriers into the profession. However, it is conceivable that physicians' fees could be set competitively even though they contain an element of economic rent.

This section is divided into two parts. First, we re-examine some of the studies reviewed in the previous section for indications of monopoly in a standard market model. In all cases, evidence pertains to individual physicians' practices. These indicators include physicians' earnings, price-setting behavior, and quality-amenities. Second, we look for possible cartels in the medical profession at the State and local levels. In view of the paucity of evidence on these latter issues, our discussion is clearly preliminary and exploratory. We consider the dispersion of fees for specific procedures within local market areas, interactions involving individual physicians, medical societies, and third party payers, and Foundations for Medical Care.

Price discrimination in an industry is a manifestation of market power. According to a very recent survey of physicians, price discrimination is no longer important in medicine even though it probably was important historically.[22]

Concentration and Physicians' Earnings

Such measures of concentration as the share of output from the four largest firms in an industry, Herfindahl, and/or Entropy indexes are certainly inappropriate for the physicians' services market.[23] Except for rural locations, the large number of physicians in a given "market area" makes this industry's output appear dispersed, certainly by contrast to many non-service industries.

A crude analog to above concentration measures in industrial sectors is the physician-population ratio. As noted above, the ratio exerts a negative impact on physicians' earnings. We have been unable to find a study showing otherwise. While the elasticities vary, one may argue that the use of OLS yields estimates biased toward zero. That is, the true negative response of earnings to changes in the physician-population ratio may be larger than the OLS results imply. Available evidence in any case does not allow one to distinguish between a temporary disequilibrium in which high returns are eventually eliminated by entry of new physicians and monopoly profits which are likely to persist.

One strain throughout the literature on monopolies is that monopoly profits are used to purchase amenities for the suppliers, such as inefficiency, discrimination in employment, plush offices, or nonprofit-maximizing prices.

Several economists have suggested, as we have already noted, that physicians' price-output decisions are dictated by the motive of achieving a target income.[24] Although consistent with supplier-induced demand, this motive could also operate when the demand curve is exogenous to the firm. The notion derives its popularity from numerous positive coefficients relating physicians' fees to the physician-population ratio. Yet, when one moves from physicians' fees to their earnings, the target theory would be much more convincing if earnings were constant. Given the obvious nonconstancy thereof, target theory proponents are forced into one of two arguments. First, the targets themselves differ, but there is no theory to explain interphysician variation in targets. Second, physicians experiencing an inward shift in their demand curves, because of in-migration of physicians into their market areas, switch from nonprofit-maximizing price (presumably in the inelastic portion of their demand curves) to the profit-maximizing price. However, the inward shift is greater and dominates the effects of changed pricing practices. Of course, the evidence *per se* cannot be used to refute these explanations, but the necessary assumptions would appear to be needlessly complex.

Monopoly Versus Competition:
Econometric Evidence on Physicians' Fees

Newhouse (1970) proposes a test for whether individual physicians are monopolists or competitors. Newhouse's Model I (the monopolist) implies that the price and physician density are unrelated, while Model II (competition) implies a negative relationship between price and the physician-population ratio. Newhouse finds a positive relation and concludes physicians are local monopolists.

Commenting on the Newhouse article, H. E. Frech and Paul Ginsburg (1972) argue that Newhouse's distinction between Model I and Model II rests on an arbitrary assumption. Specifically, Newhouse assumes that the marginal cost of physicians' services is constant in Model I but rising in Model II. Since there is no reason for assuming that cost functions (rather than demand functions) differ according to market structure, this assumption represents a conceptual error, a point Newhouse's reply (Newhouse and Sloan (1972)) recognizes.

Plausible monopolistic *and* competitive pricing models that do not explicitly permit interphysician variation in quality-amenities predict that the area physician-population ratio should have a negative partial impact. The positive physician-population coefficient in physician pricing regressions is inconsistent with *both* monopolistic and competitive models. In fact, without examining the larger picture (i.e., explicit consideration of quality-amenities), econometric research has little to say on this issue.

Newhouse (1970) proposes another test that also merits brief mention. He uses cross sectional data to regress the change in physicians' price between the years 1960-61 to 1965-66 on the change in personal per capita income during the same period and finds a very weak relationship although the levels of these two variables are closely related. According to Newhouse, price adjustments occur more slowly in monopolistic contexts, and therefore the poor results with first differences support the monopolistic alternative. Frech and Ginsburg (1972), responding to Newhouse, cite theoretical work by Armen Alchian which demonstrates that there is no necessary relationship between market structure and adjustment speed. As before, Frech and Ginsburg's argument is more compelling. The adjustment speed of prices does not constitute valid evidence on this issue.[25]

Market Structure and Quality

Although, until recently, economists have neglected qualitative aspects of physicians' services, these features merit both theoretical and policy interest. Specifically, is quality, like quantity, set lower under monopoly than under competition? Organized medicine, in proposing and successfully obtaining State bans on physician advertising and stringent medical practice acts, has essentially argued that competition lowers quality.

To assess this issue, we borrow from Michael Spence.[26] Unlike other parts of this section, we shall, following Spence, consider positive *and* welfare aspects of this question simultaneously. A stable, negatively-sloped demand curve for the services of a "representative" physician is assumed. Certainly organized medicine's original argument would have been that this demand curve is not stable, and therefore regulation is required. But presumably entry barriers to the profession brought about by the upgrading of medicial education since the 1910 Flexner Report have largley eliminated "charlatans" and "quacks" who take advantage of innocent consumers. In fact, sophisticated observers within organized medicine must realize that if they push the supplier-induced demand argument too far they will support public demands for external controls less favorable to the medical profession. Indeed, the profession is reluctant to push this line of reasoning. If entry barriers have done their job, it is appropriate to assess the effects of restraints such as advertising bans, which confer monopoly power on each physician.

As before, let price be P, per physician quantity W, and quality-amenities A. Then P = P(W,A) and C = C(W,A) are demand and cost functions.

Consumer surplus (S) is

$$s = \int_0^W P(v, A)dv - WP(W, A). \qquad (21)$$

Net revenue for the representative physician is

$$Y = WP(W, A) - C(W, A). \qquad (22)$$

The total surplus X is then

$$X = S + Y. \tag{23}$$

Then for a *given quantity,* does the monopolist produce above or below the socially optimal quality? The total surplus is maximized with respect to quality when

$$\frac{\partial X}{\partial A} = \int_0^W P_A \, dv - C_A = 0. \tag{24}$$

The physician, however, maximizes net income, holding W fixed, when

$$\frac{\partial Y}{\partial A} = WP_A - C_A = 0. \tag{25}$$

Equations (24) and (25) may not yield the same quality levels, and if not, the monopolist under- or over-supplies quality. From (23),

$$\frac{\partial X}{\partial A} = \frac{\partial S}{\partial A} + \frac{\partial Y}{\partial A} = \int_0^W P_A dv - WP_A + \frac{\partial Y}{\partial A}. \tag{26}$$

When $\frac{\partial Y}{\partial A} = 0$ which is so for the profit-maximizing physician, the sign of $\frac{\partial X}{\partial A}$ depends on the relative magnitudes of $\int_0^W P_A dv$ and WP_A. If the average valuation of quality (i.e., if $\frac{1}{W}\int_0^W P_A dv$ exceeds P_A), then (22) is positive. Social welfare could rise if the monopolist supplied more quality. The sufficient condition for $\frac{1}{W}\int_0^W P_A dv > P_A$ is that the cross-partial P_{AW} be negative. If $P'_{AW} > 0$, which implies that patients attracted as the physician moves down his demand curve have higher marginal valuations of quality. Furthermore, plausible functional forms of $P(.)$, such as $P = \gamma_0 W^{\gamma_1} A^{\gamma_2}$, imply a negative P_{AW}.

We can now extend Spence's argument to competition. For the competitive firm, $P_W = 0$ by definition and thus $P_{WA} = 0$.[27] In competition, correct levels of both W *and* A are supplied.

This analysis has two implications. First, regulations conferring a degree of monopoly power on physicians result in welfare losses in quality as well as in quantity. Second, if one could show that P_{WA} is negative, one could empirically test for relations between monopoly power and quality-amenities. As noted above, there is already some evidence that more A is supplied, *cet. par.,* in physician-dense areas.

Up to now, we have assessed the degree of competition in the physicians' services market in terms of individual physicians acting independently. It is also frequently alleged that physicians exercise monopoly power via their professional associations. We now turn to evidence from this perspective.

Activities of Professional Associations

Fee Dispersion in Local Market Areas

In a market with many buyers and sellers, there is rarely one price, regardless whether the market is competitive or monopolistic. Quality may vary, especially in the physicians' market. Furthermore, since information on prices charged by alternative suppliers is costly, consumers will choose incomplete information and take the chance of paying high prices. For these reasons, strict uniformity of offer prices in a market area has been viewed by the courts as evidence of collusion, not competition, among firms.

Evidence on the dispersion of physician prices within individual market areas is available from a few sources. Newhouse and Sloan (1972) present coefficients of variation, based on *Medical Economics* surveys, for initial and follow-up office visits, and for appendectomies. Separate calculations are shown for general practice, internal medicine, and general surgery in two cities, New York and Chicago. The coefficients of variation are about 0.2 to 0.3. These compare to the offer price coefficient for a Chevrolet in Chicago of 0.02 and bids to the Federal Government for the delivery of anthracite coal of 0.07 (George Stigler, 1961). While Newhouse and Sloan recognize that part of the within-market area dispersion in physicians' fees may reflect product differences among physicians, they contend that such differences alone cannot account for the much greater dispersion among physicians than among automobile dealers and sellers of coal. Rather, a meaningful proportion of the dispersion of fees in the physicians' services market is attributable to incomplete patient search.

From 1973 through 1975, Mathematica, Inc., conducted national telephone surveys of physicians' practices. The sample size suffices to permit precise estimates of fees in numerous metropolitan and nonmetropolitan sites. The coefficients of variations are in the 0.2's.[28]

Neither Newhouse-Sloan's nor Mathematica's evidence sheds light on Newhouse-Sloan's contention that product differences do not fully account for the observed fee dispersion. A recent study by Fred Goldman and Michael Grossman is a useful test. Goldman and Grossman estimate hedonic fee functions, using data on physicians' fees from a sample of pediatric patients living in two communities within New York City. Measures of physicians' credentials in the fee functions include experience, specialty, board certification status, location of medical school attended, and medical school faculty appointment. The highest R^2 for any of the estimated fee functions is 0.18. One could clearly argue that a higher proportion of the variance in fees could have been explained if additional "quality" variables were included.[29]

From the three studies, it appears the (1) effective price-fixing arrangements among individual physicians within a local market area are unlikely and (2) price dispersion at the local level reflects more than product differences. The first conclusion is not surprising in view of the substantial costs that would almost certainly be involved in policing price-fixing arrangements. There are often hundreds or, in some cases, thousands of individual firms offering heterogeneous products. As Jack Hirschleifer states, "Cartels have an Achilles heel. However desirable the arrangement is to the firms as a group, for a single firm it pays to 'chisel' on the agreement" (p. 296). Physicians could chisel by changing the descriptions of work performed (i.e., describing a procedure different from the one actually performed), and by varying the nature of the service itself. Also, it would be very difficult for a cartel to accommodate interphyscian variations in quality. Attempts to assign quality levels to individual members of any professional group would certainly be resisted. At most, quality differences could be measured by years of experience, board certification status, academic affiliations, and the like. But such variables have been included by Goldman and Grossman, and they explain a small proportion of the variance in fees within a local market area.

Advertising bans, both legal and those embodied in associations' codes of medical ethics, have undoubtedly made it more difficult for the medical care consumer to comparison shop and at least partly account for the market power the individual physician possesses.

Physicians' Associations and the Market for Insurance

While price fixing among individual physicians can be ruled out, physicians' associations can engage in a more subtle form of price manipulation in their dealings with third-party payers. According to S. G. Vahovich and P. Aherne (p. 146), fee-for-service physicians obtained 52 percent of gross revenue in 1970 (the only year for which these data are available) from private and government insurance sources.[30] There are important inter-specialty differences. Pediatricians derived 20 percent from third-party sources while general surgeons, radiologists, and anesthesiologists obtained 68, 74, and 75 percent, respectively. Few patients are covered in full for initial and follow-up office visits, irrespective of specialty seen. By contrast, more than one-half are fully covered for surgical procedures and hospital visits.

When revenue from third-party sources is important, physicians' associations may find it advantageous to direct cartel-like activities at third parties. We shall consider three aspects: relative value studies; relationships between organized medicine and Blue Shield; and medical society-sponsored Foundations for Medical Care (FMC).

Relative Value Studies: Relative value studies (RVS) performed by several professional associations, most notably the California Medical Association (CMA), serve:

1. as a guide to physicians in establishing fees;
2. as a guide for insurance carriers and government agencies in determining the extent of their commitment; and
3. as a guide in evaluating individual claims. (California Medical Association, 1969, p. 6.)

These studies always claim to be ratios among fees, rather than fee schedules. They further state that the ratios are based on a combination of findings of sample surveys of practicing physicians *and* "professional judgment" of physician advisors to the association. In a *strict sense,* RVS is not a set of fee schedules, since the dollar level of the numeraire procedure (the "conversion factor") is not specified. But the studies are widely used by private and public third-party payers to establish fixed fee schedules or variable fee screens when the "usual-customary-reasonable" (UCR) method of reimbursement is utilized.[31] A conversion factor is included in individual insurance contracts when RVS is used for reimbursement purposes. The relative value studies define procedure definitions and associated codes as well as relative values. The way a procedure is described and coded may affect reimbursement via a change in physicians' billing methods. The introduction of a new relative value study has potential effects via changes in terminology in addition to any effect of modifications in the unit value scales themselves.

Although we can easily envision circumstances under which changes in relative values cause fee increases, there is, to our knowledge, no "hard" evidence on this issue. According to one plausible mechanism, there is downward rigidity in the conversion factors written into insurance contracts. Thus, with a downwardly-inflexible numeraire, changes in the ratios drive insurer fee schedules up, which in turn causes fees themselves to rise. Ways in which changes in procedure terminology and coding can be altered to increase third-party payments to physicians are more subtle, and there is some evidence on this phenomenon.

Using data from California Blue Shield (CBS), the Medicare Part B carrier in northern California, William Sobaski attempts to isolate impacts on Medicare expenditures attributable to changes in RVS terminology. According to Sobaski, the California Medical Association (CMA) urged CBS to replace its 1964 RVS with CMA's more recent 1969 version for purposes of reimbursing physicians under Medicare. A major difference between the 1964 and 1969 versions is the degree of precision in terminology. The 1964 version describes procedures with four-digit codes; the 1969 uses a five-digit system. According to Sobaski, greater detail allowed the physician to upgrade his own descriptions of services performed. He concludes, "had a terminology changeover occurred nationwide (rather than limited to California by the Social Security Administration), Medicare costs would have increased by $50 million or more.[32] These increases could have been compounded over time by normal price increases (which apply to a larger base)" (p. 8).

Information Engineering (mimeo.) compares the effects of using the five-digit Minnesota Relative Value Index (MRVI) and the four-digit Minnesota Blue Shield Relative Value Index on Medicare program outlays. As in California, physicians' associations within the State lobbied for the adoption of the five-digit index. Much of the argument was couched in terms of administrative convenience to the physician, since it is difficult for the physician to use several procedure coding systems. According to Information Engineering, "the escalatory impact of the MRVI coding system on the Medicare Part B program was measured by comparing the experience of a group of providers who had converted to the MRVI coding schedule to a group of providers who had not converted. The overall escalatory impact of the MRVI was calculated as being 10% (p. 52). The report adds a few caveats of an administrative nature, but they do not reverse this basic conclusion.

Although empirical evidence is unfortunately lacking, it is reasonable to speculate that the use of RVS for purposes of obtaining third-party reimbursement could lead to a subtle form of price discrimination. Procedure codes for higher-grade visits may be used when the patient has in-depth third-party coverage. Under Medicare, the physician could upgrade his description and take "assignment of benefits," whereby he is paid directly by the Medicare carrier, and then forego collection of the coinsurance from the patient. The patient would have no incentive to resist upgrading; for that matter, he would probably not even be aware of it.

Organized Medicine and Blue Shield: There is a clear historical connection between Blue Shield plans and State and local medical societies. In 1939, the California Medical Association and the Michigan State Medical Society were instrumental in organizing the first Blue Shield plans. From the outset, Blue Shield organizations in these States and elsewhere were controlled by physicians. State Blue Cross-Blue Shield enabling acts, which have given the Blues competitive advantages over the commercials (see Frech (1974)), have typically required that plans be subject to medical society approval or that a majority of the board of directors be physicians (Louis Reed, Anne Somers and Herman Somers). The local society often advanced the initial capital for a plan (Reed). In fact, Blue Shield has been publicized as "the doctor's plan—*for the people.*" (Blue Shield brochure.

Emphasis is Blue Shield's.) A more recent historical interpretation by Odin Anderson suggests that relationships between the Blues and organized medicine, and between Blue Cross and Blue Shield, have not always been a "bed of roses."

For purposes of this paper, we are much more interested in existing functional relationships between Blue Shield and organized medicine than in formal institutional linkages. Unfortunately, only fragmentary evidence exists. It is possible, however, to raise a number of issues that can be used as a guide to future research on this important aspect of the physicians' services market. Although it is possible to make some generalizations about Blue Shield it is also important to recognize the diversity among the Blue Shield plans, especially with regard to Blue Shield market shares and reimbursement practices. Research in this area will require some analysis on a plan-by-plan basis, and a complete analysis will have to account for sources of diversity in market shares and reimbursement practices.

There are at least three ways in which organized medicine and Blue Shield *could* potentially monopolize the market for physicians' service in concert: fix physicians' fees; bar entry of physicians into a market area, or, a related activity, exclude individual physicians who fail to comply with medical society norms; and prevent health insurers from effectively monitoring individual physicians' output and price decisions. We examine each of these in turn.

To understand the potential for joint fee fixing, it is first necessary to consider a few pertinent institutional details. Blue Shield plans as a group have historically displayed an unmistakable preference for "service benefit" or "payment-in-full" contracts. Under a service benefit plan, the physician accepts the insurer's payment-in-full for covered services and does not charge the patient anything. The physician is paid directly by the plan. Alternatively, under indemnity plans, typically used by commercial insurers, the insurer pays an amount for a specific procedure. The physician may (and frequently does) bill the patient for charges in excess of the third-party payment. As a rule, under indemnity, the patient is responsible for collecting from the third party. All the physicians need to do is complete a form, describing services rendered.

The indemnity concept is popular among physicians since it preserves their independence in fee setting. Yet at the same time, to the degree that patients are slow in paying, some physicians may incur higher billing and "bad debt" costs under indemnity.[33] In spite of Blue Shield's preference, a substantial proportion of Blue Shield contracts are of the indemnity variety. According to Reed and Carr (1970), in 1968, indemnity contracts were the most *prevalent* type in 21 percent of Blue Shield plans. Many of these are located in the more politically conservative States. In the remainder, full service (19 percent) and partial service (60 percent) plans were most prevalent. Under partial service, patients with annual incomes under a specified amount are eligible for service benefit coverage; the remainder (about the upper half of the 1968 income distribution) receive indemnity benefits. Under full service, every enrollee receives service benefits.

The distinction between indemnity and service benefits has important implications for analysis of physicians' fees. Under the former, if a medical society successfully convinced its Blue Shield "partner" to provide more generous reimbursement levels, the effect would be to shift the individual physician's demand curve upward with the amount of the shift depending on the proportion of the physician's patients with such coverage.[34] Given an upward demand shift, the physician's fee would be expected to rise as well. The medical society's impact on physicians' fees would be indirect; i.e., via the shift in the physician firm demand curve. Although empirical evidence on the setting of Blue Shield fee schedules is unfortunately lacking, it appears that increases in schedules are constrained by a downward-sloping demand curve in the market for health insurance. Legally, it could not be said that medical societies and Blue Shield jointly set fees in the indemnity case, even if the former has an influence on Blue Shield schedules. Effects are indirect, and in areas where Blue Shield's market share is small, these indirect effects are correspondingly small. Fees are set according to individual physician discretion.

Service benefits are more complex. The patient is entitled to full coverage from a physician who participates in a Blue Shield plan. Agreements by physicians to participate fall roughly into two categories: those in which physicians participate on an individual basis, and those in which physicians participate through medical society membership agreement. Individual agreements are about three times as numerous as medical society endorsement (unpublished correspondence with the National Association of Blue Shield Plans). When individual physicians have the option of participating, a recent study indicates that 28 percent of office-based physicians decline to do so.[35] The nonparticipating physician is likely to lose some service benefit patients, but he can treat service benefit patients still willing to see him on an indemnity basis. Only a few plans penalize the nonparticipating physician by reducing the fee schedule payable to him as an indemnity.[36] The fact that such a high proportion of physicians opt out of service benefits programs raises important questions about Blue Shield's power (or that of any Blue Shield-organized medicine "axis").

It is reasonable to suppose that the role of the medical society is stronger when physician participation takes place through medical society agreement, but empirical evidence is lacking. One could envision the society's promising to "deliver" its member physicians for a certain reimbursement level. The society and Blue Shield would jointly set prices of services rendered service benefits patients. Analytically, a number of alternative models could describe this relationship, including one in which the medical society's monopoly power counters Blue Shield's monopsony. Although such a model contradicts the notion that Blue Shield is a "doctor's plan" (and we ourselves are not ready to endorse it), articles by physicians in their trade literature are often critical of Blue Shield, especially in regard to Blue Shield fee schedules and the ways in which service benefits programs are operated.[37]

If Blue Shield had a monopoly in the market for insurance, covered most physicians' services, and offered only service benefits, it might be easy for organized medicine-Blue Shield to withhold Blue Shield payments to physicians who fail to conform to medical society norms and/or to bar new physician entrants. With a few possible exceptions, conditions are not sufficiently favorable to Blue Shield for this type of behavior to be widespread.

A recent paper by Lawrence Goldberg and Warren Greenberg deals with the role of organized medicine and physician-sponsored insurance in barring cost-conscious insurers from the insurance market. As the authors explain, before the Oregon Physicians' Service (O.P.S.), Blue Shield's predecessor, insurance in Oregon was sold by several private for-profit associations. In the interest of profit-making, the associations made serious attempts to control benefit payments to physicians and hospitals. Physicians were employed by the associations on a part- or full-time basis. Although the cost-control feature was viewed by many practicing physicians as undesirable, association coverage did have the advantage of certainty of payment. Goldberg and Greenberg present a convincing case that by establishing its own plan, O.P.S., organized medicine created an alternative to the for-profit associations, and physicians in Oregon had less reason to cooperate with the associations. The emergence of O.P.S. literally drove the associations out of the Oregon health insurance market.

Why health insurers, the majority of whom are for-profit, have not in recent years been stricter in dealing with physicians (and hospitals) remains an unanswered, yet extremely important question. Goldberg and Greenberg discuss recent attempts by Aetna, one of the largest private insurers in the U.S. to pursue an aggressive policy aimed at reducing physician charges and limiting "unnecessary" procedures. Aetna volunteered to pay a patient's legal expenses if (1) Aetna disallowed a charge, (2) the physician and patient subsequently could not agree on a fee, and (3) the physician sued the patient for nonpayment. The authors cite an AMA resolution condemning Aetna's policy as well as threatening letters from irate physicians. After supporting a patient on this basis and losing, and facing opposition from organized medicine and individual physicians, Aetna discontinued its policy. A number of questions can be asked in response to this study. Given that commercial insurers sell coverage with rather weak controls over physicians' fees and utilization, does Blue Shield still have a special role to play in excluding cost-conscious insurers from the insurance market? We suspect that the answer is "no, in general," but perhaps "yes" when Blue Shield has a dominant market share. Alternatively, does health insurance regulation effectively bar entry of "hard-nosed" insurers? Do specific statutes at the State level make it difficult for policies such as Aetna's to prevail in the courts? To the extent that companies like Aetna force other insurers to monitor costs, can competition from HMO's accomplish the same objective?

Foundations for Medical Care: Foundations for Medical Care provide a more direct link between third-party reimbursement and organized medicine. A Foundation is a nonprofit corporation under the sponsorship of a State or local medical society, ostensibly concerned with quality and cost of medical care. According to Steinwald (1971):

> Common to all Foundations are three basic beliefs: physicians must retain responsibility and leadership in the design, administration, and delivery of medical services; medical care must be provided at a just and equitable cost to both patient and physician; and peer review conducted by medical society members must be encouraged as an efficient mechanism to control the rise of medical costs. *In addition, most Foundations view as one of their primary functions the preservation of solo fee-for-service practice. Freedom of choice on the part of the physician and patient is stressed in these Foundations along with the necessity of guarding the "time honored physician/patient relationship"* (our emphasis) (p. 5)

Havighurst (1971, 1974) pursues Steinwald's point further, arguing that Foundations are an attempt by organized medicine to restrain the growth of HMO's. As of 1971, Foundation activity was greatest in California, the State in which HMO growth has been most pronounced. Although the Foundation concept differs from State to State, the California model has received the most discussion. Our description of this concept is largely based on Steinwald (1971).[38]

In California, Foundations have (1) sponsored prepaid health insurance plans in which participating physicians are reimbursed on a fee-for-service, payment-in-full basis, and (2) established local peer review committees to monitor "the type, quality, and fees of physician care" (Steinwald, p. 7). The health insurance plan offered by the Foundation (of which there were 14 in 1971) must cover a broad range of services, and offer reimbursement above prespecified minimums; e.g.; "all surgery with maximum of not less than 200 RVS units." Plans specify fee schedules in terms of RVS; conversion factors are specified as well.

The Foundation reviews claims prior to their submission to the insurer, which may be Blue Shield or commercial (most often the latter in

California). It sets coverage standards and pays providers. The role of the insurance company or carrier is to apply its own experience rating methods to insured groups or individuals, to set and collect premiums, and to market and underwrite the program. Physicians apply for membership in the Foundation and are accepted by a two-thirds vote of the Foundation Board. The Foundation thus has potential control over physicians through claims review and its membership policies.

In principle, the Foundation is an ideal cartel, controlling price and quantity decisions of individual physicians in a market area. "Undesirable" policies of individual physicians could be thwarted by the cartel.

There is reason to question, however, whether these organizations have sufficient market power to act in this manner. Table 2 shows the number of Foundation physicians as percentages of medical society membership and the number of office-based physicians. Patient enrollment in Foundation plans as a percentage of county population, or when applicable, the population of a cluster of counties, is also shown. When a Foundation includes more than one county, it is identified by the name of the largest county.

Although 80 percent of medical society physicians belong to Foundations, a large portion of physicians do not belong to medical societies, a pertinent fact in its own right. The percentage when office-based physicians rather than medical society membership is the denominator is considerably lower.[39] Only eight percent of the population in California counties with Foundations was covered by Foundation plans in 1971. In only two, Humboldt and San Joaquin, is it possible (at least as of 1971) to see medical society control over this segment of the insurance market *per se* as a major threat to competition in the physicians' service market.

RECENT DEVELOPMENTS IN THE PHYSICIANS' SERVICES MARKET

Introduction

An analysis of competition in the physicians' services market may easily become out-of-date. Although basic behavioral relationships underlying our discussion of supplier-created demand may remain reasonably constant for decades, institutional, political, and legal features change much more rapidly. For example, the nature of organized medicine's oppostion to prepaid group practice, to the extent it still exists, has changed dramatically.[40] Organized medicine has learned to live with limited utilization review, as long as the process is physician-controlled. In fact, physicians may have learned to use utilization review to further their own interests.

Table 2 California Foundations: Physician Participation and Patient Enrollment, 1971

Foundation	Foundation Physicians as percentages of Medical Society Membership	Foundation Physicians as percentages of Office-Based Physicians	Patient Enrollment as a Percentage of Population
Fresno	95	89	8
Humboldt	95	115[d]	25
Kern	80	60	12
Monterey	100[a], 95[b], 55[c]	26	4
Orange	70	60	10
Riverside	70	57	3
Sacramento	75	75	4
San Bernadino	75	74	8
San Diego	70	49	2
San Joaquin	95	96	38
Santa Clara	75	57	4
Sonoma	85	88	7
Stanislaus	90	88	14
Tulare	85	77	7
All	80	59	8

a: for San Benito County;

b: for Monterey County;

c: for Santa Cruz County, by far the largest of the three.

d: The AMA's estimate of office-based physicians exceeds Steinwald's estimates of the number of Foundation physicians.

Sources: Steinwald (1971) and our calculations based on American Medical Association (1971) and Steinwald.

"Recent developments" may be defined in a number of ways. We have selected health maintenance organizations, Professional Standards Review Organizations, and health manpower for discussion because (1) there has been significant legislation during the 1970's in each of these areas, and (2) each has important implications for the performance of the physicians' services market. Our comments on HMO's have implications for supplier-created demand.

Health Maintenance Organizations

A small but vocal group of experts in the health care delivery field look to the competition from HMO's as a stimulus for improving the performance of the traditional fee-for-service sector. At the same time, they see a vigorous fee-for-service sector as a safeguard against quality reductions that may typify monopolistic HMO's. Recent legislation at the Federal level, the HMO Act of 1973 and the 1976 Amendments to the 1973 Act, and recently-enacted State HMO enabling acts reflect a widespread belief in the potential of the HMO model, but at the same time some apprehension that unregulated HMO's underproduce quality.

A complete analysis of HMO's would necessarily take us far afield. Given this paper's objectives, our remarks will be limited to (1) an overview of theoretical considerations related to our earlier discussion of supplier-induced demand, (2) a review of impediments to HMO growth which illustrate anti-competitive practices in the physicians' services market, and (3) a few remarks on recent legislative developments with special reference to their implications for competition in this market.

Any assessment of HMO's should distinguish between financing, production of medical services, and physician preferences for particular modes of practice. In the fee-for-service mode, two distinct parties insure and provide medical services. Consumers purchase contracts from insurers entitling them to services at reduced prices. Consequently, they demand services up to the point where the marginal expected benefit equals the reduced price. The premium payments generate a pure income effect at the time medical services are purchased; but, given that premiums constitute a small portion of total disposable income, the income effect is small. The substitution effect stimulates medical care consumption.

Insurance raises both price and quantity, and consequently reimbursements, until the market clears. The physician has no incentive to convince the patient to consume less than he desires. Not only does he benefit financially, but he might be sued for doing less than is "medically possible." Furthermore, since health insurers do not risk discriminate, both patient and physician are assured that premiums will not rise because of patient consumption. The insurer also finds it costly to police claims. In some cases, attempts by the insurer to seek additional justification for a particular expense may be seen as an attempt by the insurer to escape its contractual responsibilities.

As indicated above, insurance for physicians' services is by no means neutral; some procedures are covered in full, while others are rarely covered. Physicians have an incentive to deliver more covered services. This might explain the high surgery rates associated with U.S. fee-for-service.

In contrast to fee-for-service, the HMO provides both insurance and medical care. Once the consumer has enrolled and paid his premium, consumer incentives are essentially the same as under fee-for-service. Except for nominal copayments, care is free, and the consumer adjusts his demand accordingly.

Provider incentives, however, are markedly different. Services provided subtract from, rather than add to, net physician revenue. In fact, if premium income were exogenous, physicians would have a real incentive to "take their money and run." A milder form of this incentive is to use non-price rationing against patients who, facing a low price at the point of service, desire more care than physicians are willing to provide. Interactions between physicians and "demanding" patients within the context of prepaid group practice are described by Eliott Freidson and David Mechanic. In somewhat simplified terms, the HMO establishes a communality of interest between the insurer and the physician that generally does not exist under fee-for-service.

Several comments follow from this brief conceptual discussion of fee-for-service and HMO modes. First, observed utilization differences between the two do not necessarily reflect supply-created demand under fee-for service. The differences may reflect market clearing at low out-of-pocket prices under fee-for-service and non-price rationing by HMO's. Alleged "over-utilization" of surgical procedures may reflect extensive, non-neutral coverage, and generous fee schedules in the fee-for-services sector.

Second, the HMO can potentially improve the fee-for-service sector's performance by increasing insurers's willingness and ability to monitor utilization and prices. Consumers worry about their high health insurance premiums, and if HMO's become better "values," fee-for-service insurers and physicians face losses in their market share. Insurers may also show some backbone vis-a-vis fee-for-service physicians. Whether or not the HMO can play this important role depends on factors other than their comparative advantage in utilization control. HMO's have yet to be shown to be relatively efficient producers of health care. Furthermore, there is a serious question regarding the willingness of physicians to work in this type of setting. If expansion means dipping into the pool of physicians who stress independence, HMO's may have to pay a high price to attract physicians. Unfortunately, empirical research on the performance of the fee-for-service sector in areas with a high HMO market share is very limited. More research is needed.

The competitive potential of HMO's depends in part on barriers to HMO entry. Using the results of a 1973 survey of operational HMO's and a State-by-State legal analysis, Richard McNeil and Robert Schlenker conclude that State laws have not been a serious barrier to the growth of HMO's. Their conclusion applies only to HMO presence or absence in a State. As the authors acknowledge in a footnote, "State legal conditions could, of course, slow the growth in the number of HMO's and affect their organizational form; and this would not be revealed by our comparison. For example, Inter Study's mid-1973 survey suggests that HMOs adopt special organizational forms to avoid laws against for-profit operation. Nearly half the HMOs indicated they were 'nonprofit' but had for-profit subsidiaries" (p. 199).

Several comprehensive reviews provide an "impressive" list of potential impediments to HMO growth and to other innovations in this industry.[41] A number of States have enabling acts for the Blues that require control by local physicians. State laws directed against the "corporate practice of medicine" may affect HMO entry and organizational form. The application of some State insurance regulations to HMO's requires HMO's to maintain large financial reserves, to charge unreasonably low insurance rates, and to limit asset holdings. These regulations are applied even though HMO's provide most of their benefits in-kind rather than in cash. HMO's have been subjected to certificate-of-need laws. Thus, while fee-for-service physicians are exempted "non-institutional" providers, HMO's, considered to be "institutional providers," must often seek certification for such items as physicians' office space and major equipment. The certificate-of-need franchising system can be used to bar entry of providers whom the "medical establishment" regards as "undesirable."[42] State licensing laws may prevent certain manpower substitutions which would be desirable in large-scale practices. State laws against advertising may put HMO's at a competitive disadvantage vis-a-vis sellers of fee-for-service insurance.

Robert Holley and Robert Walker (1974a, 1974b) report that 17 States had enacted specific HMO enabling legislation by mid-1974. Most of these laws exempt HMO's from advertising and corporate practice restrictions, and provide quality of care controls, methods for processing enrollee grievances, and requirements for enrollee participation in HMO decision-making. While some of these provisions are desirable (advertising, corporate practice) and others are probably harmless (enrollee participation in governance), quality controls can potentially be manipulated in the interest of fee-for-service medicine.[43] Other negative developments in State legislation include the imposition of new financial reserve requirements in some States and the enactment of open enrollment requirements which apply to HMO's but not to fee-for-service insurers.

Since excellent reviews of recent Federal legislation exist (particularly McNeil and Schlenker (1975) and Uyehara and Thomas (1975)), there is no need for an in-depth critique here. Specifically, this legislation provides overrides of some restrictive State laws (i.e., those that require medical society approval and/or physician control, and impose certain financial reserve requirements and advertising bans) as they pertain to actual or potential federally-assisted HMO's, but does nothing about some other State requirements. Overriding States' restrictive practices should give HMO's a better chance of improving the performance of the fee-for-service sector. Federal subsidies under the 1973 Act and the 1976 Amendments are really modest, which after all is a desirable feature if fee-for-service and HMO's are to compete equitably. Less fortunate, however, are certain features that tend to place HMO's at a disadvantage. Among these are the

Act's comprehensive coverage, open enrollment, and community rating provisions which, though required of HMO's, are not required of traditional insurers. In the final analysis, they may prove to be more important impediments to HMO growth than many of the State laws.

Professional Standards Review Organizations

Concern over rising health care costs and a desire to improve quality led to the establishment of Professional Standards Review Organizations (PSRO's) on a national level under provisions of the Social Security Amendments of 1972. According to this legislation, PSRO's are to monitor care provided in hospitals, extended care facilities, and skilled nursing homes and financed under the Social Security Act (except Title V). The law requires utilization review to determine whether the care provided is (or was) (1) medically necessary, (2) of professional quality, and (3) delivered in the appropriate health care facility; i.e., on an in-patient basis only when care on out-patient basis is inappropriate. PSRO's are not to deal with the unit prices of medical services.

The law provides three principal means for ensuring conformance with PSRO decisions: (1) the PSRO's direct authority to deny approval of payments for services to physicians under Social Security Act programs; (2) a malpractice exemption protecting physicians who comply with or rely upon the PSRO norms of treatment if the physician exercises due care during the course of treatment; and (3) specific sanctions imposed by the PSRO on physicians who do not provide care that meets "professionally recognized standards." If the obligations under (3) are not met, the physician can be totally excluded from reimbursement under Medicare and Medicaid and subject to fines.

The Secretary of HEW is required to divide the U.S. into PSRO districts, States, or subdivisions within States. From January 1, 1974, to January 1, 1976, physicians were given the opportunity to organize nonprofit PSRO's in their localities and to receive funds for the operation of their organizations, once recognized by the Secretary. After January 1, 1976, the Secretary was given the authority to designate PSRO's in areas where they had not been established.[44] Although the Act provides for some overall national supervision by a National Professional Standards Review Council, each PSRO is encouraged to establish its own norms of diagnosis and treatment based on typical patterns of practice in its geographic area. The law clearly places the focus of decisionmaking at the local level.

Much could be said for and against PSRO's. We shall limit our discussion to aspects of PSRO's relating to the performance of the physicians' services market. Lest it appear that our commentary emphasizes cost to the neglect of quality, it should be emphasized that the health production function is not currently known. Quality reviews, including those performed by PSRO's, are almost always based exclusively on process rather than outcome criteria. Relationships of process to outcomes are not yet understood.[45] Furthermore, there is little empirical evidence on PSRO's, although numerous articles deduce their potential effects.[46] Our discussion relates PSRO's to supply-created demand and market performance using "standard" assumptions. It examines implications of PSRO's for HMO's and various forms of health manpower—topics developed more fully in other parts of Section III.

If physician suppliers generate their own demand, an argument can be made for suspending consumer sovereignty in this market and for substituting regulation and control systems. Since existing empirical evidence cannot rule out the "supply creates-its-own-demand" argument, it is appropriate to determine whether PSRO's are likely to be effective regulatory devices under such circumstances. PSRO's, by statute, are operated by local practicing physicians. Therefore, they might legitimize rather than police supply-created demand. In fact, they could encourage physicians delivering services below the PSRO-determined maxima to shift demand up to this level. Supply-generated utilization would be reflected in the area's "style of care," which becomes the PSRO norm. Although the National Council and the HEW Secretary are responsible for oversight of local PSRO's, stringent national regulation would largely negate the tenet that decisions should be made by local practicing physicians. In order to gain physician acceptance, Federal officials have since 1972 emphasized this tenet as well as the quality-enhancing features of PSRO, as opposed to the program's cost-reducing features (Havighurst and James Blumstein, Blumstein (1976).

Effective *national* enforcement would create some new problems. For one, the National Council must, according to law, be composed of representatives of nationally-recognized physicians' associations. Such physicians tend to represent the views of academic medicine. National standards developed by a board of this type may be sufficiently high to serve as an umbrella for supply-created demand at the local level.[47]

The PSRO concept also presents some important difficulties if physicians face a stable demand curve and medical services are covered by third-party reimbursement. There is a tendency in such circumstances to over-utilize physicians' services under the fee-for-service mode (Michael Crew, Feldstein (1973)). The review mechanism envisioned by the authors of the PSRO legislation is one method for curbing utilization. But why should a board of practicing physicians curb utilization and hence Federal payments to its locality?

The law prohibits a physician from participating in the review of (1) health services provided to the physicians' patients, and (2) any health services provided by any institution in which the physician or his immediate family has a financial interest. Thus, obvious personal conflicts of interest are unlikely. But there is a potential conflict of interest involving the group of physicians comprising the PSRO; it has no incentive under the statute to curb the flow of Federal expenditures to its area. At the level of the individual board member, a physician reviewer may reason if he is tough and curbs the utilization of another physician, the latter may get even with him sometime in the future when he becomes a PSRO reviewer. Rotation of board members can be seen as a method of ensuring that boards do not become too tough; the fact that program officials encourage rotation of the review function among practicing physicians (Alice Gosfield) probably further reduces PSRO incentives to curb costs.

Some features in the PSRO statute may stimulate utilization, even in situations where the demand schedule facing the physicians is stable. Under the malpractice provision of the 1972 statute,

> no doctor of medicine or osteopathy and no provider (including directors, trustees, employees, or officials thereof) of health care services shall be civilly liable to any person under the law of the United States or any state . . . on account of any action taken by him in compliance with or reliance upon professionally developed norms and treatment applied by a PSRO. §1167 (C); 42 USC §1320C - 16 (C).

Although untested by the courts, congressional intent in the 1972 law was to shield the physician following PSRO standards from malpractice liability unless (1) the physician selects an inappropriate norm for the diagnosis and/or age group although he applies the norm correctly and (2) if he selects the appropriate norm but applies it negligently. This provision may greatly reduce the likelihood that physicians would supply care at levels below the PSRO norms. For example, if the norm were four in-patient days for a particular condition, the physician might consider it folly to release the patient after two, even though he thinks release is medically appropriate and the patient wants out. Sanctions by the PSRO, involving the loss of rights to Medicare and Medicaid reimbursement, will probably be rare, but they, too, will encourage conformance with PSRO norms.

In spite of our negative comments about PSRO's, they have features that can improve market performance. PSRO's are seen as an educational force for improving the quality of health care (W. F. Jessee *et al.*). Once the PSRO has discovered appropriate treatments, it can improve the quality of care by disseminating its findings among physicians. Whether or not PSRO's will fully develop this educational function is an unanswered question.

Furthermore, as Gosfield notes, the PSRO-generated data bases can improve patient information.

> Profiles of practitioners and providers (and patients) will be continually generated by PSROs. These profiles can reveal much about the practice of medicine in general. Among other things, they will demonstrate which types of practitioners most often perform selected procedures—whether, for example, otolaryngologists (ear, nose, and throat specialists) perform more tonsillectomies than pediatricians. This type of information can be important to a consumer who is trying to decide whether to undergo surgery. Based on profiles, he can evaluate his use in the context of others. A patient may decide, for example, that general surgeons, such as the one he has consulted, do not perform enough pacemaker insertions to be optimally competent. He may then choose a caradiothoracic surgeon who specializes in pacemaker insertions. On the other hand, a hypertensive patient for whom a vascular surgeon prescribes surgery might choose to consult an internist instead, if from profiles he knows that vascular surgeons generally treat hypertension with surgical intervention, while an internist would be more likely to treat high blood pressure with drugs. Profiles of institutions can give consumers basic information on existing quality of care as well as trends toward improvement or degeneration of institutional practices. If an institution's profile indicates a high rate of compliance with PSRO norms and guidelines, a patient can expect a better rate of coverage for services delivered there as compared with an institution with a high rate of PSRO disallowances (p. 186).

One might go even further than Gosfield and suggest dissemination of physician-specific information to consumers. The PSRO statute specifically prohibits disclosure of information to the public at large. With adequate legal safeguards, however, the PSRO data base could greatly improve patient information.

Havighurst and Randall Bovbjerg warn that PSRO's may impede the growth of HMO's. Incentives for providing ambulatory rather than inpatient care are central to the HMO concept. If HMO's differ from fee-for-service practice on mean length-of-stays and tests or procedures for specific diagnoses, they may encounter opposition from PSRO's dominated by fee-for-service physicians. Havighurst and Bovbjerg propose that PSRO's should not regulate HMO's ("divorce on the grounds of incompatibility"). An alternative is separate PSRO's for HMO's. In any case, one of the PSRO's "sticks" (probably the most important one), denial of payment for disapproved services, has no meaning here since HMO's use capitation reimbursement.

The PSRO's impact on health manpower is uncertain. Optimistically, the malpractice immunity provision will allow physicians to delegate many tasks to non-physician personnel. However, occasional remarks in the medical literature suggest that physicians may use PSRO's to develop standards that exclude non-physician competitors.[48]

Physician and Non-physician Manpower

As Herbert Lerner notes:

> In sharp contrast to the talk of health-care "crisis" and physician manpower shortage which was prevalent only five years ago (with reference to 1974), some health leaders are now beginning to speak of a "glut" of physicians in the near future, and in some specialties even currently. . . . The increase in numbers of medical schools in this country, and of students in each medical school, along with a large increase in numbers and proportions of foreign medical school graduates among the total number of physicians in training and practice in this country, and the beginnings of implementation of some physician assistant programs, have all had effect on medical manpower needs in the United States. Some scholars have focused on new patterns of practice. . . . Other health leaders, while maintaining their concern with the quality of training in each graduate medical program, have also begun to talk seriously of how best to control the numbers of physicians entering specific specialties. Current voluntary methods of structuring the graduate medical education system are being re-examined by the voluntary associations themselves. Their efforts are intended to coordinate and integrate the entire system of graduate medical education, encompassing all the specialties, in a manner similar to that developed to control undergraduate medical education in the United States (pp. 3, 4).

The above quotation from a book which is basically sympathetic to "voluntary regulation" refers to three recent developments in the manpower field that fall within the scope of this paper. First, there is widespread belief, both within and outside the physician community, that the specialty distribution of physicians is "imbalanced." Organized medicine, previously inactive in the graduate medical field, has taken steps to limit the number of slots in residency programs in certain specialties. The Health Professions Educational Assistance Act of 1976 stipulates that a given percentage of residencies under direct control of, or affiliated with, medical schools be in the "primary" specialties (*general* internal medicine, *general* pediatrics, and family medicine) as a precondition for receiving Federal educational funds.

Second, the number of foreign medical school graduates (FMG's) has grown rapidly, particularly since the change in the U.S. immigration law in 1965 which replaced the national origins quota system by giving preference to persons in "shortage" occupations. In fact, in some years since 1965, new FMG arrivals exceeded the total number of graduates of domestic medical schools. In remaining years, the numbers are quite close (Rosemary Stevens). By eliminating preferred treatment of alien physicians, the 1976 Health Professions Educational Act will effectively restrain FMG entry.

Organized medicine has been successful in gaining legislation at the State level to regulate the influence of, and perhaps the growth in, a new type of non-physician provider, the physician extender. Our discussion of this third development completes this section.

As the Lerner quote indicates, control of graduate medical education by the medical profession has been fragmented, involving many autonomous specialty programs in hospitals. In contrast to undergraduate medical education, which consistently has an excess of applicants over places, graduate education has had excess places. While residency programs have been reviewed on a hospital-by-hospital basis, until recently (the early 1970's), there has been no concerted effort to relate program accreditation to the national physician manpower situation.

What accounts for the neglect at the graduate level? First, to the extent that organized medicine aimed to advance the financial interests of existing physicians, there was no reason to be concerned with graduate education so long as entry was controlled by regulating undergraduate slots, and immigration of alien physicians was restricted. Second, it is much easier to achieve unity required for collective action when members share common interests, which often occurs when the medical profession deals with non-physicians. The interests of the various specialties within medicine, however, do not always coincide, and control over graduate medical education cannot easily be divorced from "specialty rights."[49] Third, changes in the immigration law coincided with the introduction of Medicare and Medicaid. These financing programs had two effects: (1) They greatly increased the demand for hospital inputs of all types, including residents; and (2) they boosted earnings of practicing physicians. Political campaigns are not costless, and it is reasonable to assume that higher earnings bought off physician opposition to immigration, at least in the short run.

Although barriers to entry into specialties are not desirable, they may represent a second-best solution. Hospital-oriented medicine, including surgery, has been more fully covered by insurance than primary care. Demand for physicians in the former fields increased relative to the latter, and is reflected in the derived demand for residents. Rationing of slots may be about the only way in the short run to alter specialty entry patterns to any meaningful degree. To sanction some form of regulation, however, should not mean abrogation of society's responsibilities in this regard to the specialties.

The FMG situation is less complex from the standpoint of the professional associations, since FMG's do not hold power in these organizations. Although the case for restricting FMG entry is often based on grounds of low quality, the evidence is far from conclusive. Impressionistic and test data suggest FMG's are less competent (National Advisory Commission on Health Manpower (1967), Aaron Lowin), but research using process measures to assess the quality of care delivered by U.S. medical school graduates (USMG's) and FMG's is inconclusive, and there really is no information on outcomes (Williams and Brook (1975, 1976)). As Williams and Brook state, "Comparative studies must proceed from measures of performance, not just measures of knowledge, and FMG's should be compared with USMG's, not judged against ideal standards (on which even USMG's might be found wanting)" (p. v, 1976).

Furthermore, there are few studies describing the nature of FMG's practices. Recent evidence has shown the FMG's are more likely to participate in payment-in-full plans; i.e., Blue Shield service benefit programs and Medicaid (Sloan and Steinwald (forthcoming), Sloan, Cromwell, and Mitchell (forthcoming)). This is not surprising since the fee schedules are often insufficient to attract physicians with more impressive credentials. Thus, even if there are quality differences, to truncate the distribution of quality may be to deny access of lower income groups to physicians' services.

In defense of recently-enacted entry barriers, it must be stated that the 1976 law merely places FMG's on the same basis as most other aliens. This raises questions about international flows of labor, a subject far beyond the scope of our paper.

Finally, there is little question that a dual labor market exists in graduate medical education. Allegedly, because of their poor undergraduate education, FMG's tend to enter less desirable residency programs where they may often further the financial interests of private practitioners in the community. Subsequently, they often have trouble finding positions as practicing physicians which provide good on-the-job training opportunities. Enriching FMG's educational opportunities, rather than excluding them, is a possible option.

The physician extender (PE) is a health care professional who delivers "mid-level" services (such as medical counseling of the disabled, well-baby examinations, and routine workups), tasks which have until recently been performed exclusively by physicians. The PE concept encompasses four personnel categories, the physician's assistant (PA), the Medex, the nurse practitioner (NP), and the Primex. Although there are differences in educational preparation and orientation among the four, these are not pertinent to this paper.

Physicians have always used non-physician personnel, but mostly for administrative or technical tasks rather than for tasks involving medical judgment. Since physicians and PE's are close substitutes in some functions, the growth of PE's has elicited considerable interest within the medical community. During the past decade, the majority of States have enacted statutes that (1) identify qualifications of PE's and (2) authorize supervising physicians to delegate a broad range of tasks and responsibilities to persons so designated.

Only a few States have authorized forms of limited, independent medical practice, even though there is some evidence that PE's could adequately function in this manner (Philip Kissam, W. O. Spitzer *et al.*). To expand this role would, however, require changes in licensure and practices of third-party payers. The latter often limit payment to services performed under a physician's supervision. States would also have to give PE's authority, at least on a limited basis, to prescribe retail sales of drugs before a substantial expansion of PE's independent role could occur. Limited independent practice may be a useful option in rural areas with low physician density. Not surprisingly, physicians practicing in those areas have often opposed this option. Realistically, most State legislatures will probably not allow limited independent practice, unless pressured by consumer groups or by other large professional interest groups (such as nurses).

Even when the physician maintains his supervisory role, increasing the supply of PE's augments the supply of physicians' services. But there are many obstacles to overcome. In some States, PE's job descriptions are reviewed by administrative agencies or boards on a case-by-case basis, even though the PE is employed by a physician. A few set limits on the number of PE's a physician can employ. Medical licensing boards are entirely responsible for administrative control of PE's in more than half the States (Kissam). Exessive control by such groups reduces the profitability of PE's and hence their employment potential.[50] Kissam, who prefers simply authorizing PE's to work under a physician's supervision, suggests that State health agencies rather than medical licensing boards, should regulate PE's if one is to regulate PE credentials and the scope of practice at all. Political pressures to stifle the growth of these new professions may not be as great in State health agencies.

Extensive regulation through the licensure process is ironic when contrasted with many aspects of physicians' licensing. Once licensed, physicians are not re-examined. There are no age limits. There are no statutory limits on the qualifications of physicians performing major surgery. Hospitals are expected to regulate the quality of surgery performed in hospitals, but who controls hospitals? In other words, rigorous practice laws do not exist for physicians themselves. As a final recourse, the patient can sue the incompetent physician. But this is a patient-oriented control. It is *not* professional self-control.

Conclusions and Implications

Increased interest in regulation of health providers reflects the dramatic growth of health care expenditures. Many experts in the field of health care delivery have long abandoned any faith in the system of checks and balances of the marketplace, preferring instead to regulate health care suppliers. The conventional wisdom of consumer ignorance, juxtaposed against an all-knowing, all-powerful, and *sometimes* all-caring physician has led to numerous Government regulations. Recent literature in economics, however, has documented the shortcomings of regulation. In the health field, as in others, regulations have frequently been instituted without prior analysis of their likely consequences.

This paper, and others at this conference, question the conventional wisdom. Our ultimate objective is to select policies which strengthen the workings of the health care marketplace. Hopefully, questioning the old will not lead to uncritical acceptance of the new. Our review of the literature has, if anything, increased the scope of what we do not know. Informed public policy in this area will require a substantial investment in empirical research with a firm conceptual base.

For example, there is much justification for concern that advertising bans lead to health care consumer ignorance. Yet, empirical evidence on the effects of advertising necessary for informed policy decisions is lacking. Recent legislation appears unnecessarily to impede the growth of HMO's. Yet, there is little comparative information on the performance of alternative practice modes. We do not really know if HMO's could improve the performance of the fee-for-service sector; nor do we know if dramatic expansion of HMO's will alter their form and performance. Lack of evidence on quality of care provided by foreign medical school graduates is probably the major reason for undue reliance on opinions of the vested interests in that area.

We have devoted considerable attention to the supplier-induced demand hypothesis. There are substantial differences between economists who espouse the supply-created demand view, the B's, and the neo-clasical economists, the N's. The former stress anomalies of the health care market while the latter rely on formal theoretical methods and econometrics and emphasize similarities with other markets. Though less formal, the B's have called attention to features of the industry that the N's might miss. Frequently, the N's have met the challenges. Even so, applied econometric studies based on the standard theory often report low R^2s, and some of the variables are only proxies for the theoretical concepts.

In spite of these caveats, we use the standard framework to evaluate the physicians' services market. The B's methods are conceptually weaker. Future research should pay particular attention to quality-amenity variables. Incorporating quality-amenities into the analysis may explain the anomalies involving physician-population ratios in current studies. Empirical evidence already shows that levels of certain quality-amenities are higher in physician-dense areas. To the extent this is so, higher levels of quality-amenities provide a reason for the positive association between physicians' fees and physician density, a relationship which many have used as a justification for the supplier-induced demand hypothesis. Higher quality-amenities may also go a long way toward explaining higher patient utilization in such areas. Comparing various studies, we have been unsuccessful in fully explaining inter-area utilization differences on this basis, but empirical research on this topic is still in its infancy.

We stated earlier that it is not necessary for all consumers to possess perfect information for the demand curve to be stable. And for this reason, anecdotal comments describing situations in which consumers seem not too sufficiently knowledgeable do not constitute pertinent evidence on the supplier-induced demand issue. There has been systematic research on consumer information. (See, for example, a recent review by Institute of Medicine (1976).) Further analysis specifically linking the findings of these studies to the workings of the physicians' services market would be useful.

Supplier-induced demand is not an "all or nothing" matter in which opponents of the supplier-induced demand notion are forced to find evidence ruling out supplier-induced demand shifts entirely. Rather, at issue is whether supplier-induced demand represents a major demand determinant. We find that the B's have been much too hasty in concluding it is.

Evidence supporting the notion that physician-induced demand is a *dominant* force would be bad news for almost everyone. The rationale for Government regulation would be strengthened. Patients would be controlled by numerous imperfect non-price regulations. Physicians would also work under these rules. Radical prescriptions for restructuring the delivery system would be necessary as both fee-for-service and prepaid group practice cannot deal with supplier-generated demand. PSRO's would have particularly perverse effects. Empirical work on the demand for health and for health services would be essentially useless. Much empirical work on the supply side which assumes a demand curve constraint would, at a minimum, require reinterpretation. Regulatory mechanisms would have to be developed on a much more rigorous basis than to date.

We also examine this market from a traditional industrial organization perspective. Judging from the dispersion of fees for specific procedures within local markets, even after adjusting for major differences in physicians' credentials, we conclude that individual physicians possess a degree of monopoly power. At the same time, on the basis of this evidence and the inherent difficulty of policing the price-output decisions of large numbers of individual practitioners, we find it very unlikely that price-fixing cartels are widespread. Furthermore, empirical evidence that physcians' professional associations and third parties jointly determine fees is not at all conclusive. However, by adjusting relative value scale procedure definitions, physicians' associations have obtained additional revenue for physicians from third parties. To our knowledge, there is no comparable empirical evidence (at least in the public domain) indicating that relative value scales have been used by associations to raise fees.

Price dispersion within local market areas is in large part attributable to incomplete patient search. Third-party reimbursement of physicians is a disincentive for patient search, but a large portion of the physician's bill, on the average, remains uncovered. Insurer fee schedules are generally set below the level of fees of most physicians in a community (Sloan and Steinwald (1975)). Therefore, in contrast to purchase of hospital services, the failure of patients to obtain the lowest quality-adjusted price frequently is fully borne by patients themselves in terms of out-of-pocket payments.

Advertising bans raise search costs and reduce patient search, bestowing monopoly power on individual physicians. Current advertising restrictions do not appear to serve the public interest; while specific suggestions are beyond the scope of this paper, this matter merits careful study by researchers and policymakers.

Organized medicine has traditionally justified advertising bans on grounds that unrestrained competition among physicians would lower service quality. Using plausible assumptions, one can deduce that competition *raises* quality. This is ultimately an empirical question. But lacking empirical evidence, we support the theory that competition increases quality. Fortunately, there is currently an empirical basis for some of the assumptions underlying the theory.

We have noted the PSRO's data bases may improve consumer information. While information dissemination raises important privacy issues, these legitimate concerns should not be used to enhance the individual physician's monopoly. Certainly, adequate safeguards can be developed to protect privacy *and* the consumer's right to pertinent market information. Should not, for example, an individual contemplating major surgery be able to secure information concerning the number of times a particular surgeon performs the procedure? Or should he, as now, be "protected" from quantity and price data?

We take barriers-to-entry at the medical school level as "given." Our section on "Recent Developments" discusses various recently-instituted restrictions which often appear to serve the financial interest of physicians. Legislation has probably limited HMO growth and thereby reduced the possibility of competition between HMO's and fee-for-service physicians. PSRO's are run by physicians' groups which can force individual physicians to comply with group norms. Moreover, physicians can use PSRO's to inhibit competition from non-physician providers. The potential of PSRO's (as currently constituted) for reducing competition among physicians and between physicians and other suppliers merits further analysis.

Finally, recent developments in health manpower credentialling are really "re-runs." Patient search costs are not trivial, even in the absence of restraints on information; also, the patient is sometimes not able to make informed judgments. Thus, there is a case for public intervention in this area. Yet empirical evidence on patient outcomes provides inadequate scientific support for the current system of occupational franchising. The public should, to a greater extent than currently, place the burden of scientific proof (versus "professional opinion") on the group seeking the franchise. This applies to both physicians and other occupational groups.

APPENDIX

CORRECTING THE INTERNAL RATE OF RETURN FOR HOURS-WORKED DIFFERENCES

We follow Rosen's (1977) formulation for the internal rate of return. Let a college graduate earn Y_1 dollars per year from year S_1 to the infinite future (retirement is neglected). The present value of this income stream at discount rate r_1 is

$$V_1 = \int_{S_1}^{\infty} Y_1 e^{-r_1 t} dt.$$

A physician's annual income of Y_2 dollars, starting at S_2, has present value

$$V_2 = \int_{S_2}^{\infty} Y_2 e^{-r_2 t} dt.$$

Integrating these expressions, we get

$$V_1 = \frac{Y_1}{r_1} e^{-r_1 S_1}, \qquad V_2 = \frac{Y_2}{r_2} e^{-r_2 S_2}.$$

The internal rate of return, r, is that discount rate which equates V_1 and V_2:

$$\frac{Y_1}{r}e^{-rS_1} = \frac{Y_2}{r}e^{-rS_2},$$

which implies

$$Y_2 = Y_1 e^{rS}, \qquad S \equiv S_2 - S_1.$$

Rosen's formula is easily extended by writing income as the product of hourly wages and hours worked:

$$Y_1 = W_1 L_1, Y_2 = W_2 L_2.$$

Therefore, $W_2 L_2 = W_1 L_1 e^{rS}$, or

$$r = \frac{\ln(W_2/W_1)}{S} + \frac{\ln(L_2/L_1)}{S}.$$

The "true" rate of return, adjusted to eliminate the effect of hours worked, is the first term.

The uncorrected formula rate of return to medicine, compared to male college graduates, was 23.3 percent in 1970.[1] For physicians' hours of work, we multiply weeks practiced in 1970 by total hours during the last complete week of practice before the AMA survey in 1971, or 47.33 x 53.64 = 2,539 hours per year.[2] As Lindsay notes, there are no average hours data for college graduates.[3] However, Thomas Kniesner has recently estimated labor supply equations for married men which allow us to construct a sample with any desired properties. For a college-educated group, we predict 1891 hours per year.[4] Therefore, the hours adjustment to the rate of return, $\frac{\ln(L_2/L_1)}{S}$, equals 5.9 percent. This leaves a corrected rate of return of 17.4 percent, clearly higher than the return to a college education.

APPENDIX NOTES

1. This estimate is based on average annual earnings of $43,412 for physicians and $13,509 for college graduates (U.S. Census of Population, 1970), and an assumed S = 5 years. Medical specialists of course take longer than 5 years to train, but they also earn stipends greater than the income of equal-aged college graduates. Rosen's formula ignores these stipends. On the other hand, the 23.3 percent rate is quite close to Feldman's exact calculation of 22 percent for all physicians.

2. These are sample average data. If individual weeks and hours per week are positively correlated, the product of averages will be biased upward, and adjusted r will be biased downward.

3. Some industry-specific estimates for professional and administrative occupations put the average 1970 work-week at 39 hours (U.S. Bureau of Labor Statistics, 1971).

4. Kniesner's equation is ANNUAL HOURS = 2574.3 − 111.2 HOURLY WAGE + 27.3 YEARS OF EDUCATION + 19.4 WIFE'S WAGE − 7.7 AGE + 6.9 YEARS AT CURRENT JOB − 203.9 RACE (1 if black). For a 35-year old white college-educated man with 10 years at his current job, nonworking wife, and hourly wage of $7, we predict 1891 hours worked per year.

NOTES

1. Another study, U.S. Department of Health, Education, and Welfare (1976), using 1973 data, found that the net present value of general practice relative to a B.S. degree was $47,000 at a discount rate of 15 percent. The net present values of internal medicine and surgery at the same discount rate was $20,000 and $43,000, respectively.

2. Economists' methods for assessing the welfare implications of particular market arrangements are predicated on the assumption of consumer knowledge.

3. The negative sign of $\frac{\partial U}{\partial D}$ is important. Otherwise the physician could shift the demand curve with more D but raise price by enough to keep W constant. Therefore, would not come into play. The only thing that prevents this behavior is $\frac{\partial U}{\partial D} < 0$.

[4] $U_P = U_Y(\cdot)[\cdot] + U_W(\cdot)Rf_P = 0$, where $[\cdot]$ represents the term in (4) in brackets. Then,

$$U_{PD} = U_{YY}[\cdot](Rf_D P - C_W Rf_D) + U_{YW}[\cdot]Rf_D + U_{YD}[\cdot] +$$

$$U_Y[Rf_{PD}P + Rf_D - C_{WW}R^2 f_P f_D - C_W Rf_{PD}] +$$

$$U_{WY}(Rf_P)(Rf_D P - C_W Rf_D) + U_{WW}(Rf_P)Rf_D + U_{WD}(Rf_P) + U_W Rf_{PD}.$$

If the first order condition UP = 0 is satisfied, $[\cdot] < 0$.
If the first order condition $U_D = 0$ is satisfied, $(Rf_D P - C_W Rf_D) > 0$. which also implies $P - C_W > 0$

Then, term by term (with assumptions):

$$\overset{-}{U_{YY}}[\overset{-}{\cdot}](\overset{+}{\cdot}) \to +; \quad \overset{-}{U_{YW}}[\overset{-}{\cdot}]\overset{+}{Rf_D} \to +; \quad \overset{-}{U_{YD}}[\overset{-}{\cdot}] \to +;$$

$$\underbrace{\overset{+}{U_Y}[R\overset{-}{f_{PD}}(P \pm C_W) + R\overset{+}{f_D} - \overset{+}{C_{WW}}R^2 \overset{-}{f_P}\overset{+}{f_D}]}_{Y_{PD}} \to ?;$$

$$\overset{-}{U_{WY}}(R\overset{-}{f_P})(\overset{+}{\cdot}) \to +; \quad \overset{-}{U_{WW}}R\overset{-}{f_P}R\overset{+}{f_D} \to +;$$

$$\overset{-}{U_{WD}}R\overset{-}{f_D} \to +; \quad \overset{-}{U_W}R\overset{-}{f_{PD}} \to +.$$

All expressions are positive except the fourth, which is thus far unsigned. A plausible argument can be made that Y_{PD} is positive. To see this, assume that the physician is a profit-maximizer; i.e., he maximizes Y from equation (3), and D is any exogenous variable shifting the demand function outward. Then, $\frac{dP}{dD}$ is positive if, and only if, Y_{PD} is positive. Although the model in the text is more complex than this, there is no reason to believe that the added complexity disturbs this particular interrelationship. The restriction that fpD be negative amounts to saying that increased discretionary power makes the demand curve steeper—in much the same way that product advertising lowers the elasticity of the demand function facing the individual firm.

$$U_{PR} = \overset{-}{U_{YY}}[\overset{-}{\cdot}]\frac{\partial \overset{+}{Y}}{\partial R} + \overset{-}{U_{YW}}[\overset{-}{\cdot}]\frac{\partial W}{\partial R}$$

$$\underbrace{+ \overset{+}{U_Y}(\overset{-}{f_P}P + f(\cdot) - \overset{+}{C_W}\overset{-}{f_P} - \overset{+}{C_{WW}}R\overset{-}{f_P}f(\cdot))}_{Y_{PR}} +$$

$$U_{WY}^{-}(Rf_P^{-})\frac{\overset{+}{\partial Y}}{\partial R}+U_{WW}^{-}(Rf_P^{-})\frac{\overset{+}{\partial W}}{\partial R}+U_W^{-}f_P^{-}$$

where

$$\frac{\partial Y}{\partial R}=Pf(\cdot)-C_Wf(\cdot)>0$$

and

$$\frac{\partial W}{\partial R}=f(\cdot)>0.$$

The third term is ambiguous. But the case for R is really the same as in the above comment on Y_{PD}; Y_{PR} is also plausibly positive.

$$^5U_{DR}=U_{YY}^{-}[\overset{+}{\cdot}]\frac{\overset{+}{\partial Y}}{\partial R}+U_{YW}^{-}[\overset{+}{\cdot}]\frac{\overset{+}{\partial W}}{\partial R}$$

$$+\underbrace{U_Y^{+}(f_D^{+}P-C_W^{+}f_D^{+}-C_{WW}^{+}Rf_D^{+}f(\cdot))}_{Y_{DR}}+$$

$$U_{WY}^{-}(Rf_D^{+})\frac{\overset{+}{\partial Y}}{\partial R}+U_{WW}^{-}(Rf_D^{+})\frac{\overset{+}{\partial W}}{\partial R}+U_W^{-}f_D^{+}+U_{DY}^{-}\frac{\overset{+}{\partial Y}}{\partial R}+U_{DW}^{-}\frac{\overset{+}{\partial W}}{\partial R}.$$

The derivative Y_{DR} is ambiguous and cannot be signed by the method used in the previous footnote.

6. A few articles by physicians themselves imply this sort of behavior. See, for example, D. Haddock.

7. Kenneth Arrow's comment that the low price elasticities for physicians' services are incompatible with profit-maximizing monopolistic pricing has been cited as evidence for satisficing models (Newhouse 1970) and Newhouse and Sloan. Arrow referred to evidence on industry demand curves, not individual physician firm demand curves. The latter may in fact be substantially higher. In fact, a recent paper by Sloan and Steinwald (forthcoming) on physician participation in Blue Shield plans presents indirect evidence on marginal revenue from which one can infer that the firm elasticities are at least three. We are grateful to Ted Frech for this insight. Arrow's evidence really relates to cartelization of the industry. If local medical societies had full control over individual MD's, the elasticity of industry demand curves could well exceed unity.

8. Totally differentiating (10), $\frac{dL}{dR}=\frac{1}{R}\frac{dW}{dR}-\frac{W}{R^2}=f_P\frac{dP}{dR}+f_D\frac{dD}{dR}\cdot\frac{dW}{dR}$ may be positive, but $\frac{1}{R}\left[\frac{dW}{dR}-\frac{W}{R}\right]$ may be positive or negative even if $\frac{dW}{dR}$ is positive, depending on the relative magnitudes of the marginal impact of R on W, $\left(\frac{dW}{dR}\right)$, and services per capita $\left(\frac{W}{R}\right)$.

9. Following from footnote [1], changes in R have no impact on medical services utilization of the population if $\frac{dW}{dR}=\frac{W}{R}$. Then $dL=RdW-WdR=0$. Converting into elasticity form, $\frac{R}{W}\frac{dW}{R}-1=0$. If $dL<0, \frac{R}{W}\frac{dW}{R}-1<0$.

10. An example of this type of research is Charles Lewis and studies referenced there.

11. For a more general critique of FK's price elasticity estimates, see Joseph Newhouse and Charles Phelps (1974).

12. Data for the May study come from a 1970 study of health care utilization and expenditures conducted by the University of Chicago's Center for Health Administration Studies.

13. The appointment delay is really not a time price variable in the usual sense since a person can generally engage in other productive activities while waiting for the date of the appointment. May could have included a measure of patient waiting time in the physician's office, but apparently did not.

14. The notion that the patient has more say about his initial visit is frequently found in the literature (for example, Harold Luft (1976)). May's results are inconsistent with this view.

15. In two cases we were unable to reproduce the authors' elasticity calculation. We suspect that decimal points have been misplaced in the coefficients and assume the authors' elasticity calculations are correct.

16. British Columbia Department of Public Health (mimeo.) is the source we used for district definitions.

17. The 1974 study contains an important error in the empirical work. Therefore, our comments on NP's empirical results refer to the 1976 study.

18. Of course, we recognize that nonwage income tends to be poorly measured. Errors-in-variables would bias the nonwage income parameter estimates forward to zero.

19. Each Province had the responsibility of developing its own Medicare program.

20. Regressions are also estimated in first difference form; these results, however, are much more difficult to interpret and compare with other studies.

21. The coinsurance rate of .8 is an average for the entire population. For persons with major medical insurance, the coinsurance rate is about .2 or .25 once the deductible is satisfied, but in 1969, these persons were a minority.

22. See Kessel (1958) for historical information, and Sloan, Jerry Cromwell, and Janet Mitchell (forthcoming) for recent survey results.

23. These measures of concentration are discussed in standard industrial organization texts and books of readings. See, for example, George Stigler (1968).

24. One of the articles proposing this view is Newhouse and Sloan (1972). Frank Sloan is obviously much less sympathetic toward this view than he was six years ago when the Newhouse-Sloan article was written.

25. On the transactions cost of changing price with particular reference to the monopolist, See Robert Barro (1972).

26. Recently, M. Mussa and Sherwin Rosen and Lawrence White have analyzed the case of a monpolist who offers a "product line" of different qualities. The general result is that monopoly almost always reduces, and certainly never increases, product quality. However, the functional analysis required to reach that conclusion is beyond the scope of this paper.

27. Intuitively, imagine the opposite; i.e., $P_{WA} < 0$. Then a small increase in quality would raise price more at low levels of quality. This raises up one end of the demand curve, and the competitive firm is no longer a competitor.

28. We are grateful to Philip Held for providing us with unpublished estimates from the Mathematica surveys.

29. One might argue that the low R^2 reflects price discrimination at the level of the individual physician. But, as stated above, recent evidence clearly shows price discrimination is now unimportant. (See Sloan, Cromwell, and Mitchell (forthcoming)).

30. Fee-for-service physicians obtained a slight amount of revenue from prepaid group practice. We eliminated payments from this source before calculating the percentages.

31. The UCR method is described in Sloan and Bruce Steinwald (1975). Among published studies on the uses of relative value studies, see Agnes Brewster and Estelle Seldowitz.

32. If this additional cost were spread equally over all office-based physicians, it would amount to a payment of $196 per 1970 patient care physician.

33. See Sloan, Cromwell, and Mitchell (forthcoming) for a much more complete discussion of these points.

34. We are referring to changes in fee schedules under basic insurance. Major medical, when combined with basic, is somewhat more complex, but the essential nature of the analysis is unchanged.

35. Sloan and Steinwald (forthcoming).

36. Reed and Willine Carr, and Sloan and Steinwald (forthcoming).

37. See, for example, Robert Brenner, Cotton Lindsay (1959), *Medical Economics* (1962), E. Rosen, and Hugh Sherwood.

38. More recent publications (e.g., Richard Egdahl and Donald Harrington) lack Steinwald's quantitative details.

39. Data on American Medical Association membership may be found in American Medical Association (1972).

40. See Kessel, David Hyde *et al.* (1966), and Somers and Somers for historical accounts.

41. In addition to McNeil-Schlenker, see Ira Greenberg, Michael Rodburg, Robert Holley and Rick Carlson (1972), Institute of Medicine, and Esther Uyehara and Margaret Thomas.

42. See, for example, David Salkever and Thomas Bice.

43. Avedis Donabedian, Milton Roemer, William Shonick, and David Mechanic provide evidence, on the whole, favorable to HMO's. Empirical evidence providing a justification for special quality controls for HMO's is lacking.

44. Until January 1, 1976, if more than ten percent of physicians in a given area objected to a proposed PSRO on grounds that it was unrepresentative of area physicians, HEW was obligated to poll local physicians. If more than half the physicians voted against the proposed PSRO, it could not be designated.

45. Robert Brook.

46. For empirical evidence, see Brook, and Kathleen Williams and A. R. Nelson. Neither of these studies examines PRSO's from the standpoint of market performance.

47. Marvin Korengold discusses problems of organizing a local PSRO, including difficulties in establishing norms when styles of care differ among physician members of the PSRO.

48. See, for example, Lerner, p. 23.

49. For example, board certified surgeons would like to curb surgery by physicians without this credential. See American College of Surgeons and the American Surgical Association.

50. Recent evidence indicates some physician reluctance to employ PE's (Robert Coye and Marc Hansen). However, once the capabilities of PE's are established, they may become less reluctant. Patient and physician satisfaction with PE's is reportedly high (Gary Appel and Aaron Lowin).

REFERENCES

A. A. Alchian, "Information Costs, Pricing and Resource Unemployment," *Western Econ. J.*, June 1969, 109-128.

O. Anderson, *Blue Cross since 1929*, Cambridge, Mass., 1975.

G. Appel, and A. Lowin, "Physician Extenders: An Evaluation of Policy-Related Research," Minneapolis, Jan. 1975.

K. J. Arrow, "Uncertainty and the Welfare Economics of Medical Care," *Amer. Econ. Rev.*, Dec. 1963, 941-973.

R. J. Barro, "A Theory of Monopolistic Price Adjustment," *Rev. Econ. Stud.*, January 1972, 17-26.

L. Benham, A. Maurizi and M. W. Reder, "Migration, Location and Remuneration of Medical Personnel: Physicians and Dentists," *Rev. Econ. Statist.*, Aug. 1968, 332-347.

J. F. Blumstein, "Inflation and Quality: The Case of PSROs," in M. Zubkoff, ed., *Health: A Victim or Cause of Inflation?*, New York 1976, 245-295.

R. L. Brenner, "What Doctors Criticize Most About Blue Shield," *Medical Economics*, July 3, 1961, 58-62.

A. W. Brewster, and E. Seldowitz, "Medical Society Relative Value Scales and the Medical Market," *Public Health Reports*, June 1965, 501.

R. H. Brook, "A Skeptic Looks at Peer Review," *Prism*, Oct. 1974, 29-32.

———, and K. Williams, "Evaluation of the New Mexico Peer Review System, 1971 to 1973," *Medical Care*, Dec. 1976, 1-122.

M. G. Brown, A. Benham and L. Benham, "The Introduction of Medicare in Canada and Windfall Gains to Physician," mimeo., 1976.

R. D. Coye and M. Hansen, "The Doctor's Assistant: A Survey of Physician's Expectations," *J. Amer. Med. Assn.*, July 1969, 529-531.

M. Crew, "Coinsurance and the Welfare Economics of Medical Care," *Amer. Econ. Rev.*, Dec. 1969, 906-905.

K. Davis, and R. Reynolds, "The Impact of Medicare and Medicaid on Access to Medical Care," in R. Rosett, ed., *The Role of Health Insurance in the Health Services Sector*, New York 1976, 391-435.

A. Donabedian, "An Evaluation of Prepaid Group Practice," *Inquiry*, September 1969, 3-27.

R. H. Egdahl, "Foundations for Medical Care," *New England J. Med.*, March 8, 1973, 491-498.

R. G. Evans, "Supplier-Induced Demand: Some Empirical Evidence and Implications," in M. Perlman, ed., *The Economics of Health and Medical Care*, London 1974, 162-173.

———, (1976a) "Does Canada Have Too Many Doctors?—Why Nobody Loves an Immigrant Physician," *Canada Public Policy*, Spring 1976, 147-160.

———, (1976b) "Review of *The Economics of Health and Medical Care*, M. Perlman, ed.," *Canadian J. Econ.*, Aug. 1976, 532-537.

———, *E. M. A. Parish and F. Sully, "Medical Production, Scale Effects, and Demand Generation," Canadian J. Econ.*, Aug. 1973, 376-393.

R. Feldman and R. M. Scheffler, "The Supply of Medical School Applicants and the Rate of Return to Training," Economics Department, University of North Carolina at Chapel Hill, mimeo., 1976.

M. Feldstein, "The Rising Price of Physicians' Services," *Rev. Econ. Statist.*, March/April 1973, 251-280.

———, "The Welfare Loss of Excess Health Insurance," *J. Polit. Econ.*, March/April 1973, 251-280.

H. E. Frech, *The Regulation of Health Insurance*, unpublished Ph.D. dissertation, University of California at Los Angeles, 1974.

——— and P. B. Ginsburg, "Physician Pricing: Monopolistic or Competitive: Comment," *Southern Econ. J.*, April 1972, 573-577.

R. Freeman, "Over investment in College Education?," *J. Human Resources*, Summer 1975, 287-311.

E. Freidson, "Prepaid Group Practice and the New 'Demanding Patient,' ", *Health and Society*, Fall 1973, 473-488.

V. R. Fuchs and M. J. Kramer, *Determinants of Expenditures for Physicians' Services in the United States 1948-68*, Washington, December 1972.

L. Goldberg and W. Greenberg, "The Effect of Physician-Controlled Health Insurance: *U.S. v. Oregon State Medical Society*," *J. of Health Politics, Policy and Law*, Spring 1977, 48-78.

F. Goldman and M. Grossman, "The Demand for Pediatric Care: An Hedonic Approach," mimeo., April 1976.

A. Gosfield, *PSROs: The Law and the Health Consumer*, Cambridge, Mass., 1975.

I. G. Greenberg and M. L. Rodburg, "The Role of Prepaid Group Practice in Relieving the Medical Care Crisis," *Harvard Law Rev.*, Feb. 1971, 887-1001.

D. Haddock, "Set Proper Charges on the Basis of Your Costs," *Med. Econ.*, Oct. 1968, 75-80.

D. C. Harrington, "The San Joaquin Foundation Peer Review System," *Medical Care*, March-April 1973, 185-189.

C. C. Havighurst, "Health Maintenance Organizations and the Market for Health Serivces," *Law and Contemporary Problems*, Part II, Autumn 1970, 716-795.

———, "Speculations on the Market's Future in Health Care," in C. C. Havinghurst, ed., *Regulating Health Facilities Construction*, Washington 1974, 249-270.

——— and J. F. Blumstein, "Coping with Quality/Cost Trade-offs in Medical Care: The Role of PSRO's," *Northwestern University Law Rev.*, March-April 1975, 6-68.

——— and R. Bovbjerg, "Professional Standards Review Organizations and Health Maintenance Organizations: Are They Compatible?", *Utah Law Rev.*, Summer 1975, 381-421.

J. Hirschleifer, *Price Theory and Applications*, Englewood Cliffs, N.J. 1976.

R. T. Holley and R. J. Carlson, "The Legal Context for the Development of Health Maintenance Organizations," *Stanford Law Rev.*, April 1972, 644-686.

——— (1974a) and R. W. Walker, *Catalog of 1973 State Health Maintenance Organization Enabling Bills, Minneapolis.*

——— (1974b) and R. W. Walker, *Catalog of State Health Maintenance Organization Enabling Bills:* January through June 1974, Minneapolis.

L. F. Huang and O. Koropecky, *The Effects of the Medicare Method of Reimbursement on Physicians' Fees and on Beneficiaries' Utilization*, Washington 1973.

E. F. X. Hughes, V. Fuchs, J. Jacoby, and E. M. Lewit, "Surgical Work Loads in Community Practice, *Surgery*, March 1972, 315-327.

D. R. Hyde, *et al.*, "The American Medical Association: Power, Purpose, and Politics of Organized Medicine," in W. R. Scott and E. R. Volkart, eds., *Medical Care, Readings in the Sociology of Medical Institutions*, New York 1966, 163-180.

W. F. Jessee, W. B. Munier, J. E. Fielding, and M. J. Goran, "PSRO: An Educational Force for Improving Quality of Care," *New England J. Med.*, March 27, 1975, 668-675.

B. H. Kehrer, "Factors Affecting the Incomes of Men and Women Physicians: An Exploratory Analysis," *J. Human Resources,* Fall 1976, 526-545.

R. A. Kessel, "Price Discrimination in Medicine," *J. Law and Econ.,* October 1958, 20-53.

P. C. Kissam, "Physician's Assistant and Nurse Practitioner Laws: A Study of Health Law Reform," *Kansas Law Rev.* Fall 1975, 1-65.

T. J. Kniesner, "An Indirect Test of Complementarity in a Family Labor Supply Model," *Econometrica,* July 1976, 651-70.

M. C. Korengold, "How—and Why—We Started a PSRO," *Prism,* April 1975, 21-25, 48.

H. H. Lerner, *Manpower Issues and Voluntary Regulation in the Medical Specialty System,* New York 1974.

C. E. Lewis, "Variations in the Incidence of Surgery," *New England J. Med.,* Oct. 16, 1969, 880-884.

C. M. Lindsay, "Real Returns to Medical Education," *J. Human Resources,* Summer 1973, 331-348.

_____, "More Real Returns to Medical Education," *J. Human Resources,* Winter 1976, 127-130.

J. R. Lindsey, "Blue Shield Income Ceilings, How High?," *Med. Econ.,* Feb. 2, 1959, 151-156.

A. Lowin, *FMGs? An Evaluation of Policy-Related Research,* Minneapolis, May 1975.

H. S. Luft, Comment on "New Estimates of Price and Income Elasticities of Medical Care Services," in R. Rosett, ed., *The Role of Health Insurance in the Health Services Sector,* New York 1976, 317-320.

J. J. May, "Utilization of Health Services and the Availability of Resources," in R. Andersen, J. Kravits, and O. Anderson, eds., *Equity in Health Services,* Cambridge, Mass., 1975, 131-150.

R. McNeil and R. Schlenker, "HMOs, Competition and Government," *Health and Society,* Spring 1975, 195-224.

D. Mechanic, *The Growth of Bureaucratic Medicine: An Inquiry into the Dynamics of Patient Behavior and the Organization of Medical Care,* New York 1976.

M. Mussa and S. Rosen, "Monopoly and Product Quality," discussion paper 75-12, Department of Economics, University of Rochester, June 1975.

A. R. Nelson, "Relation between Quality Assessment and Utilization Review in a Functioning PSRO," *New England J. Med.* March 27, 1975, 671-675.

J. Newhouse, "A Model of Physician Pricing," *Southern Econ. J.,* Oct. 1970, 174-183.

_____ and C. E. Phelps, "New Estimates of Price and Income Elasticities of Medical Care Services," in R. Rosett, ed., *The Role of Health Insurance in the Health Services Sector,* New York 1976, 261-320.

_____ and F. Sloan, "Physician Pricing: Monopolistic or Competitive: Reply," *Southern Econ. J.,* April 1972, 577-580.

M. V. Pauly, "The Behavior of Nonprofit Hospital Monopolies: Alternative Models of the Hospital," in C. C. Havinghurst, ed., *Regulating Health Facilities Construction,* Washington 1974, 143-162.

L. S. Reed, *Blue Cross and Medical Service Plans,* Washington 1947.

_____ and W. Carr, *The Benefit Structure of Private Health Insurance, 1968,* Washington 1970.

U. E. Reinhardt, *Physician Productivity and the Demand for Health Manpower,* Cambridge, Mass. 1975.

M. I. Roemer and W. Shonick, "HMO Performance: The Recent Evidence," *Health and Society,* Summer 1973, 271-317.

E. Rosen, "Let's Abolish Blue Shield Income Ceilings!", *Med. Econ.*, Oct. 8, 1962, 95-97.

S. Rosen, "Human Capital: A Survey of Empirical Research," in *Research in Labor Economics: An Annual Compilation of Research*, ed. by R. G. Ehrenberg, Greenwich, Conn., 1977.

D. S. Salkever and Thomas Bice, "The Impact of Certificate of Need Controls on Hospital Investment," *Health and Society*, Spring 1976, 185-214.

H. C. Sherwood, "What Physicans Want from Blue Shield," *Med. Econ.*, January 6, 1948, 95-100.

F. A. Sloan, Economic Models of Physician Supply, unpublished Ph.D. dissertation, Harvard University, 1968.

———, "Physician Supply Behavior in the Short Run," *Industrial and Labor Relations Review*, July 1975, 549-569.

———, (1976a) "Physician Fee Inflation: Evidence from the Late 1960s," in R. Rosett, ed., *The Role of Health Insurance in the Health Services Sector*, New York 1976, 321-354.

———, (1976b) "Real Returns to Medical Education: A Comment," *J. Human Resources*, Winter 1976, 118-126.

———, "Access to Medical Care and the Local Supply of Physicians," *Medical Care*, April 1977, 338-346.

———, J. Cromwell, and J. B. Mitchell, *Private Physicians and Public Programs*, forthcoming.

——— and J. Lorant, "The Allocation of Physicians' Services: Evidence on Length-of-Visit," *Q. Rev. Econ. Bus.*, Autumn 1976, 85-103.

——— and J. Lorant, "The Role of Waiting Time: Evidence from Physicians' Practices," forthcoming, *J. Bus.*

——— and B. Steinwald, "The Role of Health Insurance in the Physicians' Services Market," *Inquiry*, Dec. 1975, 275-299.

——— and B. Steinwald, "Physician Participation in Health Insurance Plans: Evidence on Blue Shield," forthcoming, *J. Human Resources.*

W. J. Sobaski, *Effects of the 1969 California Relative Value Studies on Costs of Physician Serivces Under SMI*, Washington, June 1975.

H. M. Somers and A. R. Somers, *Doctors, Patients, and Health Insurance*, Washington 1961.

A. M. Spence, "Monopoly, Quality and Regulation," *Bell J. Econ.*, Autumn 1975, 417-429.

W. O. Spitzer, D. L. Sackett, J. C. Sibley, R. S. Roberts, M. Gent, D. Kergin, B. C. Hackett, and A. Olynich, "The Burlington Randomized Trial of the Nurse Practitioner," *New England J. Med.*, Jan. 31, 1974, 215-256.

B. Steinwald and F. Sloan, "Determinants of Physicians' Fees," *J. Bus.*, Oct. 1974, 493-511.

C. Steinwald, *An Introduction to Foundations for Medical Care*, Chicago 1971.

R. Stevens, "Physician Migration Reexamined," *Science*, Oct. 31 1975, 439-442.

G. J. Stigler, "The Economics of Information," *J. Polit. Econ.*, Oct. 1961, 213-225.

———, *The Organization of Industry*, Homewood, Illinois, 1968.

E. Uyehara and M. Thomas, *Health Maintenance Organizations and the HMO Act of 1973*, Santa Monica, Calif., Dec. 1975.

S. G. Vahovich and P. Aherne, *Profile of Medical Practice*, Chicago 1973.

L. J. White, "Market Structure and Product Varieties," *Amer. Econ. Rev.*, March 1977, 179-182.

K. N. Williams and R. H. Brook, "Foreign Medical Graduates and Their Impact on the Quality of Medical Care in the United States," *Health and Society*, Fall 1975, 549-581.

———, "Foreign Medical Graduates and Their Effects on the Quality of Medical Care in the United States," Santa Monica, Calif., 1976.

American College of Surgeons and the American Surgical Association, *Surgery in the United States: A Summary Report of the Study on Surgical Services for the United States,* Baltimore 1975.

American Medical Association, *Distribution of Physicians in the U.S., 1970,* Chicago 1971.

———, *The Profile of Medical Practice,* Chicago 1972.

British Columbia Department of Public Health, "List of Hospitals by Regional Hospital District and School District, mimeo., January 1, 1976.

California Medical Association, *1969 Relative Value Studies,* San Francisco 1969.

Information Engineering, Inc., "A Comparision of the Minnesota Relative Value Index and the Blue Shield Relative Value Index as Pertaining to the Medicare Part B Program," mimeo, 1975.

Institute of Medicine, *Health Maintenance Organizations: Towards A Fair Market Test,* Washington, May 1974.

———, *Assessing Quality in Health Care, An Evaluation,* Washington, Nov. 1976.

Medical Economics, "It Covers Too Little," June 4, 1962, 63-103.

(Report of) National Advisory Commission on Health Manpower, Washington 1967.

U.S. Bureau of Labor Statistics, *National Survey of Professional, Administrative, Technical and Clerical Pay,* Washington 1971.

U.S. Department of Health, Education, and Welfare, "Use of Present Value Calculations in Health Manpower Analysis," Manpower Analysis Branch, Bureau of Health Manpower, June 23, 1976.

Comment

Donald E. Yett*
Director of the Human Resources Research Center and
Professor of Economics, University of Southern California

At the risk of sounding like a Californian passing judgment on a highly prized French wine, it is my opinion that Frank Sloan and Roger Feldman (SF) have provided us with a good paper. Not a truly great paper, perhaps, but definitely a good paper. Indeed, given the paucity of worthy reviews of this literature, I predict it will be widely quoted in upcoming policy debates, health economics classes, and professional articles.

Since it is predictable that many persons exposed to SF's "findings" will not themselves be knowledgeable of the literature, these remarks will focus on what I consider to be the weaknesses of the paper rather than the numerous points on which we agree. My intent is to fill in certain gaps and to broaden the range of interpretations offered. It is not to diminish in any way what I consider to be a valuable contribution to the literature.

From my perspective, the two principal weaknesses of the SF paper are that (1) it is typical of the current style of developing and presenting empirical health economics studies; and (2) it contains no discussion of a major contribution to the literature on physicians' fees—one which puts a quite different light on the literature it does reveiw in this area. In what follows I will concentrate on these two points, commenting on additional topics as they come up.

Some of you may be wondering why I consider it a weakness of the SF paper that it is very much in the mainstream of contemporary health economics studies. After all, the same could be said of most of my own work. How could I possibly criticize SF for doing what most everyone else—myself included—is doing? The answer is that I am not really faulting

* I wish to express my appreciation to Richard Ernst and John Greenlees for their valuable suggestions—and to absolve them from any blame in instances where I injudiciously decided not to follow their advice. This paper was originally entitled, "Facts Versus Folklore Concerning the Market for Physicians' Services."

SF but, rather, expressing a growing convicition on my part that contemporary health economics research may not be as good as it is purported to be.

Most of us who specialize in this type of work take pride in the strides that have been made—and rightly so! [1] We are proud that the health economics literature is no longer dominated by polemic essays. Today, the emphasis is on rigor. And the term "empirical" no longer exclusively denotes case studies, illustrative tables, and anecdotal evidence. Instead, it most often stands for theoretical propositions being subjected to econometric tests. In short, there is a "scientific" aura surrounding much of our work today which was rare not so many years ago. But is it really deserved? It is this (to some, heretical) question I now want to address, using excerpts from SF to illustrate my concerns.

How scientific can a field be when an author who dichotomizes its practitioners into N's and B's on the basis of their beliefs regarding a key tenet of its analytical structure is considered to have made a contribution to the literature? Indeed, considering the possible importance of the matter,[2] one might well ask how we got into such a mess. Although no definitive answer is possible, some reasonable speculations can be made if we think back to the way things were in the late 1950's and early 1960's.

Those were the days before relatively inexpensive computer service was widely available. Data for empirical studies were even harder to come by than today.[3] Not surprisingly, the emerging health economics literature focused on the apparent structures, and unique behavioral relations believed to characterize the various health services and health manpower markets. Attention was called to the "insights" that economic analysis could provide with respect to understanding the conventional wisdom on the basis of introspection and anecdotal evidence.[4]

It was at this time that economists—mostly neophytes with respect to health services research—began to take particular note of the effect that physicians might be able to exert on the demand for their services as well as those of other health-care providers.[5] This was the beginning of a process which, as time passed, almost imperceptibly transformed speculation into "established fact."[6] The literature on the topic grew by one author quoting another until finally—its shaky empirical underpinnings obscured by the sheer weight of citations—what started out as a speculation became, all too commonly, dogma.[7]

Perhaps no proposition in the entire body of health economics literature better illustrates this process than the physician-induced demand hypothesis. Indeed, as a consequence of its haphazard development, it is quite unclear just what the issue is supposed to be. Some authors seem to be arguing that the issue is whether physicians possess "the ultimate in monopoly power—the absence of a demand constraint facing the physician firm."

Although no one has advocated that opposite extreme—namely, that physicians are akin to wheat farmers—it has been intimated that they have no more influence over their own demand than, say, plumbers, auto mechanics, and the like. Thus, only the so-called B's tend to view the matter on an all-or-nothing basis. Others take the position that unless MD's can be shown to have *unusual* influence over their own demand, regulation of this physicians' services market is unwarranted.

The matter is further complicated by the fact that the physician-induced demand hypothesis is closely tied to a related quality-of-care issue. If the so-called B's are correct—i.e., patients do whatever they are told—do physicians with insufficient workloads sell them "unnecessary," "inappropriate," or even "worthless" or "dangerous" services? That is, do physicians misuse any influence they may have over patients if it comes to a choice between their incomes and the patients' welfare? Unfortunately, this is not as simple a matter to determine as some would have us believe. There are few generally-accepted norms with respect to quality of care. And physicians—like other sellers of differentiated products—are not insensitive to patient demands. Wealthy patients demand and get a lot more attention and amenities than poor patients. But whose fault is it: the physician's or the patient's? And, more important, is it a situation requiring remedial policy action? Should we seek to limit the number of physicians, hospital beds, etc., in order to prevent health-care costs from being pushed up by greedy doctors, or would such policies consitute an unwarranted interference with consumer freedom of choice? Clearly, the answer to the last question is beyond the scope of the SF paper. It depends on quality norms and not on the signs or magnitudes of regression coefficients.

Only in the past few years have there been serious attempts to test the market power version of the supplier-induced demand hypothesis econometrically. And, contrary to SF,[8] the bulk of these efforts have been due to the proponents rather than the opponents of the hypothesis.

The literature on econometric tests of the supplier-induced demand hypothesis is illustrative of my concerns regarding contemporary health economics research. As SF pointed out, if focuses on the sign—and, to a lesser extent, the magnitude—of the estimated coefficient on the physician-population ratio in various regressions involving physician services per patient or per capita as the dependent variable.[9] The rationale being that, if all other important influences have been accounted for, the sign will be positive only if physicians in more abundantly-supplied markets are able to convince their patients to purchase more services than they otherwise would.

Given the number of alternative explanations for any observed positive coefficients on the MD-population variable, this would be an inconclusive test of the hypothesis even if the results were consistently those postulated—which, of course, they are not. As SF put it, such results could be because "... (a) the association is consistent with standard as well as supplier-induced demand models, (b) bordercrossing, and (c) physicians may locate in areas where patient demand is high." They also pointed out that differences in such omitted variables as "quality-amenities," time prices, and information costs could account for a positive coefficient on MD-population.

Following the lead of Victor Fuchs and Marcia Kramer, SF rejected the possibility that a positive partial association between the MD-population ratio and utilization could be due to "permanent excess demand for physicians' services."[10] But it is not necessary that there be a *general* excess demand for this argument to make sense. Suppose, instead, that there is excess demand only in such places as rural areas and inner-city neighborhoods (i.e., so-called "medically underserved areas"). Suppose, further, that doctors in such areas "ration" their services among patients, but those in other areas do not.[11] Under these circumstances, a positive partial correlation would be observed between physician density and utilization of services which could reflect the opposite kind of physician influence from that which concerns the proponents of the physician-induced demand hypothesis.[12]

Thus, there are substantial grounds for questioning—as do SF—that the proponents of supplier-induced demand have proven their point. But even in the absence of such strong counter-arguments, theirs would still be a very weak case. Its crucial flaw is its reliance, on the one hand, on intuition and anecdotal experiences (i.e., "common sense") and indirect statistical evidence, on the other. Indeed, in this respect, the supplier-induced demand literature reflects still another of my concerns about the direction in which empirical health economics research is going.

I would be the last to argue that we should give up trying to develop and statistically implement models of the markets for health care. What I do argue is that we should be acutely aware of what can, and what cannot, be accomplished along these lines. Specifically, we need to be more mindful of the fact that a high R^2 on a theoretically plausible equation—even one with statistically significant partial regression coefficients—does not prove causality. At best, regressions yield predictive relationships—which may or may not be due to causal associations, and may or may not be stable enough to serve as a basis for policy actions.[13] Too often it is forgotten that no matter how rigorously a theoretical proposition is deduced, it can never be sounder than its underlying assumptions—which frequently are based on causal empiricism. Likewise, the apparent precision of econometric techniques can lull us into forgetting how seldom the necessary conditions are met to produce, say, blue estimates.[14]

But perhaps the worst pitfall of all is the well-known fact—which, alas, is so easily forgotten—that a huge proportion of socioeconomic and demographic variables are related to each other, often by linkages that are not at all obvious. Thus, for example, to deduce from the sign of the partial regression coefficient on MD-population whether physicians themselves determine the demand for their own services is equivalent to saying: (1) The equation contains all of the variables determining per capita utilization and none—especially not the MD-population ratio—is really a statistical proxy for an omitted variable which is positively associated with utilization; (2) the functional form accurately reflects the true underlying relationship; (3) the data are such that they can be used to make unbiased and efficient estimates of postulated parameters; and (4) they were not collected during a period of disequilibrium (i.e., a temporary period of transition).

The several studies reviewed by SF in connection with the supplier-induced demand hypothesis illustrate how great the odds are against the foregoing conditions being met. For example, as SF pointed out, it is probably the fact that Martin Feldstein's structural equation system was under-identified—rather than the existence of "permanent excess demand for physicians' services"—which explains why his 19 data points yielded a positively sloped demand curve. By the same token, a misspecified system (e.g., SF lamented the absence of time prices) may be the explanation of why Joel May obtained the "implausible" result that the MD-population ratio has a stronger positive influence on office visits of all respondents in his sample than on only those by patients with one or more visits—despite the fact, as SF stated, that ". . . the physician-induced demand hypothesis is particularly plausible for follow-up visits [while], by contrast, the first visit is most likely to be patient-oriented."

Like SF, I am hesitant to draw any conclusions concerning physician-induced demand from the Joseph Newhouse and Charles Phelps and Karen Davis and Roger Reynolds studies given their omissions of obviously important variables. The fact that the latter included no prices may have had something to do with their finding "that increasing the supply of doctors has a negligible or even a zero impact on workload per physician." Finally, I share SF's skepticism regarding the findgings of the Robert Evans, E.M.A. Parrish, and Floyd Sully study. Recall that they took data on sparsely populated areas of British Columbia (where one must travel considerable distances to see a doctor), combined them with data from the Vancouver-Victoria area, ran a regression, and inferred from a "small negative estimated elasticity of the physician-population variable" as a regressor on the log of billings that physicians induce their own demand.

Let me emphasize again, my intention is not to be hypercritical of these particular studies. Indeed, in their support I would have to say that several are far superior to the bulk of recent empirical health economics research. Rather, what I am calling for is a re-examination of how far we are willing to push indirect results in general. I would argue that such results are best looked upon as *indicators* of possible relationships. But until direct verification is possible, we should be a lot more restrained about claiming that they verify the underlying hypotheses.

Direct tests of the supplier-induced demand hypothesis are feasible. Data could be assembled on utilization patterns for patients with the same diagnosis in areas with high and low MD-population ratios. These data could be compared with alternative medical care norms in order to distinguish the possibility of scarcity area "rationing" from possible instances of physician-induced demand. And, since neither is (as SF noted) an "all or nothing" proposition, their respective importance could be established. Such a study would shed more light on the issue than a hundred more regressions of utilization on MD-population ratios and whatever other variables are available.

Before moving on to the other points in the SF paper, I would like to discuss briefly their efforts to improve upon the theoretical basis of the physician-induced demand hypothesis. For all the mathematical sophistication of their argument, it is well to bear in mind that it hinges critically on the inclusion of the decision variable "discretionary influence on patient demand" in the physicians' utility function (with an assumed negative sign on the partial derivative). It is plausible to believe that this variable—which presumably represents guilt relating to the exercise of power—is an important argument of physicians' utility functions except in extreme cases? And if it applied only in extreme cases, should we expect to observe its effects under any sort of typical market situations? There is more than just a possibility that, despite its elegance, this SF extension of the theory underlying the physician-induced demand hypothesis has brought us no closer to having a directly testable version—the goal which I strongly endorse.

Later in their paper, SF introduced a considerably more promising extention of the theory in the form of a vector of "quality-amenities" variables (A). They then derived the interesting hypothesis that a fall in the physician-population ratio leads to what I have termed "rationing"—i.e., physicians producing lower levels of A ("e.g., more harried visits, physician unavailability by telephone, etc."). And, as they noted, "it is worth emphasizing that high volume practices, often found in rural areas, can be understood with reference to this model."

Although SF offered a time price calculation based on fragments from the literature, they—quite rightly—did not claim that it was anything other than illustrative.[15] I would like to second their call for further research on this issue—by more direct means as well as the method they developed—because I fully agree with SF that "to adequately assess the notion of supplier-induced demand, it is essential to isolate qualitative aspects of physicians' services." And, as will be abundantly clear shortly, I share their view that "possibly, as physician density increases, quality-amenities increase systematically. If so, empirical relationships seemingly inconsistent with the standard model may be explained by a *very* standard model according to which patients willingly pay for quality" in terms of physician rapport, availability, short waiting times, etc.

But setting aside for the moment such important matters as differences in consumer tastes with respect to quality-amenities, transactions costs, and the like, I wonder how SF feel about the possibility of actually testing the physician-induced-demand hypothesis given the present state of available data. What is the right measure of utilization to employ? How much sense does it make to use State-level data when almost everyone argues that markets for physicians' services are local in character? How much sense does it make to lump specialists of all kinds into aggregates? What about the role of hospital-based services, and the positive correlation between MD-population ratios and hospital availability? In short, what sense does it make to treat the production of physicians' services in Arkansas and Massachusetts, or in distinctly urban and rural areas generally, as points on the same physician services demand function?

An obvious point—and perhaps that is why it was not stressed by SF—is that even if physicians could induce consumers to buy more services than they need, in what sense would this constitute monopoly power? More specifically, what precisely is meant by the term "monopolistic elements" in the physician market? Would physicians possessing the ability to influence patient purchasing decisions be considered to have a worrisome degree of monopoly power even though—as SF pointed out—in most markets they are many in number and face quite elastic individual demand curves? If so, this would have very broad policy implications. For instance, is it likely that the FTC will soon be suing persuasive automobile salesmen who convince customers to buy more "extras" than they really need? Not likely! Thus, the issue of monopolistic elements in the market for physicians' services would seem to be critically dependent on the available evidence with respect to concentration *or* collusion in such markets. But before turning to SF's review of this evidence, I would like to pursue some further implications of their discussion of the physician-induced-demand hypothesis.

In my view, the greatest weakness of the SF paper is its treatment of physicians' fees—first with respect to the physician-induced-demand hypothesis, and later in connection with measures of fee dispersion as indicators of "monopoly power in a standard market context." Their failure to make any mention of the important work of Barbara Kehrer and James Knowles is more than a little puzzling, especially since it provides unique evidence pertaining to this issue.

Using data for 1970 on over 1,500 medical practices of all sizes from solo to large groups, Kehrer and Knowles estimated regression equations to explain fees and "mark-ups" (ratios of average revenue to average costs)[16] for 12 single specialty and 2 multi-specialty practice categories. They tested 4 alternative pricing models—atomistic competition, monopolistic competition, oligopoly, and price discrimination. They also developed a model to explain average variation in patient waiting time.

Briefly summarized, the following are their major findings:

1. The estimated mark-up regressions showed that profit margins are insignificantly related to practice size, except in the cases of (a) GP's where they were positively related to size, and (b) multi-specialty groups where they fell with size.
2. Tests of the group significance of the monopolistic competition and oligopoly variables revealed that they did not improve the explanatory power of the mark-up equations over simply assuming physician fees are determined in atomistic markets.
3. Comparison of the estimated fee and mark-up equations yielded evidence of substantial variation in either the complexity or quality-amenities of a unit of medical service from one practice to another. That is, a number of variables were found to be related to fee levels, but not to the mark-up of fees over average costs. Among the variables which appeared to be positively related to complexity or quality-amenities are: county per capita income, income of the patient population served by the practice, the degree of relative market concentration, *and the number of sellers in the market area.*
4. Physicians charge proportionately higher fees to cover higher unit costs of producing more complex or higher quality services—i.e., prices for physicians' services are "cost-sensitive."
5. *Physician-to-population ratios were typically insignificant in the mark-up equations.* In the fee regressions the results were mixed—i.e., sometimes MD-population (or close proxies) were positive and in other cases negative.

From the evidence provided by Kimbell (cited earlier) and Kehrer and Knowles as well as that reviewed by SF, the following seems to be the case. (1) There is a tendency (far from universal) for higher utilization of physician services in richer, urban areas, with high physician densities than in poorer, rural areas, with low physician densities. (2) The same conditions are sometimes associated with higher physician fees, but not with higher mark-ups over unit costs, indicating a positive correlation between costly quality-amenities differences and fees.[17] (3) Nonetheless, physicians in areas with low MD-population ratios (i.e., areas that are likely to be rural and to have low per capita incomes) do well by selling less costly "basic-model" services, at lower prices, fewer times per year, to a larger percentage of the area's population. (4) Consequently, all of the studies reviewed by SF reported a negative correlation between physician density and physician incomes, indicating a market premium in terms of income for physicians willing to produce high-volume, low-cost, basic care in sparsely-populated areas. Furthermore, the possibility that physician services are essentially atomistically priced cannot be ruled out on the basis of the Kehrer and Knowles results.

Thus, like SF, I find that the evidence provides very little support for those who would have us believe that physicians have such extraordinary powers over consumers that they "possess considerably more market power than the ordinary monopolist." But then I was never much impressed by that particular argument anyway. After all, if physicians really do have the power to raise fees and sell more of the same services to a smaller number of patients in areas where the physician density is high, why don't they do this sort of thing under all circumstances? Indeed, why would physicians not push this course of action vigorously enough to eliminate the net income disadvantage of urban doctors noted by Kimbell. Or, for that matter, what constrains them from pushing their incomes beyond existing levels in every area? If the answer is that they aim for target incomes, what determines the height of the target?

In this regard, an interesting point that SF did not pursue is why, if physicians can in fact determine their own demand, they do so by selling patients too many services rather than by charging still higher prices for a small volume of sales. In short, why is there an asymmetry between price and quantity in the physician-induced-demand hypothesis? One answer—which is consistent with the Kehrer-Knowles findings—would be that physicians are afraid of "pricing themselves out of the market." That is, their individual (quality-amenity adjusted) demand curves have very shallow negative slopes.[18] But, if that is the case, they should be able to sell as many services as is profitable without resorting to "inducing" unnecessary patient demands.

Another possibility—deserving of further study—is that third-party payers are more sensitive to fee levels than to amounts of covered services consumed. Thus, the same amount of additional net revenue may more easily be "induced" by selling unnecessary services than would be the case if the doctor simply raised his charges. Certainly, the widespread use of "prevailing," as well as "usual," reimbursement criteria suggest this may be true. But as they become more pervasive, PSRO's could change this situation, at least as far as inpatient services are concerned. Indeed, looked at in this manner, the implementation of the PSRO program may present health economists with yet another way of *directly* testing the supplier-induced-demand hypothesis.

The remainder of the SF paper is relatively easy to comment on since—notwithstanding their style of presentation—it basically states that they examined a number of other possible "monopoly elements" and found little or no evidence to substantiate their existence. And, as in the case of the physician-induced demand hypothesis, I substantially agree with their judgment.

Specifically, I agree with their observation that "such measures of concentration as the share of output from the four largest firms in an industry, Herfindahl and/or Entropy indexes are certainly inappropriate for the physicians' services market." I also join with them in rejecting Joseph Newhouse's interpretation of a positive relation between physicians' prices (unadjusted for quality-amenity differences) and the physician-to-popuation ratio as evidence that physicians are local market monopolists, as well as his use of first differences in physician price and area per capita in-come for the same purpose.

But to forestall any impression of collusion between us, I would like to part company with SF on their interpretation of the finding that coefficients of variation for physicians' fees are higher than those for automobiles and coal in local market areas. In perfect competition *and* in a homogeneous-product oligopoly one would expect to observe identical or nearly identical prices. All other cases fall into indeterminate categories, Since there are no theories that link other market structures unambiguously with dispersion in prices, I cannot agree with the implication of their statement: "judging from the dispersion of fees for specific procedures within local markets, even after adjusting for major differences in physicians' credentials, we conclude that individual physicians possess a degree of monopoly power." The issue is not whether physicians' markets are like those of wheat farmers, but whether they are like those of most small-scale businessmen selling personal serivces. It should not have been obscured by phrasing it in all-or-nothing terms. Perhaps it is worth noting that this puts me in the position of questioning virtually the only direct evidence presented by SF of a *serious* and currently active "monopolistic element" in the market for physicians' services.[19]

Indeed, their reasoning on this topic strikes me as being directly descended from that well-known proposition: Catch-22. They indicated that if the coefficient of variation for physician fees were very small, they would take this as evidence of collusive market behavior. Since, in their opinion, it was relatively large, they took that as evidence of individual monopoly power. Under the circumstances, one might well wonder if there is any value of the coefficient of variation for physician fees which they would take as evidence of reasonably competitive market behavior.

SF devoted most of the remainder of their paper to developing the *possibilities* that RVS's, FMG's, PSRO's, etc., could be used as devices to restrict competition in the physician services market. The way this material was presented, it was all too easy to lose sight of the fact they did not claim—nor did the present evidence that—these mechanisms are, in fact, being used for such purposes. Consider the following quotations from the SF paper.

> Although we can easily envision circumstances under which changes in relative values cause fee increases, there is, to our knowledge, no "hard" evidence on this issue.[20]
>
> Although empirical evidence is unfortunately lacking, it is reasonable to speculate that the use of RVS for purposes of obtaining third-party reimbursement could lead to a subtle form of price discrimination.
>
> . . . Empirical evidence that physicians' professional associations and third parties jointly determine fees is not at all conclusive. . . .
>
> If Blue Shield had a monopoly in the market for insurance, covered most of physicians' services, and offered only service benefits, it might be easy for organized medicine-Blue Shield to withhold Blue Shield payments to physicians who fail to conform to medical society norms and/or to bar new physician entrants. With a few possible exceptions, conditions are not sufficiently favorable to Blue Shield for this type of behavior to be widespread.
>
> Why health insurers, the majority of whom are for-profit, have not in recent years been stricter in dealing with physicians (and hospitals) remains an unanswered, yet extremely important question.[21]
>
> In principle, the Foundation [for Medical Care] is an ideal cartel, controlling price and quantity decisions of individual physicians in a market area. . . . There is reason to question, however, whether these organizations have sufficient market power to act in this manner.
>
> Lacking empirical evidence, we support the theory that competition increases quality. Fortunately, there is currently an empirical basis for some of the assumptions underlying the theory.[22]
>
> . . . There is little empirical evidence on PSRO's, although numerous articles deduce their potential effects.
>
> HMO's have yet to be shown to be relatively efficient producers of health care.
>
> Unfortunately, empirical research on the performance of the fee-for-service sector in areas with a high HMO market share is very limited.[23]

As the foregoing quotations indicate, SF are well aware of the inadequacies of the available evidence with respect to the *actual*—as opposed to the *potential*—effects of existing and emerging institutional arrangements on the degree of competition in local markets for physicians' services. Unfortunately, this fact is often obscured by their tendency to set forth *a priori* speculations in a manner which seems to preclude even the possible validity of alternatives. Moreover, misunderstanding on this score is further abetted by SF's proclivity for drawing conclusions which are more consistent with the title of their paper than with the empirical evidence it contains. Consider, for example, the following quotations:

> Few, our study included, question that monopolistic elements exist in [the physicians' services] market.
>
> Although some of the evidence is inconclusive, there is sufficient information to conclude that individual physicians possess some monopoly power.
>
> Advertising bans . . . at least partly account for the market power the individual physician possesses.
>
> Judging from the dispersion of fees for specific procedures within local markets, even after adjusting for major differences in physician credentials, we conclude that individual physicians possess a degree of monopoly power. At the same time, on the basis of this evidence and the inherent difficulty of policing the price-output decisions of a large number of individual practitioners, we find it very unlikely that price-fixing cartels are widespread.

Perhaps my reaction to these assertions reflects more a difference of style than of substance. If anyting, my tendency is to emphasize that there are two sides to *a priori* hypotheses, and to stress that final judgment should be withheld in cases where existing evidence is fragmentary or inconclusive. I realize that such words as "tentative" and "preliminary" have historically been over-used by academics, and that these days editors look more favorably on papers that "prove something." But, given the danger of misleading policymakers with studies that really do not prove what they say they do, I believe that we need to reconsider the virtues of old-fashioned academic conservatism in presenting the results of health economics research. Thus, I would restate the conclusions of the SF paper along the following lines.

SF have warned us of potential sources of monopoly power which may play a role in the physicians' services market. But—and this point should be emphasized—they have not produced a single piece of convincing evidence that "monopolistic elements" are currently *important* factors in the market for physicians' services, or even that such "elements" constitute a "clear and present danger."

Finally, I would like to endorse strongly what I take to be SF's least controversial conclusion. Namely, that "This paper, and others at this conference, questions the conventional wisdom. Our ultimate objective is to select policies which strengthen the workings of the health care marketplace. Hopefully, questioning the old will not lead to uncritical acceptance of the new. Our review of the literature has, if anything, increased the scope of what we do not know. Informed public policy in this area will require a substantial investment in empirical research with a firm conceptual base." Amen!

NOTES

1. See, for example, Herbert Klarman.

2. As SF put it: "[The B's] arguments imply the ultimate in monopoly power—the absence of a demand constraint facing the physician firm." Furthermore, "evidence supporting the notion . . . would be bad news for almost everyone. The rationale for government regulation would be strengthened. . . . Radical prescriptions for restructuring the delivery system would be necessary. . . . . PSROs would have particularly perverse effects. *Empirical work on the demand for health and health services would be essentially useless* [emphasis mine]. Much empirical work on the supply side which assumes a demand curve constraint would, at a minimum, require reinterpretation. Regulatory mechanisms would have to be developed on a much more rigorous basis than to date."

3. Another serious weakness of the body of empirical health economics research is the extent to which its development has been dictated by the availability of data. Can anyone seriously doubt, for example, that the ease with which data can be obtained from publicly available sources is the explanation for the plethora of hospital cost studies--while there is such a dearth of cost studies for all other types of health services? Perhaps when the number of such "targets of opportunity" has been still further reduced—and there are few alternatives to the dreary task of collecting and processing the data one needs—health economics research may at last enter into a period of relatively balanced growth.

4. One of the best known examples of this genre is Reuben A. Kessel.

5. A landmark in this regard was the discovery that when an upstate New York hospital expanded its bed capacity local physicians hospitalized more of their patients and increased lengths of stay. Thus, was born "Roemer's Law" that in the hospital sector "supply creates its own demand" (see: Joseph Newhouse and Milton Roemer). The alternative view that suppliers are responsive to demand pressures has received much less attention.

6. Given the tendency for a speculation to become an "established fact" if it is repeated enough times, there are quite a number of worrisome speculations in the SF paper. These include the following:

> In principle, the Foundation [for Medical Care] is an ideal cartel, controlling price and quantity decisions of individual physicians in a market area.
>
> . . . physicians may have learned to use utilization control to further their own interests.
>
> . . . quality controls [on HMOs] can potentially be manipulated in the interest of fee-for-service medicine.
>
> [PSROs] might legitimize rather than policy supply-created demand.
>
> Legislation has probably limited HMO growth and thereby reduced the possibility of competition between HMOs and fee-for-service physicians.

SF clearly indicated these, and other similar comments, to be taken as *speculations* deserving of study. But if their paper attracts the amount of attention I suspect it will—and if past experience is repeated—in a short while they will be referenced as a source of these "facts." The only way this unfortunate behavior pattern can be broken is to emphasize knowledge of the literature as a major qualification for manuscript referees. I am not optimistic this will happen.

7. I recall an instance which aptly illustrates this point. It occurred at the "International Conference on Health Costs and Expenditures" sponsored by the John E. Fogarty Center at NIH in June 1975. The final speaker summed up what was then known on the topic. And, according to him, one of the established facts was that physicians determine the demand for their own services. In the discussion which followed, I expressed skepticism that it had really been proven they have anything like total control over demand. Not only was I unconvinced by the statistical evidence (see below), but I wondered aloud why, if this were the case, there is such a good market for books and articles on approaches physicians can employ to get patients to comply with instructions that just might save their lives! I asked why psychologists and sociologists put considerable effort into studying factors relating to patient compliance if physicians have so much control over patient behavior that patients consume whatever amounts of services doctors tell them to. The discussion died because, in a conference room full of health economics specialists, no one else expressed reservations about the validity of this proposition.

A potentially major contribution of SF is the perspective they placed on this issue after a critical review of the evidence. As they put it, "supplier-induced demand is not an 'all or nothing' matter in which opponents of the supplier-induced demand notion are forced to find evidence ruling out supplier-induced demand shifts entirely. Rather, at issue is whether supplier-induced demand represents a major demand determinant. We find that the Bs have been much too hasty in concluding it is." I could not agree more.

8. According to SF "the [Bs] stress anomalies of the health care market while the [Ns] rely on formal theoretical methods and econometrics and emphasize similarities with other markets. . . . The Bs' methods are conceptually weaker."

9. In fairness, it should be pointed out that SF failed to call attention to some evidence which can be interpreted as providing support to the supplier-induced demand proposition. For example, John Holahan found that Medicaid expenditures on medical services *per user* are positively related to the ratio of office-based physicians to total population. (His estimated elasticities for the disabled, AFDC children, and AFDC adults are .39, .33, and .40, respectively.)

However, an even more unpleasant interpretation of Holahan's findings would be that Medicaid reimbursement levels are often so low that such patients receive too little care, having to rely on doctors who are willing to produce services of a low enough "amenities-quality" level that they can profitably sell them at the prices established on a "take-it-or-leave-it basis" by many State Medicaid programs. If this is the case, it has no greater monopolistic implications than the discovery that the makers of most consumer goods produce more than one "line." It does, however, have less sanguine implications with respect to the quality of care for the disadvantaged.

10. Recall that both sets of authors dismissed this possible interpretation because of its links to what they believed to be an econometrically-flawed study by Martin Feldstein.

11. Evidence that this may, in fact, be the case has been provided by Larry Kimbell. Using a crude definition of a relative scarcity area (i.e., a county with a MD-population ratio below the national average), Kimbel found that physicians in such areas: "[1] work . . . a few more hours per week . . . , use more aides and more rooms . . . , and tend to delegate more tasks to ancillaries . . . ; [2] have substantially more patient visits in every location—office, hospital, and other . . . , and gross more [if they are in solo practice] . . . ; [3] [charge] fees [which] are lower . . . ; [and, perhaps most illuminating, their] patients wait more days to get an

appointment and wait longer upon arrival . . . ; [4] see more patients per practice hour . . . , [and] see a slightly higher percentage of White patients, but the major socioeconomic contrast is that they see more poor patients."

These findings suggest that product differentiation and "rationing" in low-income, physician-scarce areas is a more important factor acting on the relationship between utilization and physician density than is positive supplier-induced demand. Otherwise, if they have the power to do so, why would MD's in high-income areas with high MD-population ratios not induce sufficient demand to make their average net incomes at least equivalent to those in scarcity areas? (This point is discussed further below.)

12. I would be even more inclined to stress the welfare and policy implications of the causal uncertainties relating to the statistical association in this case. That is, norms are required to determine whether patients are getting too few or too many services, but such norms would require professional expertise, and, if one takes the attitude that physicians are "guilty until proven innocent," it is impossible to obtain such norms. But suppose, for the sake of argument, that acceptable norms could be agreed upon. Suppose, further, that when they were applied these norms disclosed that 80 percent of all physicians neither ration their services nor generate unnecessary demands, but 15 percent ration their services and 5 percent induce "over-utilization." Clearly, such results would not support the same remedial policies as a finding that all physicians manipulate demand. It is to SF's credit that they stressed "supplier-induced demand is not an 'all or nothing' matter . . . , and the [real] issue is whether supplier-induced demand represents a major demand determinant."

13. As discussed below, the SF reformulation of the Evans model of physician-induced demand is critically dependent upon physicians' finding it distasteful to induce patient demand. Suppose that (as is not likely) this could be verified beyond any reasonable doubt. Should it then be embodied in remedial public policy? What if a few months after such a policy were initiated, medical schools, physicians or both decided to revise their professional ethics positions—perhaps, in response to the policy itself? Should we base longrun policy—which may involve major structural changes in physicians' services markets—on behavior patterns which can be altered at will by producers?

14. My views on this matter and those in the SF paper differ only in terms of emphasis. Recall, they cautioned that " . . . applied econometric studies based on the standard theory often report low R^2s, and some of the variables are only proxies for the theoretical concepts."

15. The evidence proved by Larry Kimbell (discussed earlier) is also clearly supportive of this hypothesis.

16. Average costs in their analysis include an imputed annual labor cost for self-employed physician labor. Thus, when they use the term "profit margin," it is exclusive of the value of the physician-entrepreneur's labor input.

17. I.e., because urban patients demand higher levels of quality-amenities—and because factor prices are higher in urban areas—per unit costs of physician services are higher in urban areas. Therefore, with relatively constant mark-ups over unit costs, fees are higher in the types of areas physicians (as well as other people) find most attractive.

18. As SF noted: " . . . it is conceivable that physicians' fees could be set competitively even though they contain an element of economic rent." They also cited a forthcoming paper by Sloan and Bruce Steinwald which ". . . presents indirect evidence on marginal revenue from which one can infer that the [physician] firm elasticities are at least three."

19. Recall that SF attributed "price dispersion within local market areas . . . in large part . . . to incomplete patient search." In turn, they contended that "advertising bans raise search costs and reduce patient search, bestowing monopoly power on individual physicians." However, they presented no empirical evidence on either assertion, but, instead, advocated (as I do) that "this matter merits careful study."

20. SF did cite two studies—one by William Sobaski and one by Information Engineering —which purported to prove that "... by adjusting relative value scale procedure definitions, physician associations have obtained additional revenue for physicians from third parties."

Here, as in other instances, my view is that there is a plausible alternative explanation of these findings—which means that the issue should be considered unsettled. Specifically, an equally tenable explanation of the findings is that the use of RVS *held down* price increases that would have occurred in its absence, much as a 3-, 4-, or 5-year collective bargaining agreement may temporarily hold down wages in some industries during periods of rapid inflation—at least until it is renegotiated. The longer any job description or fee schedule is in force, the more out of date it becomes. New discoveries are made, and new techniques come to the fore. In science-based industries (like medicine) these changes usually result in more complexity, rather than simplification. As tasks increase in complexity, their prices will naturally rise. In the absence of an RVS, this rise will start right away and proceed piecemeal. However, the billing convenience of not discarding an RVS will entice some physicians to delay relative price adjustments longer than they otherwise would. But eventually the pressure for adjustment builds up. It becomes a matter of either updating the RVS or seeing it widely disregarded. When the update does occur, it is the *effect* of increasing complexity of the services covered, and it permits price adjustments that reflect the increase in complexity. Certainly, this view is as plausible as the cause-and-effect scenario posited by SF. Which is "true" (or to what degree) requires better empirical analyses than are currently available.

21. The wording here conveys the impression that health insurers have been passive claims processors. Although it is a matter of judgment whether or not they should have been "stricter," it is not correct that they have been passive. All "Blue" plans have charge screens, and many have pre-admission certification and other forms of utilization review for private as well as Medicare and Medicaid patients. Several commercial insurers are justly proud of their cost-containment programs. Aetna, for example, reported that it renegotiated half a million claims in 1976—reducing them on the average by $50 each. Employers Insurance of Wausau pioneered the concept of a "Medical Foundation Without Walls" which has achieved utilization levels comparable to HMO's for subscribers in several Wisconsin cities. See Kimbell and Yett.

22. The section in SF's paper entitled "Market Structure and Quality" contains a detailed theoretical analysis of this issue (based on the work of A. M. Spence), but no mention of "an empirical basis" other than the evidence discussed earlier "... that more A [quality-amenities] is supplied, *cet. par.*, in physician dense areas."

23. In my original remarks I noted that Warren Greenberg and Lawrence Goldberg at the FTC were engaged in a study which, hopefully, would shed light on this issue. That study has since been completed, and a summary of the statistical results presented at the June 1977 meetings of the Western Economic Association.

Greenberg and Goldberg employed regression analysis and found a significant negative relationship between number of hospital days per thousand for Blue Cross Plan subscribers and the HMO share of the same health insurance market. However, the significance of this relationship depended upon the inclusion of the western States where HMO market shares are highest.

The Assistant Director of the FTC's Bureau of Economics, as quoted in the *Wall Street Journal,* claimed that "this study shows that alternative health-delivery systems can have a competitive influence on non-profit and commerical health insurance organizations, hospitals, medical societies and physicians." Although his claim is not warranted by the evidence, it does vividly illustrate the dangers of making inconclusive findings available to policymakers. What, in fact, the study showed was that something in the western States was correlated negatively with Blue Cross hospitalization rates. It may have been the HMO market share, or almost anything positively correlated with it—e.g., the effect of a mild climate on the need for health care. What should be done is to follow up and see if Blue Cross plans in areas with high HMO market shares took any steps (e.g., stricter utilization monitoring) which could have caused the statistical relationship. Until it has been directly tested, the effect of HMO market share on private insurer behavior must be considered an unresolved issue. Certainly it would be injudicious to use evidence of this sort as the basis for a policy of still more Federal subsidies for HMO's.

REFERENCES

K. Davis and R. Reynolds, "The Impact of Medicare and Medicaid on Access to Medical Care," in R. Rosett (ed.), *The Role of Health Insurance in the Health Services Sector,* New York, 1976, 391-435.

R. G. Evans, "Supplier-Induced Demand: Some Empirical Evidence and Implications," in M. Perlman (ed.), *The Economics of Health and Medical Care,* London, 1974, 162-173.

______, Review of "The Economics of Health and Medical Care," M. Perlman (ed.), *Can. J. Econ.,* Aug. 1976, 532-537.

______, E.M.A. Parish and F. Sully, "Medical Production, Scale Effects, and Demand Generation," *Can. J. Econ.,* Aug. 1973, 376-393.

M. Feldstein, "The Rising Price of Physicians' Services," *Rev. Econ. Statist.,* May 1970, 121-133.

V. R. Fuchs and M. J. Kramer, *Determinants of Expenditures for Physicians' Services in the United States, 1948-68,* Washington, D.C., 1972.

W. Greenberg and L. Goldberg, "The Health Maintenance Organization and Its Effects on Competition," presented at the meetings of the Western Economic Association, June 1977.

J. Holohan, "Physician Availability, Medical Care Reimbursement and Delivery of Physician Services: Some Evidence from the Medicaid Program," *J. Human Resources,* Summer 1975, 378-402.

B. Kehrer and J. C. Knowles, "Economics of Scale and Pricing of Physicians' Services," in D. E. Yett (Project Director). *An Original Comparative Economic Analysis of Group Practice and Solo Fee-for-Service Practice—Final Report: Analyses from the Seventh Periodic Survey of Physicians,* PB-241 546, Springfield, Va., 1974, 422-521.

R. A. Kessel, "Price Discrimination in Medicine," *J. Law Econ.,* Oct. 1958, 28-53.

L. J. Kimbell, "Physician Behavior in Scarcity Areas," in D. E. Yett (Project Director), *An Original Comparative Economic Analysis of Group Practice and Solo Fee-for-Service Practice—Final Report: Analyses from the Seventh Periodic Survey of Physicians,* PB-241 546, Springfield, Va. 1974, 179-200.

______ and D. E. Yett, *An Evaluation of Policy Related Research on the Effects of Alternative Health Care Reimbursement Systems,* PB-244 400, Springfield, Va., 1975.

H. E. Klarman, "Trends and Tendencies in Health Economics," in H. E. Klarman (ed.), *Empirical Studies in Health Economics,* Baltimore 1970.

J. J. May "Utilization of Health Services and the Availability of Resources," in R. Andersen, J. Kravits, and O. Anderson (eds.). *Equity in Health Services,* Cambridge, Mass., 1975, 131-150.

J. Newhouse, "A Model of Physician Pricing," *Southern Econ. J.,* Oct. 1970, 174-183.

______ and C. E. Phelps, "New Estimates of Price and Income Elasticities of Medical Care Services," in R. Rosett (ed.), *The Role of Health Insurance in the Health Care Sector,* New York, 1976, 261-320.

M. I. Roemer, "Bed Supply and Hospital Utilization: A Natural Experiment," *Hospitals*, Nov. 1961, 36-42.

F. A. Sloan and B. Steinwald, "Physician Participation in Health Insurance Plans: Evidence on Blue Shield," *J. Human Resources*, forthcoming.

W. J. Sobaski, *Effects of the 1969 Relative Value Studies on Costs of Physician Services under SMI*, (S.S.A.) 75-11702, Washington, D.C., 1975.

A. M. Spence, "Monopoly, Quality and Regulation," *Bell J. Econ.*, Autumn 1975, 417-429.

Information Engineering, Inc., "A Comparison of the Minnesota Relative Value Index and the Blue Shield Relative Value Index as Pertaining to the Medicare Part B Program," mimeo., 1975.

Wall St. Jnl., August 5, 1977.

Comment

Uwe E. Reinhardt*
Associate Professor of Economics and Public Affairs, Princeton University

During the past decade or so, the number of active physicians in the United States has grown at a much more rapid rate than the Nation's population. The increase reflects in part a steady influx of foreign-trained medical graduates and, for the rest, an enormous expansion in the capacity of American medical schools. This upward trend in the supply of physicians can be expected to continue for at least three to four more decades. Current forecasts place the number of active physicians per 100,000 population at between 190 and 200 by the year 1980 and between 220 to 225 by 1990.[1] The comparable number in 1970 was 155.

What impact this trend will have on the nature and cost of health care in this country is as yet an open question. At least two distinct schools of thought have emerged on this question, with various shadings in between.

One school of thought takes its inspiration from neoclassical economic theory according to which an increase in the supply of something relative to the prevailing demand for it tends to depress its price. In the context of medical practice, this thesis leads one to predict decreases in physician fees as a result of increases in the physician-population ratio, other things being equal, and probably also decreases in hourly and yearly physician income.[2] Central to this thesis is the assumption that, in setting their fees and rates of output, physicians are subject to a rigid market constraint over which they have no control or even influence. Economists refer to this constraint as a "stable market demand function."

The second school of thought takes its inspiration from Parkinson's famous law that work, in some contexts, tends to expand to fill the time available, even if some of that work is of dubious value. According to this view, an increase in the physician-population ratio tends to increase the number of services (tests, revisits, medical procedures) physicians prescribe for given medical conditions, and neither fees nor physician incomes are

* The author wishes to thank Roger Feldman, Victor Fuchs, Joseph Newhouse, and Frank Sloan for helpful comments on an earlier draft.

likely to fall. Central to that thesis is the assertion that, once a patient has decided to present a given condition to the health–care sector, the decision of how to treat the condition is dominated by one or several physicians and the patient loses much of his/her sovereignty in the matter. Extreme versions of the theory accord the individual patient virtually no discretion in determining the treatment for given conditions. Moderate versions acknowledge that patients often do participate in these decisions, but that physicians play a dominant role. In either case, the demand for physician services is said to be "unstable."

The Parkinsonian thesis itself has little to say about the relationship between physician-population ratios and fees for particular procedures. Parkinson's law is assumed to operate even if the individual physician had no discretion whatever over the levels of these fees.[3] But in the United States, those who espouse the Parkinsonian view almost always espouse also the allied "target-income hypothesis" according to which physicians set their fees so as to attain some desired target income. In its extreme form, the thesis imputes to physicians complete discretion over their fees, which implies that the latter can be set so as to attain any desired target income. A more moderate version of the thesis is that there ultimately are external limits to the fees physicians can charge but that, for a variety of reasons, fees tend to fall short of that limit so long as a market area is not over-doctored. Support for the "target-income hypothesis" is drawn from observed positive first-order correlations between regional physician-population ratios and prevailing fees.

From the viewpoint of policy analysis, neither of these theories is completely satisfactory.

The neoclassical prediction does have the virtue of emerging from a rigorous analytic structure. Its detractors, however, argue that this analytic structure rests on an overly narrow conception of human behavior. Chief among the suspect assumptions are (1) that in the conduct of their medical practice, physicians are motivated solely to maximize their net income per hour worked, and (2) that consumers of physician services act as well-informed rational decisionmakers. The critics of the neoclassical thesis further assert that predictions from the neoclassical theory often do not square with observable facts—for example, with the observed positive correlations between physician-population ratios and fees. These critics are not easily dismissed.

The Parkinsonian school claims to derive its intuition primarily from first-hand experience with the operation of the health-care sector. Its detractors argue that the thesis lacks a rigorous analytic underpinning and thus is suspect from the outset. In particular, argue the critics, the thesis fails to explain what, if anything, does ultimately constrain physicians' decisions concerning their fees, the service-intensity of their treatments, and the target-incomes they seek to attain. Obviously, those critics are not easily dismissed either.

This paper presents a lengthy comment on the issue of physician-induced demand for health services. The comment is structured as a review of Frank Sloan's and Roger Feldman's "Competition Among Physicians." Against the backdrop of a rigorous economic model of physician behavior, Sloan and Feldman survey the existing econometric research bearing directly and indirectly on the issue of supply inducement. Noting that the conceptual underpinnings of the Parkinsonian theory are weak and that the empirical evidence is inconclusive, the authors appear in the end to favor the standard neoclassical view of the issue. The thrust of my comment will be that the standard neoclassical framework, although rigorous, is much too narrow to come to grips with this phenomenon, thus rendering the economists' traditional research strategy on the issue rather impotent. As one tending toward the Parkinsonian view, I see no evidence persuading me to reject that view. My comment ends with the suggestion of a potentially more yielding research strategy.

First, a prefatory remark seems in order. The Sloan-Feldman paper treats not only the issue of physician-induced demand, but encompasses the market for physician services as a whole, including the effect of market structure on the quality of physician services and the role of professional organizations, of Professional Standards Review Organizations (PSRO's) and of health maintenance organizations (HMO's) on the performance of that market. In short, the paper represents a rather ambitious effort and strikes me as a fruitful starting point for economists interested in the market for physicians' services. At the same time, a paper of such enormous length defies thorough review of all of its parts. I shall therefore exercise the reviewer's license to emphasize points of disagreement.

THE ECONOMIC THEORY OF PROVIDER-INDUCED DEMAND

Price-Induced Demand vs. Provider-Induced Demand

Much confusion surrounds the phenomenon of provider-induced demand for health care. This confusion reflects, in part, a failure to appreciate the economist's distinction between "price-induced" and "supply-induced" increases in utilization.

Since Sloan's and Feldman's treatment of this issue is in mathematical notation—it may be useful to illustrate the economists' distinction between "price-" and "supply-" inducement diagrammatically.

Figure 1 depicts the total demand for and supply of some hypothetical commodity in a given market area. The demand schedule (D_0) represents the

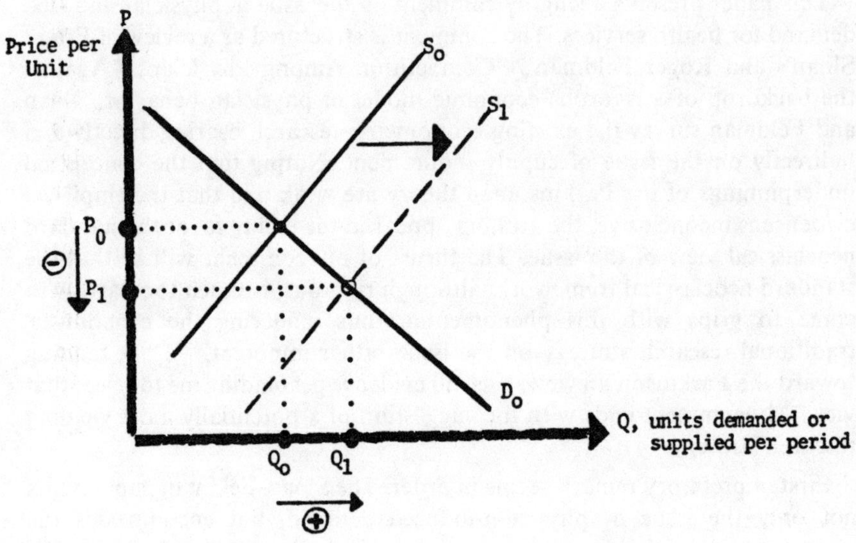

Figure 1

number of units of the commodity consumers would demand at alternative, given price levels. It is assumed that total demand decreases as price increases. Similarly, the supply schedule indicates the total number of units of the commodity that would be offered for sale by the providers in the area at alternative, given price levels—more being offered as price increases. Competition drives the market to an equilibrium market price P_0 and an associated utilization rate Q_0.

Suppose now the supply curve shifted from its original position to the dashed line S_1. At each given price level more is being offered in the market than had been the case before. This development might reflect some cost-saving innovation in production or simply the immigration of additional producers into the market area. If the market were competitive, the additional supply would drive down the price of the commodity. As the demand schedule suggests, a lowered market price would induce consumers to increase their utilization of the commodity. A new market equilibrium would be reached at price level P_1 and utilization rate Q_1. In other words, the increase in supply did ultimately result in an increase in the observed utilization. *This result, however, is standard fare in neoclassical analysis. It would be observed in any normally functioning market; that is, one in which the position of the demand schedule is not influenced at all by producers.*

A casual observer might read into the positive association between the change in supply and the change in utilization the working of Parkinson's law; that is, of "supply-induced demand." When economists speak of supply-inducement, however, they have in mind a *direct* influence of providers over consumers' decisions through a mechanism *other than price changes.* In terms of figure 1, they have in mind a rightward shift of the entire demand schedule in response to a rightward shift in the supply schedule, or at least in response to some deliberate act by providers. Figure 2 illustrates this case.

In figure 2 it is assumed that the supply curve shifts to the right for some reason, and that thereafter providers, singly or jointly, induce consumers to

---

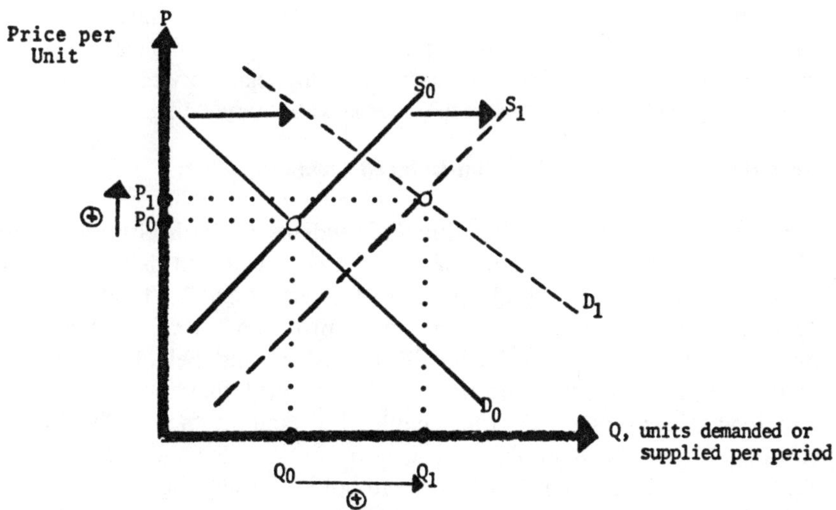

Figure 2

demand more of the commodity at any given price level—hence, the rightward shift of the demand schedule to position D_1. Ordinary business firms could attempt to do this through a vigorous advertising campaign. Professionals often can achieve this through more subtle forms of "persuasion."

In the case modeled in figure 2, an increase in supply is, once again, seen to be associated with an increase in utilization, although the equilibrium price in this case is seen to have *increased* from P_0 to P_1. It may be thought that this movement in price furnishes a simple characteristic for distinguishing the case modeled in figure 1 ("price-inducement") from that depicted in figure 2 ("provider-inducement"). Unfortunately, the equilibrium price need not always increase under provider inducement, as is illustrated in figure 3.

In figure 3, the supply curve is, once again, assumed to shift to the right for some reason, pulling along with it the demand curve to a new position D_1. In this illustration, however, the power to induce demand is more limited. Consequently, a new equilibrium is reached at a higher utilization rate but at a *lower* price. Simple correlations between supply changes on the one hand and utilization or price on the other could not distinguish this case from that modeled in figure 1 where the power to induce has been assumed away. In both cases, an increase in supply leads to an increase in utilization and a *decrease* in price, and one would have to know the precise shape and position of the demand and supply curves to distinguish between the cases empirically. This illustration highlights the difficulty economists encounter in econometric research on the market for physician services and is one reason why such research has been so remarkably unyielding.

Empirical Evidence on Physician-Induced Demand

As already noted in the introduction, students of the health sector are divided on the question whether or not physicians can shift the demand for their services in the manner illustrated with figures 2 and 3. This division of opinion carries over into the economics profession itself. Following a nomenclature proposed by Robert Evans, Sloan and Feldman therefore divide the profession into two groups: the so-called "narrow economists," identified by the symbol N's (which could also stand for "no shift"), and the so-called "broad economists," who believe that the demand curve can be shifted and who are identified by the symbol B's (which the authors might well be inclined to translate in the well-known American vernacular "BS").

By way of introduction, the authors remark that "the arguments of the B's imply the ultimate in monopoly power—the absence of a demand constrant facing the physician firm" (p. 61)—that is, the absence of any constraint on the number of services that can be foisted on patients. If this were the

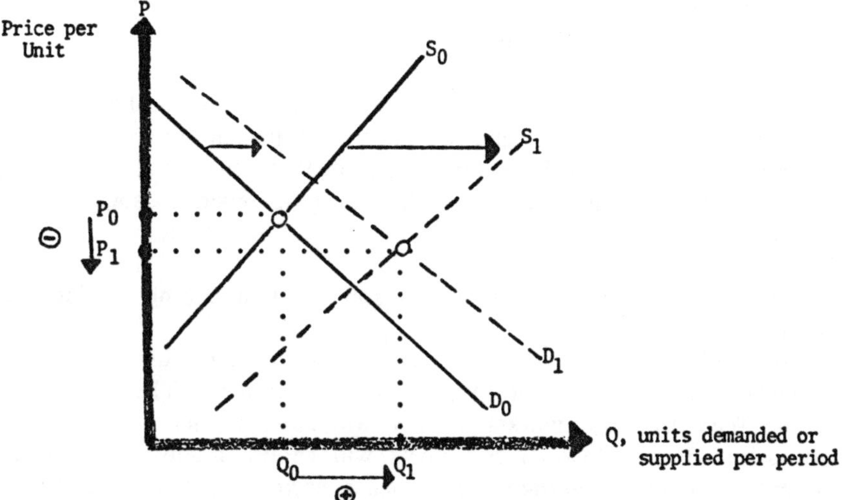

Figure 3

foundation of the Parkinsonian view, one could indeed write it off as conceptually untenable. Actually, no sensible observer would or could go that far, for the power to induce demand is apt to have limits and is apt to vary across medical specialties and market contexts.

For uninsured, routine services such as check-ups or well-baby care, for example, the market undoubtedly imposes fairly narrow limits on the physician, as it may do for some fully insured services placing heavy demands on the patient's time. Similarly, there are bound to be real physical limits to per capita rates of surgery, regardless of patients' insurance status. The thrust of the B's argument is simply that physicians typically have much leeway in determining the treatment modality for particular conditions—especially in complex cases—and that, for some reason, the economic potential of this leeway is not invariably fully exploited, especially when the supply of physicians is taut.

Next, Sloan and Feldman address the Parkinsonian's assertion that consumer ignorance is the foundation for supply-induced demand in health care. They point out, correctly, that "standard theory does not require that *everyone* possess perfect information—only that there be a sufficient number of marginal consumers both able to assess output and willing to seek it out at its lowest price" (p. 61). Sloan and Feldman buttress this point by quoting Mark Pauly's observation:

> I know even less about the works of a movie camera than I know about my own organs; yet I feel fairly confident in purchasing a camera for a given price as long as I know that there are at least a few experts in the market who are keeping sellers reasonably honest (p. 61).

Employed in this manner the quotation is somewhat misleading, a point that warrants elaboration.

Pauly is obviously referring to the market price of a particular model in a particular line of cameras (or TV sets, or stereo systems). The question is whether the existence of market prices for alternative models automatically assures one that individual consumers will choose intelligently among alternative models, *given their own particular requirements.* To drive home this point, I present below a set of rather bewildering technical properties of two stereo amplifier-tuners offered by the same manufacturer at substantially different prices:

	MODEL A	MODEL B
Audio Section		
Continuous Power	25/35W (4Ω) 28/28W (8Ω)	43/43W (4Ω) 35/35W (8Ω)
Power Amplifiers Section		
Frequency Response (at normal listening level)	15-40000Hz±1dB	10-50000Hz±1dB
Preamplifier Output	.8V (at rated input) 3V (max.)	.5V (at rated output) 2.5V (max.)
Power Amplifier Input Voltage	.8V (at rated output)	.5V (at rated output)
Tuner Section		
FM Sensitivity	1.6μV (20dB quieting) 2.0μV (IHF)	1.4μV (20dB quieting) 1.8μV (IHF)
Capture Ratio	2.5dB	1.0dB
Image Frequency Rejection	Better than 85dB	Better than 90dB at 98MHZ

and so on . . .

Consider now a consumer without knowledge of electronics, with an only moderately sensitive ear. It can be wondered how our consumer would necessarily be driven to select the right model from these and other models *for his or her particular circumstances* simply because true experts in the market have established reasonable prices for these models, *given these experts' predilections and circumstances.* Chances are that our consumer would rely on expert advice in making the selection; chances are that the *vendor* would offer such advice freely; and chances are that the consumer will take home a model that may not be the most appropriate for his or her particular circumstances, especially if the vendor is overstocked on a particular model or if profit margins differ among models. It could happen even to an economist! This illustration is somewhat closer to the analogy we seek.

Even more apropos would be the case where a stereo system breaks down. Although the price of a new unit would limit the degree to which the service-intensity of repairs could be varied—a constraint usually absent in repairs on the human body—the market usually leaves room to vary that intensity for given technical malfunctions, especially for complicated gadgets.

In short, then, the issue of consumer sovereignty seems not adequately laid to rest by the analogy offered in the Sloan-Feldman paper.

After commenting on these conceptual issues, Sloan and Feldman turn to the empirical evidence on the issue. To that end they explore the predictions from a model that specifically attributes to physicians the power to induce demand for their services. Since the unit of analysis in that model is the individual physician (and not the entire market, as in figures 1 to 3), it is necessary to specify clearly the physician's professional goals and the constraints under which these goals are pursued. This specification is borrowed from Evans who calls himself a "B" and is of the Parkinsonian school.

It is assumed in Evans' model that the physician conducts his or her practice so as to maximize an objective described mathematically as

$$U = U(Y, W, D). \qquad (1)$$

Economists refer to this equation as a "utility function." It is more aptly called a "happiness production function." The function states that the physician's happiness (indexed by U) depends somehow on net practice income (Y), on the rate of output from the practice (W), and on an index (D) denoting the degree to which the physician has induced demand. It is assumed that, other things being equal, increases in income (Y) make the physician happier; increases in output (W) detract from happiness because that implies added hours of work; and increases in D detract from happiness, presumably because the physician is basically reluctant to apply medical procedures of only marginal benefit, especially if that visits added fiscal burdens on patients.

It is further assumed in Evans' model that in the pursuit of happiness the physician is constrained by a downward sloping demand curve that can be described mathematically as

$$W = R \cdot f(P,D). \tag{2}$$

In this expression, P denotes the price per unit of physician output; R is the physician-population ratio; and function f(P,D) is the demand for care by the "representative" patient in the area. It is assumed that, for a given physician density (R) and degree of inducement (D), consumers demand more services if physician fees (P) decline; that for a given R and P, consumers demand more services if they are persuaded to do so (if D increases); and finally, that for given values of P and D, an increase in physician density (a decrease in R) would lower the demand for each physician's output (W) proportionately. Function f(P,D), incidentally, equates the physician's power to induce demand for additional services *at a given fee level* with the power to *raise fees for given procedures* at will. As was noted earlier, the validity of this assumption is not to be taken for granted.[4]

Neoclassical economists naturally wonder why a physician with these objectives and with these powers would not immediately shift up (to the right) the demand for his services as much as possible even prior to any increase in the physician-population ratio. In Evans' model, this question is answered by the assumption that the physician finds it discomforting to prescribe services of marginal medical benefit, especially if the individual patient has to pay for them, but that this reluctance erodes when added physicians compete for a given patient pool and the physician's income is threatened.

To explore the implication of this "provider-inducement" model, Sloan and Feldman put it through the paces of comparative statics, a technique enabling one to derive mathematically the direction of the change in particular dependent variables (fees, physician income, output, and so on) in response to a change in, say, the physician-population ratio in the physician's market area. Table 1 overleaf presents these predictions (also known as "impact multipliers"). To facilitate comparison, table 1 includes analogous predictions from a purely neoclassical model—one in which physicians are assumed to face a rigid demand curve that cannot be shifted by them.[5] Since that model is not explicitly developed in the Sloan-Feldman paper, it is presented in the technical appendix to this comment.

The impact multipliers in table 1 reflect the mathematical properties of very general models of physician behavior, which in turn reflect a set of assumptions expressed at a very general level. This circumstance must be kept in mind in interpreting the entries in the table. For example, the very general specification of the inducement model suggests that an increase in

Table 1 Predicted Direction of the Effect of an Increase in the Physician-Population Ratio on Per-Capita Utilization of Physician Services, and on Physicians' Fees, Output and Income

Dependent Variable		**NEOCLASSICAL MODEL** **Assuming Physicians *Cannot* Induce Demand for Their Services**		**PROVIDER-INDUCEMENT MODEL** **Assuming Physicians *Can* Induce Demand for Their Services**
1. SERVICES USED/ CAPITA				INCREASE
(impact inferred from the impact		INCREASE	*or*	DECREASE*
multiplier dL/dR)			*or*	NO CHANGE*
2. PHYSICIANS' FEES				INCREASE
(impact inferred from the sign of		DECREASE[a]	or	DECREASE
impact multiplier dP/dR)			*or*	NO CHANGE
3. OUTPUT/PHYSICIAN		INCREASE		INCREASE
(impact inferred impact multplier	*or*	DECREASE	*or*	DECREASE
dw/dR)	*or*	NO CHANGE	*or*	NO CHANGE
4. INCOME/PHYSICIAN		INCREASE*		INCREASE*
(impact inferred impact multiplier	*or*	DECREASE	*or*	DECREASE
dy/dR)	*or*	NO CHANGE	*or*	NO CHANGE

[a] If one makes the plausible *assumption* that Y_{pr} is positive.

the physician-population ratio may increase per capita utilization of physician services, or decrease it, or leave it unchanged (see row 1 of table 1). This is not to say that each alternative would occur with equal probability; the comparative-statics exercise is silent on this point. The exercise merely indicates that, *in terms of the general model from which the impact multiplier is derived,* one cannot rule out a priori the possibility that an increase in the physician-population ratio in an area might *decrease* per capita utilization in the area. One's intuition may suggest that such an outcome would be *improbable.* Indeed, one's intuition may lead one to replace the very general demand and utility functions in the model with more specific versions that would rule out such improbable outcomes in a comparative-statics exercise. At this general level of the model, however, one is to take the results from the exercise at face value and can at best offer some opinions on the relative likelihood of each possible outcome. In table 1, for example, an asterisk has been placed next to predictions that seem improbable.[6]

The main purpose of deriving the so-called "impact multipliers" implicit in an economic model is to contrast them with empirical data, thus to test the hypothesis embodied in the model. In the case at hand, such tests tend to take the form of multiple regression analyses in which the dependent variables "fees," "physician income," "physician output" or "per capita utilization of physician services" in some region or at some time are regressed on the relevant physician-population ratio and other control-variables that may influence the dependent variable. Of interest is the estimated coefficient associated with the physician-population ratio. For example, if a regression of fees on the physician-population ratio and other variables yields a positive coefficient for the ratio, the inducement model would be said to be "maintained" or "compatible" with the empirical data, while the neoclassical model would have to be rejected (unless one had reason to believe that the entire regression equation is misspecified and that the coefficient estimates are not reliable).

With this background, table 1 leads to some disturbing conclusions. First, unless the various functional relationships implicit in the inducement model are more fully articulated, the model is compatible with literally any sign of the coefficient-estimate for the physician-population ratio in a regression of per capita utilization, fees, output per physician, or income per physician on that ratio (although, as noted, some signs would be expected with low probability). It is therefore not possible to reject the general inducement model with empirical tests of this sort.

Second, it is apparent from the table that multiple regression analyses of the sort described above can help one distinguish the inducement from the neoclassical model unambiguously only if physician fees are the dependent variable; the criteria "per capita utilization," "output per physician," and "income per physician" are not helpful for this purpose. If a *properly specified* regression of fees on the physician-population ratio and other pertinent variables yielded a positive coefficient on the ratio, then one could reject the neoclassical model and maintain the inducement hypothesis. (If the coefficient were negative, both hypotheses would, of course, be maintained.) Unfortunately, researchers can never be quite certain that their regression equation in such a test *is* properly specified, and not merely because it is so difficult to devise a reliable, one-dimensional measure of the individual physician's fees. Adherents to the neoclassical view can therefore always write off a positive coefficient on the ratio as the product of misspecification. For it is true, regretably, that only God would be completely immune from specification error in econometric research, and that single terrestrial studies of this sort almost always become essays in persuasion. One tends to be persuaded one way or the other by such studies only after numerous replications on independent data sets have yielded consistently similar results.

It would have been legitimate for the authors to rest on their analytic results, as summarized in table 1. They do, however, proceed to examine the existing empirical research on the issue. This survey serves a useful purpose, for it reminds the adherents to the inducement theory (myself included) that some of the studies they have cited in support of their theory also support the standard neoclassical view. For example, as the authors correctly point out in their section C.1 (pp. 67-74), a positive correlation between the physician-population ratio and per capita utilization of physician services supports *both* rival theories and not just the inducement theory, as is sometimes pretended by Parkinsonians. By the same token, one must observe in connection with Sloan's and Feldman's Section C.3 on "Physicians' Earnings" that the generally observed negative correlation between the physician-population ratio and physicians' incomes is consistent with both rival theories, too, and not just with the neoclassical theory as is sometimes pretended by adherents to that point of view (see row 4 of table 1).

As is indicated in table 1, the potentially most useful criterion on which to test the two rival theories with the standard econometric research reviewed by Sloan and Feldman is "physicians' fees". A *positive* partial correlation between physician fees and the physician-population ratio (after proper adjustment for other variables determining fees) is incompatible with the neoclassical theory, but fully compatible with the inducement theory. On the other hand, an observed *negative* correlation between fees and the ratio is fully compatible with *both* theories.

In their section C.2 on "Physician Fees," Sloan and Feldman cite earlier work by Sloan and Bruce Steinwald in which it was found that:

> For general practitioners and general surgeons, increases in the number of competing physicians per-capita lowers fees in *most* of the regressions [though not in all of them]. *But the opposite is obtained for internists, pediatricians and obstetrician-gynecologists* (p. 76). (Emphasis and comment in brackets added.)

In other words, results from the Sloan-Steinwald study are fully consistent with predictions from the inducement model (as they must be) but are not always consistent with the neoclassical theory—in fact, not for three of five specialties.

In a subsequent study by Sloan, this pattern appears to have reappeared, although results for pediatricians and ob-gyn specialists were apparently not presented. From these two studies, Sloan and Feldman then conclude that:

> Both studies report signs for [the coefficient of] the demand-shift variables [i.e., physician density] that are fully consistent with the Ns' interpretation of physician behavior [i.e., with the neoclassical theory] (p. 76). (Remarks in brackets added.)

Further on it is noted that:

> . . . the supplier-induced demand argument contains numerous weaknesses. Yet current evidence cannot rule it out completely (p. 83). (Emphasis added.)

I am puzzled by this interpretation of the available evidence. Surely a more appropriate conclusion would have been that the inducement theory is alive and well—that the econometric evidence on fees and physician-population ratios has not at all ruled out the inducement theory (because it cannot do so) while there is considerable evidence contradicting the neoclassical theory. Presumably, the only reason why one would not rule out the neoclassical theory on this evidence is that regression equations indicating a positive correlation between fees and the physician-population ratio can always be written off as misspecified and, hence, unreliable.

One reason why Sloan and Feldman give little weight to observed positive correlations between fees and physician density (physician-population ratios) appears to go back to their formal analytic framework. Drawing on the impact multipliers derived from that framework, the authors observe on page 65 that:

> . . . several empirical studies of physician pricing behavior report a negative dP/dR, and the authors have often been quick to attribute this finding to physician-generated demand. . . . *dP/dR may be negative* in an inducement world, *but it must then be negative for all variables shifting the demand curve outward.* Patient income and insurance, for example, would operate on price in the same manner as a change in R. However, estimates of patient income in physician price equations have without exception been positive.

Variable R in the Sloan-Feldman paper denotes the population-physician ratio. Translated to the more familiar physician-population ratio, the statement implies that observed positive correlations between that ratio and fees support the inducement theory only if increases in patient income or insurance coverage are found to *decrease* fees. The implication appears to be that, because patients' income and insurance coverage are generally found to have a positive effect on physicians' fees, one ought not to adduce positive correlations between physician density and fees as evidence for the inducement theory. I find this conclusion troublesome, even within the confines of the authors' formal analytic framework.

First, one may ask just how one is to interpret positive coefficients on physician density in regressions of fees on density, for such evidence clearly is not compatible with the neoclassical model either. Second, the model in question is highly non-linear, and the effect of a change in a so-called "shift variable" (patients' income, insurance coverage, the physician-population ratio) on equilibrium price depends on the size of the demand-shift thereby induced. Third, if one wishes to use tests of this sort for purposes of practical policy analysis—as distinct from economic analysis—there remains the question whether the demand-inducement issue as seen by policymakers is at all well modeled by a shifting demand curve. This is a matter to which I return in the concluding section of my comment.

Extensions of the Inducement Model

Implicit in the inducement model reproduced by Sloan and Feldman is the assumption that increases in the output from a physician's practice require proportionate increases in the input of the physician's time. Taken by itself, any increase in output is, therefore, assumed to detract from the physician's happiness.

Actually, one should think of the output from a physician's practice as a composite of two broad classes of services:

1) those requiring relatively substantial inputs of the physician's own time; and
2) ancillary services produced primarily by non-physician personnel and requiring little or no input of the physician's own time.

For the first type of service, the availability of the physician's own time represents a strong, natural constraint to physician-induced demand. By prescribing the second type of service, however, physicians can increase their net revenues without having to work additional hours. Their own time constraint will not come into play. A formal model incorporating this modification is easily constructed (and available from the author); but it is not necessary at this point.

Table 2 presents data from the Canadian Province of Quebec whose residents have been covered, since 1970, by a comprehensive universal health

Table 2 Secular Movements of Health-Care Statistics Province of Quebec, Canada
1971-1974
(Figures in parentheses are index numbers with 1971 = 100).

	1971	1972	1973	1974
1. Per capita cost of physician services	$45.4 (100)	$49.9 (110)	56.1 (124)	59.4 (131)
2. Average number of physicians services paid for, per capita	5.34 (100)	5.76 (108)	6.41 (120)	6.66 (125)
3. Average cost per service	$8.50 (100)	$8.65 (102)	$8.75 (103)	$8.93 (105)
4. Average remuneration per physician:				
(a) All General Practitioners	$33,047 (100)	$32,217 (97)	$34,236 (104)	$36,379 (110
(b) Cohort of 1,850 fulltime GPs	$47,409 (100)	N.A.	$49,938 (105)	N.A.
(c) All Specialists	$43,645 (100)	$44,376 (102)	46,827 (107)	$47,597 (109)
(d) Cohort of 2,770 Specialists	$53,586 (100)	N.A.	$56,132 (105)	N.A
5. Consumer Price Index (Canada)	100	105	113	124
6. Physicians per 100,000 population	116 (100)	128 (110)	136 (117	140 (121)

Sources: Government of Quebec, Regie de l'assurance-maladie du Quebec, *1974 Annual Statistics,* various tables. Lines 4b and 4d from A.P. Contandriopolous (1976), Table 1, p. 165.

insurance program. Under the program physicians are reimbursed, on a fee-for-service basis, according to a negotiated fee schedule. *The schedule had remained unchanged during 1970-76. Physicians in the Province generally do not operate their own laboratory facilities and typically refer such services to hospitals which, in turn, are reimbursed for them under their budgets.* For the most part, the revenues earned by physicians reflect services whose production requires heavy impact on physician time.

It will be noted from line 6 of table 2 that the physician-population ratio in the Province rose by 21 percent during the three-year period 1971-74. The average "number of physician services" per capita rose by 25 percent during the same period. It is, of course, not apparent whether these trends reflect satisfaction of hitherto unmet demand by patients or physician-induced demand.

Of particular interest are lines 4a to 4d of table 2. These data indicate that the average gross billings per practitioner remained more or less *constant* in nominal terms during 1971-74; they actually decreased in real terms. It is doubtful that physicians would passively have tolerated this erosion of real income if they possessed, as *individuals,* near unlimited power to induce demand for their services. The question is, then: Precisely what has been the constraining factor? As noted, the fee schedule used for reimbursement remained unchanged during the period. To alter the traditional practice style in Quebec—for example, to acquire laboratory equipment and to hire technicians—may not have been feasible in the short timespan under consideration. Quite possibly, then, physicians in Quebec *had* to accept the decline in real income because the only shortrun measure to combat it would have implied added hours of work. Medical practice in Quebec may thus approximate the assumption in the Sloan-Feldman model that added output per physician always implies added hours of work. The constraint on inducement created by this practice may be of great interest to policymakers with influence over the number of physicians admitted to practice.

Consider, in contrast, table 3 presenting data from the comprehensive, universal health insurance program in West Germany. *The typical West German practitioner owns a laboratory or is a member of a physician-owned lab-cooperative* and can therefore increase revenues substantially without substantial input of physician time. Private medical practitioners are reimbursed for their services on a fee-for-service basis, on fee schedules negotiated between associations of physicians, and on fee schedules of insurance companies.

During the period 1965-74, average gross income per physician in ambulatory practice and from the social insurance program rose by about 12 percent per year; during the period 1970-74, the average annual increase was 13 percent.[7] These growth rates substantially exceeded the rate of general inflation in the country and the growth of average employee compensation and gross national product. Table 3 suggests that much of this growth in revenue has come from technical procedures not generally requiring a heavy input of physician time per unit of revenue.

One gathers from the West German press and from the trade literature[8] that neither the public nor administrators of the insurance system doubt any longer that diagnostic procedures are used by physicians to regulate the annual growth of their income. In 1975, for example, the physician

Table 3 Mix of Services Reimbursed per "Case"[a] Local Sickness Funds in West Germany

Service Category	Fourth Quarter 1965		Fourth Quarter 1974		Percentage Change 1965-74
	DM	%	DM	%	%
Consultations	7.70	31.2	7.31	20.0	−5.1
Visits	2.06	8.3	1.55	4.2	−24.8
Minor Medical Procedures	7.53	30.5	10.42	28.5	+38.5
Medical Supplies	1.33	5.4	1.69	4.6	+27.1
Diagnostic Procedures	2.56	10.4	9.13	25.0	+256.6
X-Ray Procedures	2.45	9.9	4.65	12.7	+89.3
Total Per "Case"	24.68	100.0	36.59	100.0	+48.3

[a] "Case" in this context means "patient treated by a given physician during the quarter" and is not to be confused with a medical case.

Source: Th. Siedbeck, "Zur Kostenentwicklung der Krankenversicherung, "*Die Ortskrankenkasse,* April 1976, Table 11, p. 276.

associations consented to a mere 2.5 percent increase in fee schedules "as a contribution toward cost containment." Prior years' experience had shown the service intensity per case to increase by about 7 percent per year, so that the increase in overall expenditures per patient were expected to stay below 10 percent during 1975. As it turned out, however, in that year the number of services per case rose by as much as 12 percent, raising overall expenditures per case by 14 percent. Few observers believed that this increase was mere happenstance. Indeed, to prevent a recurrence of this phenomenon, an overall limit to total national expenditures on physician services was recently adopted in West Germany.

The preceding illustrations were presented to suggest that the individual physician's power to increase revenue through induced demand is apt to be a function of his/her ability to produce and prescribe ancillary services. The latter generally requires little input of physician time. Moreover, they can often be applied in the sincere belief that the quality of treatments is thereby enhanced, or the probability of a malpractice suit is thereby reduced.

Admittedly, these illustrations are drawn from the context of complete insurance coverage and can, therefore, not readily be grafted onto the semicovered market for physician services in the United States. But this brings me to yet another point. Virtually, all of the models or empirical studies reviewed by Sloan and Feldman evoke the image of a primary-care physician dispensing well-patient care to sensible patients with little or no insurance coverage. As the authors acknowledge, these models may not, for much longer, represent adequately the market for physician services in the United States. In terms of the Evans model, the physician's reluctance to induce demand (to increase D) is apt to diminish as insurance reduces or eliminates the fiscal burden demand-inducement visits on patients. Even if one could demonstrate—as has not been done—that in the absence of insurance coverage physicians cannot induce demand for their services, national health insurance may nevertheless soon be upon the Nation. The time is at hand for policymakers—and for researchers as well—to attune their thinking to this new market context.

OTHER POINTS IN THE SLOAN-FELDMAN PAPER

I have dwelled at some length on the issue of supply inducement in this comment because it is a dominant theme in the Sloan-Feldman paper, because this is one of the more important questions confronting health policy makers at this time, and because I take issue with the authors' interpretation of the available evidence. It behooves me to mention, however, that the paper contains numerous points that I found instructive or that confirmed my own preconceptions.

I concur, for example, with the authors' contention that the internal rate of return to medical education is not an informative index of monopoly power. Much too much seems to be made of that statistic in the literature. In the presence of barriers to entry into the medical profession, the internal rate of return to medical education, could, in principle, be high even if the market for physician services were perfectly competitive. Besides, as students in corporation finance are taught regularly, as an investment criterion the internal rate of return is conceptually flawed from the outset.[9]

I also concur with the authors that "observed utilization differences between [Health Maintenance Organizations and the fee-for-service model] do not necessarily reflect supply-created demand under fee-for-service" and that "the differences may [simply] reflect market clearing at low out-of-pocket prices [to insured consumers] under fee-for-service and non-price rationing [on the part of physicians] by HMOs" (p. 103)[10] The point that the physician's economic incentives under the HMO mode is just the obverse of those (s)he faces under fee-for-service is not sufficiently acknowledged by proponents of the HMO concept. Where the incentive to underserve is acknowledged by these proponents, they add that such underservicing would drive members away from the HMO and would thus not be in the HMO's economic interest. That assertion, however, is not a fact but merely a hypothesis—one in need of sustained empirical testing.[11]

Finally, I share the authors' jaundiced views on the existing system of professional licensure. The ostensible objective of the system is to protect patients from incompetent health professionals. At the same time, such a system cannot help but slice up economic turf among the various health professions, a point surely not lost on the professions. In view of this added effect, Sloan and Feldman refer to licensure as "occupational franchising," (p. 120) evoking images of CHICKEN DELIGHT and DAIRY QUEEN.

American medicine has been blamed recently for virtually every shortcoming in our health system. Sensible observers have begun to wonder whether matters can really be as simple as that. In connection with professional licensure, however, the profession's posture is truly puzzling. As Sloan and Feldman hint on page 87 of their paper, it seems rather inconsistent for American physicians to argue, as they often do, that the market for health services would work well if only the Government ceased to intrude into it, all the while enlisting the powers of Government to restrict the professional activities of potential competitors—for example, of independent paramedical practitioners. If consumers are deemed too ignorant to protect themselves against, say, an independently practicing nurse practitioner, then one can hardly blame public officials for carrying that argument to its logical conclusion by seeking to monitor the professional practice of, say, general practitioners or of any other physicians. At the very least, the argument calls for periodic relicensing of physicians.

The debate over professional franchising is likely to heat up in the years ahead as the number of health professionals per capita continues to climb. A useful exercise for organized medicine would, therefore, be to reexamine its current position on professional licensing and to develop a position based on internally consistent reasoning. Given the profession's long-professed preference for free, competitive markets, it really ought to favor a move away from *mandatory licensure* to *permissive licensure.*

An interesting development in a closely related area is the brewing struggle between dentists and denturists over the right to replace dentures. As an economist, I am not qualified to comment on the medical aspects of this issue. Since the driving force behind the struggle may well be mere concern over economic turf, however, the dental profession might be asked why permissive rather than mandatory licensure would not serve society well in this case.

CONCLUDING REMARKS

Policy makers pondering the economic consequences of their health-manpower policies are apt to be discouraged by the Sloan-Feldman paper and by my review thereof. For some time now these policymakers have wondered whether it is wise to encourage a sustained secular growth in the physician-population ratio—whether, in other words, such a policy would serve to curb the rapid secular rise in health-care costs and expenditures, or perhaps even aggravate them.

For their part, economists have explored this question by following the economic footprints left behind by physicians and by inferring from these footprints the "typical" physician's motives and behavior. With rare exceptions, the results from this econometric sleuthing have been meager and ambiguous. If policymakers wished to take initiatives in this area—as they may soon have to—they would have to fall back on casual empiricism, andecdotal evidence, or educated hunches. To advocate inaction until economists have explored the matter satisfactorily may be too much to ask. As Sloan and Feldman wryly observe in their review of the literature:

> The reader lacking a vested interest in econometric applications may (perhaps, legitimately) question whether economic theory and applied econometrics will ever settle this matter [of supply inducement] (p. 83).

I consider this one of the more valuable insights offered in the authors' paper.

Part of the problem has, of course, been the paucity of robust data on private medical practices. Typically, these data have come from secondary sources or telephone and mailed questionnaires. In connection with the issue of physician-induced demand, however, the main problem may well have been that economists have barked up the wrong tree, so to speak.

Barking up wrong trees is one of the hazards attending a certain dialectic social scientists favor in exploring issues in social policy. As part of this dialectic, the process at issue is modeled in terms of small sets of extreme assumptions, individual researchers develop vested intellectual interests in one or the other of the implied models, and then the search is on for empirical evidence that might support the favored analytic structure. Choice of the latter, incidentally, does not invariably reflect political ideology. Just as often it is dictated simply by disciplinary allegiance. As Richard Nelson has observed on this point:

> Powerful analysis requires strong analytical structure. . . . However, an intellectual tradition of the sort required to develop a strong analytic structure usually develops an explicit or implicit commitment to a particular point of view. . . . [In other words], intellectual traditions tend to involve a greater commitment to particular structures, which may or may not obtain, than their practitioners believe (pp. 15 and 23).

Economists have a strong commitment to the standard neoclassical economic theory of human behavior and of markets. It is a theory that has much intuitive appeal to begin with, but one whose technical mastery requires years of hard study that breed a special kind of loyalty to this particular view of the world. Given this heavy investment, it is legitimate—or at least understandable—that economists begin their exploration of perceived social problems strictly in terms of the familiar theory, if only to ascertain how far that theory can carry one in explaining observed behavior.

One ought not to belittle the advantages of this approach. First, the neoclassical theory furnishes a shared set of sophisticated and rigorous ground rules by which arguments can be settled at the conceptual and empirical levels. Proper application of the theory also reminds researchers that more than meets the eye may lurk behind simple (first-order) correlations. The ideologically charged literature on health policy, in particular, is rife with instances in which even distinguished observers rush to infer entire causal structures from simple correlations or even anecdotes. Viewed in this light, the ambiguities sometimes resulting from economic research can be powerful insights rather than signs of failure.

At the same time, the formal analytic approach preferred by economists does carry with it certain risks, and these ought to be acknowledged. The most important among these risks is what may be called "model-induced myopia." To illustrate from another context, I recently came across a paper in which an economist seriously proposed that a longer payoff period to investments in child health-care was the "most ready explanation" why children between the ages of one and five receive relatively more well-child pediatric visits than children between ages five and eight.[12] I view this as an advanced stage of model-induced blindness. Economists may similarly straightjacket their inquiries into physician behavior by refusing to attribute to physicians motives other than unbridled maximization of hourly profits. To begin one's analysis on that assumption seems, as noted, legitimate. To write off alternative explanations as *ad-hocery*—as, incidentally, the authors appear to do on page 80 of their paper—may not be helpful in the end, and seems unwarranted in the face of the low explanatory power so far achieved with the standard neoclassical model.

A related danger is that by forcing perceived social problems into their standard analytic framework, economists may cease to be responsive to the questions originally raised by policymakers. In connection with the inducement issue, policymakers wonder whether under certain circumstances marginally beneficial or dubious medical procedures are applied by physicians to particular medical cases, and if so, whether the penchant to prescribe such services tends to increase with physician density. Their intuition and occasional experience as patients appears to suggest to policymakers that a substantial fraction of the procedures received by patients cannot be technically evaluated by patients. Given their intuition and experience, policy-makers naturally wonder how anyone could deny the physician's ability to manipulate the number of his or her services patients will accept for particular medical cases.

As is apparent from equation (2), in the Sloan-Feldman paper, the standard approach taken by economists to this question has been to define the physician's power to induce demand as his or her ability to shift the demand function:

$$Q = f(P; X_1, \ldots, X_N) \tag{3}$$

Here Q denotes the number of "physician services demanded" by the representative consumer per period, P denotes the "price paid per unit of service," and X to X denote non-price factors influencing the rate Q demanded by the consumer.

As a guide to thinking, this characterization of the issue is undoubtedly a good point of departure. From Sloan and Feldman's review, however, I gather that so far no attempt has been made to link this conceptual framework carefully to the policymaker's original concern. Indeed, neither in the Sloan-Feldman paper, nor apparently in the literature it reviews, is much thought given to the precise definition of Q in the demand function: Yet therein lies the very heart of the matter.

For example, does variable Q in equation (3) represent output actually *demanded* by the patient on his or her initiative, or does it merely represent output *accepted* and paid for, after consultation? From the viewpoint of analysis this distinction need not always be important—it might not be, for example, if one were interested merely in the question whether the volume of services utilized by patients is responsive to the price they pay per unit of service.[13] The distinction does become important, however, in an analysis of physician-induced demand.

Next, does Q in equation (3) represent "cases treated" or "sets of medical procedures"? This distinction is important because patients may not react in quite the same manner to changes in the prices of particular procedures as they would to changes in the total cost of managing a particular medical condition. For example, parents might willingly accept a pediatrician's recommendation to bring in a child for a third revisit (at a given price per visit) for an upper respiratory condition, but resist an increase in the visit fee from $15 to $20.

Finally, is the standard neoclassical version of equation (3)—one which imples that physicians *cannot* shift the function at all—based on the proposition that the physician does not have much discretion over the composition of medical treatments to begin with? Or, is it assumed by the proponents of this version that the representative physician will, at all times, have fully exploited any available profit potential, so that no further demand-inducement could profitably take place should the physician-population ratio increase? If the latter is the case, does the treatment modality chosen by this profit-maximizing physician possibly include procedures of dubious or zero medical value? And, if the latter were the case, is it a proper use of language to refer to such a situation as one of "no inducement (technically speaking)"?[14]

In short, it would be helpful if the proponents of the standard neoclassical demand function took somewhat greater pains to articulate in more detail the scenarios thought to drive their analytic structure, and preferably to do so in language compatible with the policymaker's perception of the issue. For, what the Parkinsonian school lacks in conceptual rigor, the neoclassical school lacks in plausible detail. Indeed, failure to furnish this detail is really a lack of conceptual rigor as well.

One research strategy falling out of this recommendation is the so-called "tracer analysis" by which one attempts to trace the entire treatment of well-defined tracer conditions in alternative health-care settings.[15] Such analyses can reveal how the composition and the cost of medical treatment responds to differences in physician density, in the financing of health care, and in the organization of health-care delivery. One may even be able to identify differences in the quality of treatments.

Tracer analyses go beyond the comparative advantage of a single discipline. At the very least, they require the involvement of physicians both in design and implementation. They are also expensive. And although tracer analyses are by no means inconsistent with standard economic theory, it may be difficult to fit the analysis neatly into the standard, compact version of that theory and it may not even yield the unequivocal, compact conclusions social scientists like. One suspects, however, that tracer analysis will be one of the more cost-effective approaches to an understanding of the issue of physician-induced demand.

TECHNICAL APPENDIX

A Neoclassical Model of Physician Behavior

Using notation employed by Evans and adopted by Sloan and Feldman, a neoclassical economic model of physician behavior would have the physician maximize an objective function

$$U = U(Y, W), \qquad U_Y > 0, \qquad U_W < 0; \qquad [1]$$

subject to the demand constraint

$$W = R \cdot f(P), \qquad f_P < 0 \qquad [2]$$

and the definition of net income

$$Y = P \cdot W - C(W), \qquad [3]$$

where Y = the physician's net income per period
W = an index of the physician's rate of "output" per period (however defined)
P = the average fee per unit of the output index
R = the population-physician ratio in the physician's market area
C(W) = A cost function representing the *minimum* practice cost (excluding the value of the physician's own time) at alternative output rates (W).

The central assumption distinguishing this model from Evans' supply-inducement model is that the demand function f(P) cannot be influenced by the physician.

Embedded in the model is a production function and a set of input supply functions that need not be articulated for present purposes. Given this compact form of the model, there is only one decision variable—either P or W.

Maximization of [1] with respect to P, and subject to [2] and [3], implies the equilibrium condition

$$\frac{\partial U}{\partial P} = U_Y[PRf_p + Pf(P) - Rf_pC_W] + U_WRf_p = 0 \qquad [4]$$

which can be written more compactly as

$$\frac{\partial U}{\partial P} \equiv U_p(P; R) = 0 \qquad [4']$$

Equation [4] is, of course, identical to Sloan and Feldman's equation [4].

Displacement of equilibrium condition [4'] to a new equilibrium in response to a change, dR, in physician-density implies

$$0 = U_{pp}(P; R)dP + U_{PR}(P; R)dR \qquad [5]$$

or

$$\frac{dP}{dR} = -\frac{U_{PR}(P; R)}{U_{PP}(P; R)} \qquad [6]$$

If net income is maximized at the new equilibrium, then U_{pp} (P; R) must be negative. As Sloan and Feldman argue convincingly, a reasonable assumption is that U_{PR} (P; R) is positive at that point. It follows that impact multiplier dP/dR must be positive. *In other words, according to the neoclassical assumptions, the average fee level (P) decreases as the physician-population ratio (1/R) increases.*

From equation [2], *above, it follows that*

$$\frac{dW}{dR} = f(P) + Rf_P\frac{dP}{dR} \qquad [6']$$

Since f_p is negative and dP/dR is positive, the sign of dW/dR is not unambigously given. *In the purely neoclassical model, then, the physician's rate of output may either increase, decrease, or remain unchanged as the physician-population ratio changes.* The direction of the impact depends crucially on the price-elasticity of the demand for physician services.

The change in equilibrium net income in response to a change in the physician-population ratio is indicated by

$$\frac{dY}{dR} = [P - C_W]\cdot\left[f(P) - Rf_P\frac{dP}{dR}\right] + W\frac{dP}{dR} \qquad [7]$$

For dP/dR>0, this change may be either positive, zero, or negative. Once again, of crucial importance is the price-elasticity of demand.

Finally, since the function of f(P) represents the per capita demand for physician services at fee level P,

$$\frac{df(P)}{dR} = f_P\frac{dP}{dR} \qquad [8]$$

is negative for $f_p <_h 0$ and dP/dR>0. *In other words, in response to an increase in the physician-population ratio, observed per capita utilization is predicted to increase according to the purely neoclassical model.*

In sum, one obtains from the purely neoclassical specification the *impact multipliers:*

$$dP/dR > 0 \qquad dW/dR \gtreqless 0$$

$$df(P)/dR < 0 \qquad dY/dR \gtreqless 0$$

where R, it will be recalled, is the inverse of the physician-population ratio. Empirically, the neoclassical model cannot be distinguished from the inducement model by the response of the physician's workload or income to changes in physician density (unless the precise shape of equations [1] to [3] were known, as they never can be). A negative response of per capita utilization to physician density (1/R) *is* inconsistent with the neoclassical theory, as is a positive response of fees (P) to density.

NOTES

1. See, for example, U.S. Department of Health, Education, and Welfare and Reinhardt (ch.2).

2. If consumers elected to increase their utilization of physician services substantially in response to a decrease in fees—that is, if their demand were highly "price-elastic"—then physician incomes might actually increase as fees decline. Empirical evidence suggests price elasticities much below the level required for this possibility.

3. It should not be taken for granted that the power to prescribe more procedures for a given condition necessarily implies the power to charge more per procedure. In this connection, see section III of this Comment.

4. The model could be operated with a fixed level for P. Sloan and Feldman assume P to be variable in their analysis framework.

5. This assumption need not mean that physicians do not ever have the power to induce demand. It simply implies that every physician will automatically have exploited such power to the fullest under any market condition. That is the core of the neoclassical argument.

6. I am indebted to Victor Fuchs for bringing the point made in this paragraph to my attention.

7. In 1965, the figure stood at DM 72, 995; in 1974, at DM 199,263. The figures exclude income from private patients. In this connection, see G. Wollny.

8. See, for example, *Die Ortskrankenkasse,* a biweekly publication of one of the largest insurance pools.

9. In using the criterion to evaluate alternative investments with differently timed outlays and receipts, one implicitly assumes that all intermediate receipts from a project are reinvested at precisely the internal rate of return from the project. This is a highly unrealistic assumption.

10. In a similar vein, the mere fact that rates of surgery per capita in the United States far exceed those in England and Wales does not indicate that American physicians operate too much. There *may* be physician-induced demand for surgery of dubious merit in the United States, but there may also be too few operations performed in the United Kingdom.

11. I offer these remarks as one who is not at all opposed to the concept of the HMO. One problem in comparing HMO's with the fee-for-service mode is that one rarely, if ever, can do so under conditions of a controlled experiment. Instead, the observed utilization records are left behind by patients and physicians who have deliberately chosen one or the other mode. An anlysis based on such data may be subject to serious preselection bias, or bias that is difficult to detect.

12. Since this paper was part of a great application, I am not at liberty to disclose its author. Suffice it to say that this is not an isolated case. Many similar illustrations could easily be culled from the published literature in economics.

13. In an environment in which patients pay for all or a substantial part of physician services they receive and in which physicians are concerned about the impact of their treatment on the patient's fiscal position, the volume of services utilized (demanded and/or accepted) by patients may respond inversely to price even if the physician dominates the decisionmaking.

14. One strictly neoclassical acquaintance of mine, for example, recently described to me the following situation as one of no-inducement: "In an environment in which patients enjoy first-dollar health insurance coverage and physicians are reimbursed on a fixed fee schedule, a technological change reduces the cost of performing a particular test hitherto not performed by physicians because the corresponding marginal revenue (fee) was below marginal cost. The patient willingly accepts the test although, unbeknownst to him/her, the test is not at all

medically indicated, a fact known to the profit-maximizing physician. This is not a case of demand-inducement because the demand curve has not shifted; marginal cost simply moved below an unchanged marginal revenue." I suspect that the representative policymakers would be flabbergasted by this characterization of the inducement issue, and the attendant application of the English language.

15. There have been a number of such studies, and I am informed that the Rand Corporation will conduct such analyses as part of its Health Insurance study. It is to be hoped, however, that additional research of this sort will be funded in the years ahead.

REFERENCES

C. G. Archibald, "The Quantitative Content of Maximizing Models," *J. Polit. Econ.* Feb. 1965, 27-36.

A. P. Contandriopolous "Change l'Organisation du Systeme de Sante Plutot que Limiter le Nombre de Medecins: Un Commentaire de l'Article d'Evans," *Canadian Public Policy Analyse de Politiques,* Spring, 1976, 161-168.

R. G. Evans, "Supplier-Induced Demand: Some Empirical Evidence and Implications," in M. Perlman (ed.), *The Economics of Health and Medical Care,* London 1974.

R. Nelson, *The Moon and the Ghetto,* New York 1977.

M. V. Pauly, "Is Medical Care Different?", paper presented at the Federal Trade Commission Conference "Competition in the Health Care Sector: Past, Present and Future," Washington, D.C., June 1-2, 1977.

U. E. Reinhardt, *Physician Productivity and the Demand for Health Manpower,* Cambridge, Mass., 1975.

T. Siebeck, "Zur Kostenentiwicklung der Krankenversicherung," *Die Ortskrankenkasse,* Apr. 1976, 276.

F. Sloan, "Physician-Fee Inflation: Evidence from the 1960's," in R. Rosett (ed.), *The Role of Health Insurance in the Health Services Sector,* New York 1976, 321-354.

——— and B. Steinwald, "Determinants of Physicians' Fees," *J. Bus.,* Oct. 1974, 493-511.

G. Wollny, "Arzthonorar und Bruttosozialproduct," *Die Ortskrankenkasse,* Oct. 1975, 718.

Government of Quebec, "Regie de l'assurance-maladie du Quebec," *1974 Annual Statistics,* Table 1, 165.

U.S. Department of Health, Education, and Welfare, Bureau of Health Resources Development, *The Supply of Health Manpower: 1970 Profiles and Projections for 1990,* Washington, D.C., 1974.

Competition Among Hospitals

*David S. Salkever**
Associate Professor of Health Services, School of Hygiene and Public Health,
The Johns Hopkins University

My remarks today will focus on two major issues. First, I shall review the economic literature on the present degree of competition in the hospital sector as indicated by market structure and supplier conduct within this sector. Particular emphasis will be placed on the implications of competitive behavior for the level of hospital costs. Second, I shall comment on the prospects for increasing the degree of competition among hospitals. It will be argued that changes in financing arrangements are the most effective means of increasing price competition and that altering other structural aspects of the hospital services market will have only modest effects. Problems posed by increases in price competition will also be noted.

Both actual competition among existing hospitals and potential competition from new hospitals entering the market will be considered. We should, however, bear in mind that non-hospital providers—such as HMO's and ambulatory surgical facilities—also may exert competitive pressures on hospitals. Since this is being considered by other speakers at this conference, it will be ignored here.

Basic economic theory suggests that market structure can usefully be defined (in part) in terms of the numbers of sellers and buyers engaging in arm's-length transactions. A competitive market is characterized by many sellers and many buyers; a monopolistic market, by one seller and many buyers; a monopsonistic market, by many sellers and one buyer; and so on. But the application of this approach to the market for hospital services is complicated by the recognition that transactions typically involve more than two parties. While the patient is in a legal sense the buyer of hospital services, his private or public insurance generally pays most of the bill. And the patient's decision to purchase services is clearly influenced by the recommendations of his physicians. Moreover, the fact that physician and hospital services are purchased jointly leads us to consider the physician's role on the sellers' side of the market as well.

These unusual institutional features of the market for hospital services have important implications for our discussion of market structure. For example, the functions of insurers need not be strictly limited to the

---

* Comments on an earlier draft by Phillip D. Bonnet, M.D., are gratefully acknowledged.

collection and disbursement of funds. If they enter into direct contractual relationships with hospitals and negotiate with them over the cost and nature of services to be provided to their policyholders, their influence on the buyers' side of the market cannot be entirely disregarded. The same can be said for the physician whose own preferences may influence the recommendations he makes to his patients. Furthermore, the joint purchase of hospital services and physician services implies that the structure of the market for physicians' services may influence the degree and nature of inter-hospital competition. For these reasons, physicians and insurers will figure prominently in this discussion.

THE STRUCTURE OF THE MARKET FOR HOSPITAL SERVICES

A number of different economic models have been constructed to explain the behavior of hospitals. These models vary considerably in their postulated objectives for the hospital and in the roles which they assign to the medical staff and hospital administrators in the decisionmaking process. According to some, the preferences of the hospital are defined in terms of the quantity and quality of its output. Others view the maximization of staff physicians' incomes as the hospital's primary objective.[1] However, virtually all these models share the presumption that the structure of the market for hospital services deviates from the standard of perfect competition and hence that the hospital is a price-setter rather than a price-taker. The bases for this presumption will be examined in the description of hospital market structure offered here.

Entry Barriers

There is general agreement in the literature on hospital economics that high entry barriers are an important limitation on competitive market pressures. These entry barriers include legal requirements for licensure, particularly the requirement in most States that certificate-of-need approval be granted by the relevant planning agency. Even in those States which have not yet passed certificate-of-need laws, disapproval by areawide or State planning agencies may still obstruct potential entrants into the market by making it difficult to obtain public (State or Federal) construction subsidies or donor capital. Such disapproval may also preclude participation in Blue Cross contracts and Federal reimbursement for capital costs under Medicaid and Medicare. Accreditation standards, administered by the Joint Commission on Accreditation of Hospitals and by State agencies, are also important since they determine eligiblity for participation in governmental insurance programs. Concerted opposition from established physicians and hospitals can also block entry by discouraging support from local private or public capital sources and by deterring local physicians from staff participation. I suspect that vigorous and open opposition from local providers has been encouraged by governmental reluctance or inability to apply antitrust statutes in this area.

There is reason to believe that entry barriers are particularly high for proprietary facilities. Non-profit hospitals are keenly aware of the danger that proprietaries will engage in price competition and lure away their most profitable patients. (This is the well-known cream-skimming argument.) Thus, they are especially likely to oppose vigorously entry of proprietaries into their market area. Recent descriptive studies (Lewin and Associates, Inc., Joel May, 1974a) also indicate that State and areawide planning agency personnel tend to be biased against for-profit providers and hence it seems probable that these providers are at a disadvantage in attempting to obtain agency approval for new facilities. This is supported by Joel May's (1967) statistical comparisons of investment and market share trends for proprietaries in areas with and without areawide planning which revealed a lesser growth of proprietaries in the presence of planning.[2] In addition, several States have laws which prohibit the ownership of for-profit hospitals by public corporations. Since recent national trends have indicated a shift toward corporate ownership and away from sole proprietors or partnerships (Bruce Steinwald and Duncan Neuhauser), one may speculate that the negative effects of these legal prohibitions on entry and investment have been considerable.

Market Concentration and Economies of Scale

Another aspect of markets for hospital services which departs from the competitive model is the small number of hospitals typically found within a single market area. Data reported by the American Medical Association (1975) for the 288 SMSA's and "potential" SMSA's with less than 2 million inhabitants in 1974 indicate that the mean number of non-Federal, short-term, general and other special hospitals per area was 8.04. Furthermore, in each of 84 of these areas, fewer than 4 such hospitals were reported. Admittedly, these figures are imperfect indicators of market concentration since, as I noted at the outset, competition from non-hospital providers can also be important. Moreover, the market for hospital services may extend beyond the boundaries of an SMSA so that the degree of concentration is overstated by these data. But in spite of these qualifications, I think it is clear that the hospital markets in these areas are highly concentrated.[3] This is probably even more true of non-metropolitan areas but somewhat less true of the 12 SMSA's with over 2 million population in 1974 for which the mean number of hospitals was 8.06.

Several different factors may explain this oligopolistic market structure. For example, it might be the result of tight restrictions on entry. More frequently, however, it is viewed as the result of economies of scale. The conventional wisdom is that hospitals with much fewer than, say, 150 beds cannot economically provide a wide range of services because the necessary special services and equipment will be underutilized. Statistical cost and production function studies tend to support this conclusion although contrary results are not uncommon and inadequacies in the data and techniques employed in these studies have often been noted.[4] Of course, if economies of scale are due primarily to indivisibilities in specialized services, it might seem that very small hospitals could contract for access to these services at other institutions and that this arrangement would reduce the degree of seller concentration in the market. However, there are several obstacles to this mode of operation, including accreditation standards which require that certain services and specialized personnel be present in a hospital, the additional risk to patients in emergency situations if specialized services are not present and immediately available, and the inconvenience to attending physicians if their patients must frequently be transferred to other facilities (at which they may not have staff privileges) to obtain these services.

Other Aspects of Market Structure

As I have already noted, the structure of the hospital service market is not fully described by crude seller concentration measures (numbers of hospitals, concentration ratios) because of this market's peculiar institutional features. Other aspects of the market that have received attention in the economic literature include medical staff arrangement, insurance, and restrictions on the flow of information.

In the context of the present discussion, the most significant point to be made about medical staff arrangements is that private physicians tend to confine their active staff participation to a very small number of hospitals (E. D. Rosenfeld). This seems efficient from the viewpoint of the individual physician since his scheduling problems and travel time involved in providing in-hospital services are minimized when all his patients are concentrated in one or two hospitals. The administration of the hospital may also prefer this arrangement for a variety of reasons. For instance, it may foster a physician's commitment to his responsibilities as a staff member. It ensures that physicians practicing in the hospital are familiar with its standard operating procedures. It also may diminish competition from other hospitals since staff physicians have limited opportunities to take their business elsewhere. Indeed, Milton Roemer and J. W. Friedman's case studies of medical staff organization revealed that, as a condition for active staff membership, hospitals may even require the staff physicians send them a substantial portion of their hospitalized patients.

The implication of this arrangement for the patient's scope of choice is clear. If the patient has already selected his physician, his options, in terms of the hospital at which he could receive care are at best limited to two or three institutions. Of course, if the market for physicians' services is competitive and the patient has many options in terms of choosing his physician, medical staff arrangements will not restrict his choice of hospital. However, analyses of the structure of the physicians' services market by Sloan and Feldman (1977) and by Newhouse and Sloan (1972) point to the conclusion that this market is non-competitive. The implication for our analysis of the hospital services market is that seller concentration measures based on hospital data typically understate the degree of concentration when medical staff arrangements conform to the situation I have described.

A similar conclusion is reached in discussions on the effect of insurance and restricted information flows on consumer behavior. It is often pointed out that roughly 90 percent of hospital costs are paid for by third parties (Martin Feldstein and Amy Taylor). Roughly three-fourths of these third-party payments are made under public and private service benefit plans in which consumer cost-sharing at the margin is virtually eliminated, while the private indemnity plans, which account for the remaining one-fourth of payments, typically involve limited coinsurance provisions.[5] For the great majority of consumers, little is to be gained by shopping around to find the hospital which provides the desired quality of service at the lowest price. Furthermore, it is difficult if not impossible to obtain the relevant information by shopping around. The multitude of separate fees for specific services makes the task of comparing prices complex. And much information relating to important dimensions of quality, such as expected outcome, is simply unavailable. In short, because of present insurance arrangements and the inaccessibility of pertinent information, consumer search activities are minimal (H. E. Frech and Paul Ginsburg). The result is that, even if there are so many hospitals in a community, each hospital will have some monopoly power since its potential customers would generally be ignorant of opportunities to purchase comparable care at a lower cost elsewhere.

Thus far, I have considered the options facing the individual patient and concluded that his choices among sellers will be restricted to one or two hospitals. But is it not possible that all hospitals in a community compete indirectly with one another for patients by seeking to attract physicians to their medical staff? My impression is that such competiton does indeed occur, particularly for physicians in specialities that are much in demand. However, it is also clear that shifting of physicians among hospitals can be limited under closed staffing arrangements. If a hospital's capacity is being utilized intensively, its medical staff would probably be reluctant to grant privileges to physicians seeking to migrate from other hospitals. Of course, its staff may be more accommodating in the long run if expansion of capacity is possible.

CONDUCT AND PERFORMANCE

What are the implications of the structure of the hospital services market for conduct and performance, and particularly for the level of hospital costs? A definitive answer to this question is not possible because the available evidence is quite limited. But a brief review of this evidence and of some plausible hypotheses about the relationship of market structure and conduct may at least point to some tentative conclusions.

Analyses of the impact of entry restrictions have been primarily concerned with effects on costs and prices. Sol Shalit has argued that entry restriction raises the price of medical and surgical services by enabling physicians to control the supply of medical services through constraints on available hospital resources. In support of his hypothesis, Shalit presents cross-sectional regression analyses in which the relationship between an index of surgical procedure prices and the ratio of hospital beds to doctors (which he presumed to vary inversely with the degree of entry control) is significantly negative. Similarly, the analysis of certificate-of-need programs by David Salkever and Thomas Bice (forthcoming) suggests that legal restriction of entry and investment reduces the volume of hospital services while increasing their average unit cost. May's (1973) analysis of the impact of planning agencies in the period prior to the enactment of certificate-of-need laws points to the same conclusions although his results are somewhat equivocal.

The idea that entry by proprietaries has been particularly restricted may also have implications for market performance. If Herbert Klarman (p. 113) and Steinwald and Neuhauser are correct in their thesis that investment in proprietaries responds more quickly to growing demand in communities lacking adequate hospital facilities, then entry barriers will presumably retard this market response. Effects on costs and prices may also occur if proprietaries are more likely to compete on the basis of prices rather than quality and if proprietaries are more efficient producers than voluntaries. However, it should be noted that the evidence supporting these conjectures is not very substantial.[6]

The implications of seller concentration for conduct and performance are not obvious. Standard theory suggests, of course, that prices should be higher in highly concentrated markets. With a small number of sellers, informal arrangements to prevent price competition become feasible. These arrangements are also encouraged by the fact that the risk of antitrust sanctions is minimal or non-existent. A further obstacle to price competition is the extensiveness of third-party coverage, which renders patients relatively insensitive to inter-hospital price differentials. On the other hand, non-price competition among hospitals may be vigorous even within concentrated markets. The notion has frequently been advanced that hospitals compete with one another for patients by offering highly sophisticated equipment and services to attract business from staff physicians.[7] Large urban hospitals that have many salaried staff physicians and that serve populations with little access to private practitioners may also compete for inpatients by expanding their emergency services, walk-in clinics, or other ambulatory care facilities. Obviously, this non-price competition has the potential for increasing costs and necessitating higher charges to cover these costs. The implications for service quality are less clear. For example, the addition of highly sophisticated equipment and services, which are rarely or inappropriately used could actually decrease quality.

However, one might plausibly argue that in extremely concentrated markets, served by only one or two hospitals, pressures for higher costs and prices are not as great because of the absence of non-price competition. The conclusion reached by E. M. Kaitz in his interview study of a small sample of Massachusetts hospitals is consistent with this view. He notes that:

> . . . the position of the noncompeting rural-hospital board vis-a-vis the physician is stronger. The rural physician cannot threaten the hospital with a decrease in its patient load, since he has no other hospital in which to place his patients. He either accepts what the hospital has to offer, or he treats his patient on an ambulatory basis (or at home). Consequently, the community is in a strong position vis-a-vis the physician and can more effectively control the flow of resources into the hospital (p. 80).

Admittedly, this conclusion may be less applicable to the urban teaching hospital in a monopolistic or duopolistic market if the hospital's board and administration share the staff physicians' desires for high-technology medicine. But Kaitz's observations at least suggest the possibility that the relationship between seller concentration and price is non-monotonic, with prices in moderately concentrated markets being higher than those in highly concentrated markets.

Econometric evidence on the relationship between costs, prices, and market structure is very sparse and inconclusive. In the most thorough study of this question, Carolyn Watts employed three different market structure variables: the number of hospitals within a county, the ratio of physicians to hospital beds (which was intended to measure hospital market power vis-a-vis staff physicians), and the ratio of physicans to population (used as a measure of competition in the physicians' services market). She reports positive but not highly significant effects for all three variables on revenue per day and revenue per admission. An analysis of State data on total (physician plus hospital) price per admission by Mark Pauly (n.d.) used the number of hospitals as a measure of competition and found no significant effect. Other measures of market power that have been used by Karen Davis (1972, 1974) in her work with individual hospital data are the hospital's percentage share of all beds in its county, the number of hospitals per square mile in the county, and the ratio of the hospital's active staff physicians to its bed complement. The latter variable was positively and significantly related to the level of average unit costs per admission and per day. The first two variables were used in a mark-up model of pricing but did not show that greater market power increased prices relative to costs.

The recent study of registered nurse staffing in individual hospitals by Sloan and Richard Elnicki (n.d.) is also relevant since nursing costs are an important component of total costs. In particular, it is noteworthy that the hospital's percentage share of all beds in its county was not significantly related to the level of RN employment in their analysis. Finally, a number of studies[8] have examined the possibility that market concentration also results in a monopsonistic situation in the labor market for nurses and other highly trained hospital workers. Results generally indicate that greater concentration has a small but significant negative impact on wages.

REGULATORY EFFECTS ON COMPETITION

We are all aware that the economic behavior of hospitals is currently constrained by a variety of regulatory mechanisms such as licensure and accreditation requirements, certificate-of-need, surveillance by Professional Standards Review Organizations (PSRO's), and rate or revenue regulation. In concluding this review of current competition in the hospital services market, let us briefly take note of the implications of regulation for competitive behavior.

The main effect of licensure or accreditation standards is to preclude the offering of less expensive (and perhaps lower quality) styles of care. Hence, these devices tend to obstruct price competition from lower-cost providers. It has been noted (Clark Havighurst and James Blumstein) that PSRO reviews may have a similar result, although they can also restrict more expensive styles of care by finding the provision of certain services to be unnecessary.

Rate regulation clearly has the potential for restricting price competition (as in other industries), although with the current emphasis on cost containment most regulators would probably be happy to approve a hospital's request for reductions in its rates. However, the method of regulation and its incentive effects are also important. If rates are set restrictively, and volume adjustments make it impossible to circumvent financial pressures by generating additional utilization, acquisition of high-cost equipment and services for competitive purposes will be curtailed. But this effect will be offset somewhat if rates are set by a formula based on previous years' costs.[9]

Controls on capital expenditures have the potential for restricting some forms of non-price competition but there is little evidence that this has occurred in practice. Indeed, an indirect result of these controls may have been to encourage investment in more sophisticated services (Salkever and Bice, 1976).

INCREASING COMPETITION IN THE HOSPITAL SERVICES MARKET

The major conclusion which emerges from the foregoing description of the hospital services market is that competition among hospitals is based primarily upon the availability and sophistication of services and facilities rather than price. This lack of price competition is most frequently explained by the current structure of insurance arrangements. Virtually complete coverage makes consumers insensitive to price considerations while third parties have made only limited efforts to control the prices paid by their enrollees. Clearly, these insurance arrangements must be modified if price competition is to be encouraged.[10]

Because hospital services and physician services are purchased jointly, competition in the physicians' services market influences the economic behavior of hospitals. But for the reasons just stated, changes in insurance arrangements may also increase price competition among physicians. Even under current staffing arrangements which somewhat restrict physicians' choice of hospitals, this would probably result in greater pressures for hospitals to hold down costs and prices.

While a change in financing arrangements is probably the most powerful way to influence competitive behavior, other structural changes may have at least marginal effects. For example, ending restrictions on proprietaries and increases in the availability of information on costs may generate slightly more price competition. Open-staffing arrangements for use of highly specialized equipment could perhaps diminish competitive pressures for every hospital to offer a full range of services (Gerald Rosenthal), although the inconvenience to the physician of hospitalizing his patients at many different institutions argues against this (Rosenfeld).

Finally, we should also take note of the difficulties involved in moving to a hospital system with greater price competition. The creation of more competitive markets may be hindered by several factors. The present high degree of seller concentration in many local markets may be larely due to economies of scale and thus not easily diminished. Also, we have already noted the possibility that minimum quality regulation can impede competition. Assuming that such regulation is desirable for protecting the public and should be maintained, the political problem of preventing misuse of this regulatory instrument to further providers' interests is formidable. The creation of more competitive markets further implies a need to develop new financing mechanisms for various public goods and "community services," such as stand-by capability for emergency care, treatment of individuals not covered by private or public insurance who are unable to pay their hospital bills, and clinical training of health professionals. The present mode of financing—through cross-subsidization and prices in excess of costs for more "profitable" services—will be difficult to maintain in the presence of greater price competition. In summary, the transition to a more competitive market for hospital services is not a simple matter. It involves a series of major institutional changes whose feasibility and desirability must be carefully examined.

NOTES

1. For a review and comparison of these models see Philip Jacobs (1974) and Carolyn Watts (1976).

2. However, it should be noted that May's (1974b) subsequent analysis of changes in bed supplies and market shares in planned and unplanned areas did not strongly confirm this result.

3. It is also reasonable to expect that the use of a more sophisticated and sensitive measure of seller concentration, such as the Herfindahl index, would not alter this conclusion.

4. Critiques of the methods employed in these cost studies may be found in Mark Pauly (1974) and in Sylvester Berki (1972, chapters 3 and 5).

5. Note that the distribution of payment by source referred to here is for short-term hospital care. Detailed breakdowns of third-party payments for short-term hospital care by third party are not available. My rough estimate of three-fourths for service benefits (Medicare, Medicaid, and Blue Cross-Blue Shield) and one-fourth for commercial plans is based on benefit payment statistics given in Marjorie Mueller and Paula Piro and Mueller and R. H. Gibson. I have not included direct Federal, State, or local government expenditures for services in governmentally-operated hospitals.

6. C. Bays's cost and production function estimates indicate that chain-operated proprietaries are more efficient than non-profit hospitals but that other proprietaries are not. Behavioral differences suggestive of greater efficiency are also reported in Kenneth Clarkson (1972). Other cost function studies (Will Manning, Ralph Berry) do not find significantly lower costs for the proprietary ownership form per se (although Manning's results indicate that smaller medical staff size in proprietaries results in greater efficiency). Of course, because of difficulties in controlling for inter-hospital differences in output mix and quality, these statistical comparisons must be treated with caution.

7. See, for example, M. L. Lee, May (1971), and David Mechanic.

8. Davis (1973); Richard Hurd, Charles Link and John Landon (1975 and 1976); and Sloan and Elnicki (1976).

9. See William Dowling for a systematic review of incentive effects under various prospective reimbursement mechanisms.

10. For a detailed discussion of possible changes in insurance arrangements, see Havighurst.

REFERENCES

C. Bays, "Cost and Efficiency Comparisons of For-profit and Non-profit Hospitals," unpublished paper, University of Illinois at Chicago Circle, (n.d.).

S. Berki, *Hospital Economics,* Lexington, Mass. 1972.

R. Berry, "Cost and Efficiency in the Production of Hospital Services," *Milbank Memorial Fund Quart./Health and Society,* Summer 1974, 291-313.

K. W. Clarkson, "Some Implications of Property Rights in Hospital Management," *J. Law Econ.,* Oct. 1972, 363-384.

K. Davis, "An Empirical Investigation of Alternative Models of the Hospital Industry," paper presented at the American Economic Association Meeting, Toronto, Dec. 30, 1972.

———, "Theories of Hospital Inflation: Some Empirical Evidence," *J. Human Resources,* Spring 1973, 181-201.

———. "The Role of Technology, Demand and Labor Markets in the Determination of Hospital Costs," in M. Perlman (ed.) *The Economics of Health and Medical Care,* New York 1974.

W. Dowling, "Prospective Reimbursement of Hospitals," *Inquiry,* Sept. 1974, 163-180.

M. Feldstein and A. Taylor, "The Rapid Rise of Hospital Costs," Harvard Institute for Economic Research Discussion Paper No. 531, 1977.

H. E. Frech and P. B. Ginsburg, "Imposed Health Insurance in Monopolistic Markets: A Theoretical Analysis," *Economic Inquiry,* March 1975, 55-70.

C. C. Havighurst, "Controlling Health Care Costs: Strengthening the Private Sector's Hand," *J. Health Policy, Politics, Law,* Winter 1977, 471-498.

———, and J. F. Blumstein, "Coping With Quality/Cost Tradeoffs in Medical Care: The Role of PSRO's," *Northwestern Univ. Law Rev.,* Mar.-Apr. 1975, 6-58.

R. W. Hurd, "Equilibrium Vacancies in a Labor Market Dominated by Nonprofit Firms: The 'Shortage' of Nurses," *Rev. Econ. Stat.,* May 1973, 234-240.

P. Jacobs, "A Survey of Economic Models of Hospitals," *Inquiry,* June 1974, 83-97.

E. M. Kaitz, *Pricing Policy and Cost Behavior in the Hospital Industry,* New York 1968.

H. E. Klarman, *The Economics of Health,* New York 1965.

J. Landon and C. Link, "Monopsony and Union Power in the Market for Nurses," *Southern Econ. J.,* April 1975, 649-659.

———, "Market Structure, Nonpecuniary Factors, and Professional Salaries: Registered Nurses," *J. Econ. Bus.,* Winter 1976, 151-155.

M. L. Lee, "A Conspicuous Production Theory of Hospital Behavior," *Southern Econ. J.,* July 1971, 48-58.

W. Manning, "Comparative Efficiency in Short-Term General Hospitals," Studies in Industry Economics, No. 30, Department of Economics, Stanford University, 1973.

J. J. May, *Health Planning—Its Past and Potential,* Chicago 1967.

———, "Economic Variables in Hospital Mergers," in D. B. Starthweather (ed.), *Analysis of Hospital Mergers: Conference Proceedings,* Springfield VA. 1971.

———, "The Impact of Health Planning," unpublished paper, Center for Health Administration Studies, University of Chicago, 1973.

———, (1974a), "The Planning and Licensing Agencies" in C. C. Havighurst (ed.), *Regulating Health Facilities Construction,* Washington, D.C., 1974.

———, (1974b), "The Impact of Regulation on the Hospital Industry," unpublished paper, Center for Health Administration Studies, University of Chicago, 1974.

D. Mechanic, Commentary on the papers, in C. C. Havighurst (ed.), *Regulating Health Facilities Construction,* Washington, D.C., 1974.

M. S. Mueller and R. M. Gibson, "National Health Expenditures, Calendar Year 1974" Office of Research Statistics, Social Security Administration, U.S. Dept. of Health, Education, and Welfare, Research and Statistics Note No. 5, 1975.

——— and P. A. Piro, "Private Health Insurance in 1974: A Review of Coverage, Enrollment, and Financial Experience," *Soc. Sec. Bull.* Mar. 1976, 3-30.

J. Newhouse and F. Sloan, "Physician Pricing: Monopolistic or Competitive: Reply," *Southern Econ. J.,* April 1972, 557-580.

M. Pauly, "The Behavior of Nonprofit Hospital Monopolies: Alternative Models of the Hospital," in C. C. Havighurst (ed.) *Regulating Health Facilities Construction,* Washington, D.C., 1974.

———, "Doctors, Hospitals, and the Market for Hospital Care: A Good Bit of Theory and a Few Empirical Results," unpublished paper, Northwestern University, (n.d.).

M. I. Roemer and J. W. Friedman, *Doctors in Hospitals: Medical Staff Organization and Hospital Performance,* Baltimore 1971.

E. D. Rosenfeld, "Problems of Multiple Staff Appointments," in *Collected Papers from the Hospital Medical Staff Conference, October 2-6, 1967,* University of Colorado School of Medicine, Denver 1967.

G. Rosenthal, "The Operating Structure of the Medical Care System—an Overview," in U.S. Congress, Joint Economic Committee, *Federal Programs for the Development of Human Resources,* Washington, D.C., 1968.

D. S. Salkever and T. W. Bice, "The Impact of Certificate-of-Need Controls on Hospital Investment," *Milbank Memorial Fund Quart./Health and Society,* Spring 1976, 185-214.

———, "Certificate-of-Need Legislation and Hospital Costs," in M. Zubkoff, I. Raskin, and R. Hanft (eds.), *Hospital Cost Containment: Selected Notes for Future Policy,* New York, forthcoming.

S. S. Shalit, "Barriers to Entry in the American Hospital Industry," unpublished Ph.D. dissertation, University of Chicago, 1970.

F. Sloan and R. Elnicki, "Determinants of Professional Nurses' Wages," paper presented at the Atlantic Economic Association Meetings, Washington, D.C., 1976.

———, "Professional Nurse Staffing in Hospitals," in F. Sloan, *Equalizing Access to Nursing Services: The Geographic Dimension,* Final Report on USDHEW Contract No. 1-NU-24264 (n.d.).

F. Sloan and R. Feldman, "Competition Among Physicians," paper presented at The Federal Trade Commission Conference "Competition in the Health Care Sector: Past, Present, and Future," Washington, D.C., June 1-2, 1977.

A. M. Spence, "Product Differentiation and Welfare," *Amer. Econ. Rev.,* May 1976, 407-414.

B. Steinwald and D. Neuhauser, "The Role of The Proprietary Hospital," *Law and Contemporary Problems,* Autumn 1970, 817-838.

C. A. Watts, "A Managerial Discretion Model for Hospitals," unpublished Ph.D. dissertation, Johns Hopkins University, 1976.

American Medical Association, *Physician Distribution and Medical Licensure in the United States,* Chicago 1975.

Lewin and Associates, Inc., *Evaluation of the Efficiency and Effectiveness of the Section 1122 Review Process,* Washington, D.C., 1975.

Comment

John Rafferty
Senior Research Manager, Division of Intramural Research, National Center for Health Services Research, U.S. Department of Health, Education, and Welfare

Two tasks are identified as the objectives to be achieved by this paper. The first is to review the economic literature pertaining to competition in the hospital industry, a task which Dr. David Salkever very competently carries out. The second is to comment on the prospects for increasing the degree of competition in the hospital industry, a task which is more difficult, and which therefore warrants further discussion below.

In addition to these specified tasks, another purpose also exists. In fact, this objective underlies all of the papers commissioned for this Conference. Although it was not explicitly expressed, the Federal Trade Commission is clearly interested in whether or not it should be intervening in the health care industry. Its intent, should it intervene, would be to enhance competition, and the papers presented here are meant to provide information bearing on that issue. This is a broader issue than those which the author specifies as his tasks, but it is an important one to consider if his contribution is to be appreciated: Unless this general policy interest on the part of the FTC is kept prominently in the reader's mind, much of the importance of Dr. Salkever's message is easily missed.

Specifically, throughout the paper the author points out questions that policymakers need to have anwered, and he is repeatedly forced to state that limitations in existing research place the definitive answers out of reach. This does not have an impressive ring; if it rings pleasantly at all, it is only in some other researcher's ear. But the importance of these observations by the author—here, in the crucial context of potential actions by Government—should not be underestimated. To state with authority what should be known, and to show that at present it cannot be known is, especially in the context of policymaking, a most valuable contribution. The fact that a survey of the research produces few clear answers is disappointing, but this knowledge—that such is the state of the art—could not be more important to the principal audience for this paper.

In addition to this, of course, the paper offers a number of specific observations about the nature of hospital markets that are interesting and significant in and of themselves.

The major conclusion reached in this paper is that competition among hospitals does in fact exist, but that it is not competition in the usual sense. That is, hospitals do not appear to compete on the traditional basis of price, but they compete on the basis of availability and sophistication of facilities and service. The evidence for these conclusions is more or less circumstantial, but the conclusions seem to be incontrovertible.

From the perspective of FTC policy, the reason for this limited degree of price competition in hospital markets is of special interest. As Dr. Salkever indicates, the peculiarity of hospital markets is the involvement, in each transaction, of more than two parties: in addition to the patient there is the hospital, the physician, and usually an insurer as well. And, of this triumvirate, we are told, it is the current structure of insurance arrangements, in particular, that explains the absence of price competition. Thus, it is these financial arrangements which provide the logical target for any FTC efforts at increasing competition by price.

The paper therefore draws attention to an interesting paradox involving the competitive character of the hospital industry. As mentioned above, hospitals do appear to compete, but they do so primarily on the basis of investments in capital stock—sophisticated facilities—rather than on the basis of price. As explained in the text, the nature of this activity involves competition among hospitals for medical staff. Moreover, the degree of competition is inversely related to the degree of market concentration. However, while in casual parlance enhanced competition is usually associated with lower prices and cost, the result of this kind of competition among hospitals is just the reverse. That is, the deeper the competitive activity, the greater the incentive to adopt sophisticated technology, which is generally understood to be a major source of rising hospital costs.

Financial factors involving health insurance arrangements are thus identified as the primary target for FTC policy, if intervention is to occur: Insurance arrangements must be changed if competition is to be enhanced. This conclusion is important. Even if the general notion is itself hardly novel, the degree of emphasis it commands as a result of Dr. Salkever's paper should be of considerable interest in a number of quarters. But the conclusion does lead, directly and immediately, to other questions which remain unanswered, and it is these gaps that suggest limitations in the paper.

In particular, we begin with the very broad question of how to enhance competition, and we are competently led to the relatively specific conclusion that changes in financial arrangements provide the key, but the potential nature or range of these changes is not dealt with at all. It should be stressed—immediately—that this limitation is inherent in the Conference structure, since insurance/financing topics were reserved for other sessions. This is unfortunate, in a sense, because Dr. Salkever's policy conclusion, since it is so narrowly focused, would warrant further discussion within the same analytical context in which it was derived. This, unfortunately, is not the case here.

A second limitation deserves at least brief mention. One problem that exists implicitly in any discussion of competition and pricing in the hospital sector is the dual problem of measuring output and the quality of care. Any FTC activities aimed at affecting price competition will at some point have to deal with this problem, and perhaps painfully—especially the problem of differences in quality. These are additional matters on which sufficient research has not been done, but the inherent difficulties and dangers of price-oriented policies are significant and real; policymakers should be cautioned, so as to be prepared to recognize these realities.

Dr. Salkever's paper deals directly with the question of how competition among hospitals might be stimulated, and as a byproduct he very explicitly indicates the kinds of difficulties such policies would face. This provides at least a suggestion of some social costs that might be involved. Another question, one that is related to that, is the question of what it would be worth: what social benefits would really be likely to result? This question may not readily arise among economists, among whom the benefits of competition—at least in some settings—are well appreciated, but the question should not be overlooked by the FTC.

One result of this paper—as is true of many other papers presented along with it—is to suggest that perhaps more research should be conducted before decisions on policy initiatives take place. This is probably true. One may hope, however, that further initiatives in health services research that are undertaken under FTC sponsorship will occur in a climate of continued open interaction and coordination with other Federal programs which are already involved in research in this field.

Competition Among Health Insurers

H. E. Frech III
Associate Professor of Economics, University of California, Santa Barbara
And
Paul B. Ginsburg
Associate Professor of Policy Sciences, and Director,
Center for the Study of Health Policy, Duke University

An overwhelming proportion of families in the United States have insurance to protect them from some of the financial implications of ill health. For the under-65, non-poor population, virtually all of this insurance is purchased from one of two types of private companies. Blue Cross and Blue Shield plans, organized by hospitals and physicians, respectively, and controlled by these providers, are legally non-profit public service firms. Their only business is the financing of health services. "Commercial" insurers are organized on either a for-profit (stock) or nonprofit (mutual) basis, and often sell other types of insurance as well as health insurance. Commercial insurers are controlled either by stockholders or (nominally) by policyholders rather than by medical providers or public representatives.

Blue Cross and Blue Shield plans have important cost advantages over their commercial competitors as a result of various tax exemptions and different regulatory treatment. On the basis of simple economic theory, one would expect that commercial insurers would not be able to compete with Blue plans, and ultimately would leave the health insurance business. However, this has not occurred. An explanation of the persistence of commercial insurers is essential to an understanding of competition among health insurers and is the stimulus for this paper. We will argue that Blue plans "spend" their potential cost advantages on inducing the purchase of more complete insurance (less co-payment) and on administrative slack and inefficiency.

The paper brings together the results of previous empirical research by the authors and others, and new results from ongoing research by the authors. First, we discuss in more detail the structure of the health insurance market, the tax and regulatory advantages of Blue plans, and the policy relevance of completeness of insurance. Then we review survey data to show that Blue plans have a preference for selling relatively complete insurance. Next, we develop a model of Blue Cross-Blue Shield administrative costs and market share and estimate it with data on Blue plans. Then, in a separate analysis the effect of Blue Cross market power on hospital prices (including both the effect of expanding insurance and the possible cost control benefits of a powerful Blue Cross plan) is explored. Following that, we examine the extent to which State regulatory advantages for domestic over foreign commercial insurers affect market shares in this segment of the market and shed some light on our assumption that the commercial insurers are essentially competitive. Lastly, implications for antitrust policy, national health insurance, and useful future research are discussed.

INDUSTRY STRUCTURE AND ENVIRONMENT

A Description of the Firms

American health insurance is characterized by two major types of firms. First are the commercial health insurers, both profit-seeking and mutual, who make up about one-half of the private insurance market. The commercial market is populated by a large number of firms, currently over 300. Entry appears to be easy since during the period 1958 to 1973, over 50 firms entered the market (*Argus,* various years). Unpublished work by Ronald Vogel of the Social Security Administration shows low concentration ratios in this market. Over 85 percent of individuals insured for hospital expense are covered under group policies, implying that the market is dominated by informed buyers. Indeed, it is best to think of the commercial insurers as competitively providing a schedule of prices for various types of insurance. From this competitively determined schedule, the consumer, or more commonly his representative, chooses. Thus, the commercial part of the market seems to be characterized by conditions favorable to approximately competitive behavior.

The other half of the industry comprises the Blue Cross and Blue Shield plans, organized by hospitals to provide hospital insurance and by physicians to provide physician services insurance, respectively. The Blues are organized as legally nonprofit public service firms. These firms are controlled by boards of directors with heavy representation of hospital and physician interests, in contrast to nonprofit mutual insurers which are nominally controlled by the policyholders. Further, in many States, the Blues are organized under special enabling acts so that additional entry is not allowed. This contrasts sharply with the situation of commerical insurers, where entry is relatively easy.

The Blues collude almost perfectly. Blue Cross and Blue Shield plans agree upon geographical market areas with the assistance of their national associations. Further, with few exceptions, the local Blue Cross plan agrees not to sell physician service insurance, while the local Blue Shield plan agrees not to sell hospital insurance. This means that, from a national antitrust perspective, we can treat the entire Blue Cross/Blue Shield complex as one firm. Doing so leads to a different picture than one gets from examination of the commercial sector only, for the one-firm concentration ratio is nearly fifty percent from this point of view. However, due to State regulations and historical accident, the market power of the local Blue plans varies immensely across States. There are States with almost no Blue Cross or Blue Shield insurance and some where the Blues have market shares upwards of 80 percent. Thus, the health insurance industry as a whole cannot be characterized as a competitive one, but as one with monopoly and competitive segments. As long as the Blues do not use their cost advantages to lower prices for all types of insurance, the situation can persist. The welfare implications of this structure are discussed below.

Interactions with Medical Care Costs

The effects of this high concentration may be more serious than is indicated by the standard industrial organization analysis because of the linkage of the policies of the Blue plans to the cost of health care. As is argued by H. E. Frech (1974, 1976b), the Blue plans prefer more complete[1] insurance. There are two reasons for this. First, more complete insurance raises the demand for medical care. The medical providers who control the Blue plans obtain higher revenues as a result.

It is important to note that the Blues cannot simply use their market power in a profit-maximizing manner and return the funds to the medical providers in the form of dividends or overpayments for services. The regulatory and tax advantages of these firms hinge on their nonprofit status which rules out such transfers. So, increasing the demand for medical care is virtually the only major way in which the firms can benefit the providers.

A second reason for the preference of the Blue plans for complete insurance is ideology—the belief that there should be no "financial barriers" to medical care. However, it is not important to determine the motivation of the preference at this point. Its effects on economic efficiency are the same regardless.

The mechanism by which more complete insurance is induced is a special kind of discriminatory (in the economic theory sense) price—an all-or-nothing price. Consumers are confronted with an attractive price because of the regulatory advantages, but only very complete insurance is offered. One cannot buy the entire possible menu of insurance plans from the Blues. Large deductibles (say $500-$1000) are especially rare. Given the lack of variation in the completeness of the typical Blue insurance policy (Louis Reed and Willine Carr), this goal of increasing the completeness of insurance can be pursued through market share. Since it can be measured at the plan level, market share is used in some of the empirical work below as a proxy for average completeness of insurance in a market area.

Economists have criticized the use of overly complete insurance because of its subsidy effect. When the patient pays only a small fraction of the cost of medical care, there is an inducement to utilize more care, and pay a higher price for it. Consumers wind up demanding medical care that is not as valuable to them as what it costs to produce it. Martin Feldstein (1973) has studied the additional health insurance use induced by the personal income tax and estimates a welfare loss in the billions from the use of overly complete health insurance. If Blue plans are successful in inducing purchase of more complete insurance, large welfare losses of this type may occur. Thus, the social problem of monopoly here is not the standard one of restriction of output but, rather, the inducement of an overexpansion of an aspect of output—completeness of health insurance. Since it is likely (e.g., Feldstein (1973)) that insurance is already over-used for health care, Blue inducement of more complete insurance aggravates a serious social problem.

Another link between Blue market power and medical care costs is through restrictions on cost control (claims review) activities. Lawrence Goldberg and Warren Greenberg have documented a case of Blue Shield's using its market power to prevent commercial insurers from implementing an activist claims review process.

Regulation—A Source of the Blue Cross/ Blue Shield Market Power

Insurance regulation is performed on the State level, and in various ways, regulation favors the Blue plans. Usually, they pay less in premium taxes.[2] The difference is large, often two percent of premiums or more.[3] In some States the Blues are exempt from other taxes, such as property taxes. In some States commercial insurance policies sold to individuals are regulated as to minimum benefit/premium rates, thus precluding sales of certain types of insurance with high selling costs. Required reserves are lower or nonexistent for the Blue plans in most States. Some States also regulate Blue Cross and Blue Shield rates, but in terms of the overall premium rather than the benefit-premium rate. Regulations on benefit/premium ratios, overall premiums, and required reserves are expensive to enforce and often are not. We do not have precise knowledge of the extent to which they are enforced.

One might expect these regulatory advantages to lead directly to a complete monopoly for the Blue plans. However, this is not what one observes. In fact, the Blues' share of the national health insurance market has been markedly stable in recent years. This is shown in table 1, where market share is defined as the proportion of insured persons covered. There are several explanations of this anomaly. One is that it is more convenient for employers to deal with one insurance firm or agent for all of their insurance needs. This would give commercial insurers, who usually sell many types of insurance, an advantage which offsets some of their sizable disadvantages due to taxation and regulation. It is unlikely that this is important. If it were, we would expect Blue plans to make agreements with insurance agents enabling their health insurance to be sold as part of a package.

Some more interesting explanations are the subject of ongoing research by the authors. (See Frech, 1974, 1976a, and 1976b; and Roger Blair, Ginsburg and Ronald Vogel, 1975.) As shown in the results below, the regulatory advantages conferred on the Blue plans are used to "purchase" two items of value to (or goals of) those controlling and influencing the plans. The first good purchased is administrative slack or inefficiency. By this, we mean more executive staff, attractive and spacious offices, a less harried pace, more congenial personnel, salaries higher than necessary to attract staff, and

Table 1 Blue Cross and Blue Shield Market Share

Year	Regular Medical Insurance	Hospital Expense Insurance
1940	0.066	0.488
1945	0.276	0.589
1950	0.512	0.489
1955	0.517	0.466
1960	0.504	0.437
1961	0.483	0.431
1962	0.478	0.432
1963	0.463	0.428
1964	0.449	0.427
1965	0.441	0.427
1966	0.436	0.428
1967	0.434	0.427
1968	0.434	0.429
1969	0.425	0.429
1970	0.421	0.433
1971	0.426	0.433
1972	0.428	0.432
1973	0.421	0.435
1974	0.416	0.435

Source: Sourcebook of Health Insurance Data, 1975-1976. Based on numbers of individuals insured.

so on (see Armen Alchian and Reuben Kessel, 1962). The absence of a residual claimant and consequent pointlessness of earning a profit means that the cost of these non-pecuniary aspects of compensation is low. The second item of value purchased is more complete insurance. While all-or-nothing prices do induce some consumers to purchase insurance more complete than their optimum, others will still choose to purchase a policy with large deductibles, and will only purchase such insurance from commercial insurers. In sum, we argue that commercial insurers have survived because (a) their Blue competitors are inefficient and (b) the Blues leave to them a portion of the market by refusing to sell insurance with large deductibles and coinsurance.

COMPLETENESS OF INSURANCE

In this section, we examine empirical evidence that Blue Cross and Blue Shield have a preference for more complete insurance. There are a number of methods that can be used to analyze the extent of systematic differences in product mix between Blue plans and commercial insurers. Perhaps the simplest is to compare characteristics of actual policies sold by the Blues with those sold by commercial insurers. Unfortunately, there are not sufficient data reported by insurers on characteristics of policies to perform such an analysis. Instead, we turn to survey research. The periodic Surveys of Health Services Utilization and Expenditures conducted at the Center for Health Administration Studies, University of Chicago, by Ronald Andersen and Odin Anderson provide data on characteristics of individuals' health insurance policies. These data are verified by the insurers, and information is obtained as to whether the insurer is a Blue plan or a commercial insurance company.

Regrettably, and incredibly, the published analysis of the 1970 survey (Andersen, Joanna Lion, and Anderson) does not tabulate insurance coverage variables by type of insurer. Thus, we concentrate on the analysis of the 1963 survey (Andersen and Anderson) which does focus on that distinction.[4]

For hospital insurance in 1963, Blue Cross plans had 43 percent of the market, and commercial insurers had 50 percent of the market.[5] There was no clear-cut difference with regard to income level of insured families, but Blue Cross tended to have a higher penetration in urban markets.[6] The ratio of group to nongroup coverage was approximately the same for the two types of insurers.

The first variable related to completeness of insurance is the percentage of the hospital bill covered by insurance for admissions that were insured.[7] Andersen and Anderson reported these percentages by category: 1-69 percent, 70-89 percent, and 90 percent or more. For group insurance, 8 percent of Blue Cross insured admissions had 1-69 percent of the bill covered, while 18 percent of those insured by commercial companies were in this category. Nineteen percent of the Blue Cross insured admissions and 23 percent of the commercially insured admissons had 70-89 percent of the bill covered. Most importantly, 90 percent or more of the bill was covered for 73 percent of the Blue Cross admissions and 59 percent of the commercially insured admissions.

This pattern of more complete insurance among those served by Blue Cross continues for nongroup policies. Here, 26 percent of Blue Cross admissions and 42 percent of commercially insured admissions had 1-69 percent of the bill covered. Thirty-nine percent of the Blue Cross admissions and 26 percent of the commercially insured admissions had between 70 and 89 percent of the bill covered. Finally, 90 percent or more of the bill was covered for 35 percent of the Blue Cross admissions and 32 percent of the commercial admissions.

Similar results on the proportion of the bill paid are seen for surgical insurance. For group and nongroup categories, one sees that 1-69 percent of the surgical bill is covered by insurance for 35 percent of the Blue Shield covered procedures and 39 percent of the commercially covered procedures. Seventy to 89 percent of the bill is covered for 15 percent of the Blue Shield procedures and 20 percent of the commercially covered procedures. Lastly, 53 percent of Blue Shield covered procedures and 41 percent of commercially insured procedures have 90 percent or more of the bill covered by the insurance.

While the foregoing analysis is informative, one would not label it as definitive. There are demand-side differences between populations insured by Blue Cross-Blue Shield on the one hand and by commercial insurers on the other hand that might also influence completeness of insurance. For example, Blue Cross is relatively more prevalent in urban areas. If urban or rural location influences demand for complete insurance, the cross tabulation could give a biased impression of the effect of type of insurer on completeness of coverage. A fully specified regression model should give a more definitive judgment on the effect of type of insurer on completeness of insurance.

Frech (1974) has estimated such regressions for completeness of coverage. Using a cross-section of those States which had Blue Cross plans in 1969, he regressed the proportion of hospital expense paid by insurance in the State on price of insurance,[8] income, price of hospital care, and Blue Cross market share (proportion of insured individuals). Using simultaneous equation techniques,[9] he found that States with a larger Blue Cross market share had a greater proportion of hospital expenses paid by insurance. Quantitatively, Frech found that a change in market share of 12 percent (one standard deviation) would change the percentage of hospital expenditures covered by insurance by 4 percent.[10]

The foregoing is evidence of preferences on the part of Blue plans for relatively complete insurance. If hospitals were willing to subsidize Blue Cross (e.g., by granting discounts), Blue Cross plans would be able to influence the average completeness of insurance purchased in the absence of regulatory advantages. But, to the extent that regulation gives Blue plans a cost advantage, they can further induce people to purchase insurance coverage more complete than they would have desired. Blue plans are offering a smaller loading charge than their competitors, and some buyers undoubtedly will find it attractive to buy a more complete policy in order to obtain the smaller loading charge—as in a quantity discount. Data available to us at the time of this study did not permit testing of this relationship at a micro level.[11] However, the authors plan to examine this relationship with data from the 1970 CHAS survey.

BLUE CROSS-BLUE SHIELD ADMINISTRATIVE COSTS AND MARKET SHARE

Roger Blair, P. Ginsburg, and Ronald Vogel estimated cost functions for Blue Cross and Blue Shield plans. Administrative costs per enrollee and per dollar of claims were the dependent variables, and the independent variables included the size of the plan (number of claims), a proxy for area wages, and a large number of output mix adjustments. The focus was on scale economies, which did not show up for either Blue Cross or Blue Shield plans, in contrast to evidence of scale economies found for commercial insurers by Blair, Vogel, and J. R. Jackson.

For this conference, we have extended this analysis to include regulatory variables and market share. The theoretical basis of this work is straightforward. It is a two-good consumption model. Administrators of Blue Cross and Blue Shield plans are assumed to maximize a utility function defined over two non-pecuniary goods, administrative slack and market share. Administrative slack is defined as those costs over and above the minimum necessary to produce a given output. Harvey Liebenstein has used the term "X-inefficiency" to describe this concept, while Oliver Williamson has used the term "emoluments" in his work. Examples of administrative slack might include plush offices, salaries for executives that are higher than those necessary to attract and retain them, overstaffing, lack of search effort into techniques to reduce costs, and avoidance of hiring capable people who don't "fit in" because of sex, race, or other characteristics. It is not difficult to imagine how some of these "goods" encompassed under administrative slack would be desired by executives.

There are two arguments as to why higher market share might be sought.

Among Blue Cross plans, there is a great deal of standardization in provisions of insurance policies relating to cost-sharing. Most policies are full-coverage—they have no deductible or coinsurance. Thus, if market share is larger, then completeness of insurance in the market may be greater. We already indicated the preference for more complete insurance among Blue executives, so market share may be desired to further this goal.

A different argument states that market share is desired for itself. Many scholars of the modern corporation claim that growth of the firm is a more important goal to managers than profits, as their personal welfare (salary, prestige) is more closely associated with firm size than with profitability. In a non-profit firm, growth goals may be even stronger, as there are no profits to be sacrificed, and no residual claimants to object.

While both administrative slack and market share are sought-after goods, achievement of them is constrained by the marketplace. If administrative slack is high, high premiums will have to be charged for health insurance, and market share will fall. Thus, executives must trade off administrative slack against market share along the locus CC in figure 1. The optimal combination, Z, is the point where the marginal rate of transformation between administrative slack and market share is equal to the marginal rate of substitution in consummation between them. Graphically, this point lies at a tangency between the indifference curve V^2 and the constraint CC.

Regulation enters the analysis as a variable that shifts the constraint. If a regulatory advantage, such as a lower premium tax rate, is obtained, the constraint shifts outward, as to C′C′ in figure 1. A new optimum, Z′, is obtained. In the way figure 1 has been drawn, both administrative slack and market share increase as a result of the regulatory advantage.[12]

If regulatory advantages are varied, the series of optimum combinations of administrative slack and market share trace out an expansion path, which is labeled EE in figure 1. This function shows the impact of regulatory advantages on administrative slack and market share, and is directly relevant to policy. The empirical analysis reported below is an attempt to quantitatively measure this expansion path.

The major problem involved with estimation of such an expansion path is the lack of direct measurement of administrative slack. We do have data on administrative costs, however, and experience in estimating cost functions for Blue Cross and Blue Shield (Blair, Ginsburg, and Vogel, 1975). Thus, instead of using administrative slack, we employ administrative cost as a dependent variable, and add, as independent variables, those factors which we have found to be significant as explainers of administrative cost variation. In this way, we will hold constant variables such as output mix and wage rates which explain variation in minimum costs, so that we will be able to infer that a relationship between administrative cost and regulation is really one between administrative slack and regulation.

We estimate the expansion path by estimating reduced form equations for administrative costs and market share. Exogenous demand function variables are included because they shift the constraint. Cost function variables are also included for the reasons discussed above.

Figure 1 The Relationship Between Regulatory Advantages and Choice of Non-Pecuniary Benefits for Blue Cross or Blue Shield Plans

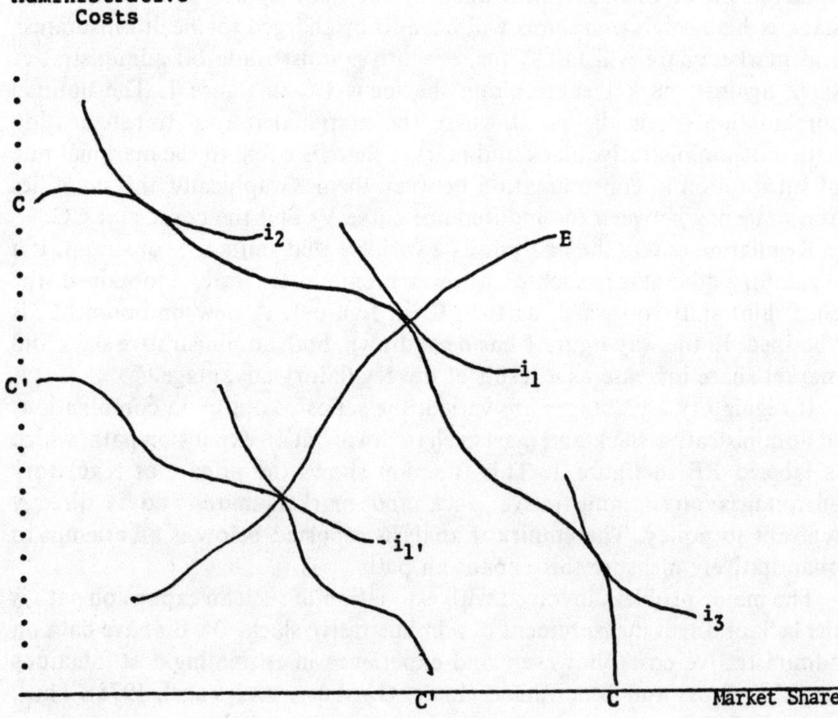

This model was estimated separately for Blue Cross and Blue Shield with data by plan for 1971.[13] The equations were estimated with ordinary least squares using a linear functional form.[14] The results appear in table 2.

The dependent variable in equation (1) ENCOST is administrative costs net of premium taxes per enrollee. While there is a choice of output units to use in the denominator, enrollee appeared superior to the number of claims or dollars of benefits as it is a more likely decision variable. Blue plans are more likely to envision themselves as producers of insurance for enrollees than insuring a certain volume (claims or benefits) of medical care. The dependent variable in equation (2) BMSR is the market share of the Blue plan. It is calculated by dividing the number of enrollees in a Blue plan by the population in its market area, and then dividing by the proportion of the population in the State that is covered by the relevant type of health insurance. To the extent that the proportion insured varies across Blue plan areas within a State, BMSR will be measured with error. However, any such errors should only reduce the efficiency of estimation and not result in any bias.

The number of enrollees (ENROLL) is used as an independent variable to reflect size, although the number of claims (CLAIM) and the dollar volume of benefits (BENEFITS) are included as output mix adjustments. Other product mix adjustments are GROUP, the proportion of policies sold to groups, MEDS, a dummy indicating whether Blue Cross plans sell medical insurance or whether Blue Shield plans sell hospital insurance, and FEHB, the proportion of policies sold under the Federal Employees Health Benefits program.[15]

NCLAIM reflects the number of claims processed for non-enrollees (Medicare, Medicaid, Champus). Since the administrative cost variable includes only those costs attributed to servicing the Blue policyholders, NCLAIM reflects any economies of scale realized from contract claims processing and errors (intentional or not) in cost accounting. SMINC is per capita income in the SMSA in which the plan is headquartered, a proxy for labor costs.

The above were cost function variables. Exogenous demand variables (facing Blue plans) include STINC, State per capita income, POP, the population of the area served by the plan, URB, the percentage of the State population living in urban areas, and PINS, the price of insurance which is the statewide ratio of premiums to benefits in health insurance.

There are three regulatory variables. DIFTAX is the difference in premium tax rates between foreign (headquartered outside of the State) commercial insurers and Blue plans. In certain States, domestic commercial insurers are taxed more lightly than foreign companies, but we judged the rate on foreign insurers to be the relevant one to the Blues as they tend to dominate the commercial market. We expect that larger premium tax differences will lead to higher administrative costs and larger market shares. COMREG is a dummy for whether loading charges on commercial insurance policies are regulated. This type of regulation may bar commercial insurers from selling certain types of individual policies—thus giving Blue plans a competitive advantage. Finally, BCREG indicates whether (total) premiums on Blue Cross-Blue Shield policies are regulated. This type of regulation should decrease administrative costs and increase market share, unless it is correlated with other (unmeasured) regulatory measures which are favorable to the Blues.

The results for Blue Cross were the more striking. The reduced form equation for administrative costs (ENCOST) explained 82 percent of the variation. DIFTAX was positive and statistically significant. A typical 2 percent differential in the premium tax is estimated to cause a 54 cent increase in costs per enrollee. Since the mean plan cost per enrollee was $4.10, this effect is quantitatively important. The presence of loading charge regulation of commercial insurers increased Blue Cross administrative costs by $1. Such an effect is larger than expected, and may be caused by other types of regulation hostile to commercial insurance or favorable to the Blues that is correlated with this type of regulation. Regulation of Blue Cross premiums is seen to reduce administrative costs per enrollee by 62 cents, although the t-statistic is only marginally significant.

Turning to the equation for Blue Cross market share (BMSR), 64 percent of the variation is explained. DIFTAX was positive and statistically significant. A 2 percent premium tax difference increases market share by 6.7 percent. Neither of the other regulatory variables were statistically significant.

Results for Blue Shield were somewhat less favorable to our hypotheses. The equation for ENCOST explained 75 percent of its variation. The coefficient for DIFTAX was statistically significant, although only at the 10 percent level. A 2 percent premium tax difference is expected to raise costs by 80 cents. Neither of the other regulatory variables was statistically significant. Fifty-three percent of the variation in market share was explained for Blue Shield. The only regulatory variable that was significant was COMREG. It had the wrong sign, but was quantitatively very small (0.1 percent).

There are a number of possible explanations for the weaker results for Blue Shield. One is that there is more variation in completeness of insurance across plans and policies in Blue Shield than in Blue Cross. As a result, market share is not as good a proxy for completeness in Blue Shield as it is in Blue Cross. Another explanation is based on the fact that Blue Shield is controlled by physicians, who are residual claimants in their practices, while Blue Cross is controlled by hospitals, which are also non-profit organizations. The property rights theory of the firm would predict that physicians

Table 2 Reduced Form Estimates: Administrative Costs and Market Share, 1971

	Blue Cross		Blue Shield	
	(1)	(2)	(1)	(2)
VARIABLE	ENCOST	BMSR	ENCOST	BMSR
DIFTAX	27	335	40	−1.6
	(2.0)	(1.9)	(1.7)	0.0)
COMREG	1.0	−1.5	.44	−12
	(3.3)	(.36)	(.65)	(1.9)
BCREG	−.62	.36	−.47	2.8
	(1.5)	(.66)	(.67)	(.42)
MED	4.6	−16	3.6	−10
	(10.2)	(2.7)	(4.4)	(1.3)
BENEFITS	−.0015	.13	.014	−.076
(millions)	(.21)	(1.4)	(.68)	(.37)
# CLAIMS-P	.22	11	.30	−.037
(millions)	(.37)	(1.4)	(.32)	(0.0)
ENROLL	.012	−2.7	−1.7	24
(millions)	(0.0)	(.44)	(1.9)	(2.9)
GROUP	.21	21	2.7	19
	(.11)	(.79)	(.72)	(.54)
SMSA-INC	−5.9	34	1.2	5.4
(thousands)	(.91)	(.96)	(1.1)	(.53)
FEHB	1.4	34	4.1	−45
	(.47)	(.83)	(1.3)	(1.5)
# CLAIMS-O	.22	1.4	.23	.62
(millions)	(1.0)	(.51)	(1.7)	.49)
POP	.0082	−3.7	3.4	−1.1
(millions)	(0.1)	(2.7)	(1.0)	(3.4)
URB	−2.4	−34	−5.4	25
	(2.0)	(2.1)	(1.7)	(.80)
ST-INC	.16	14	.30	−2.3
(thousands)	(.33)	(2.1)	(.24)	(.20)
PINS	1.4	−5.8	−2.9	−7.4
	(1.9)	(.57)	(1.8)	(.48)
CONSTANT	4.1	29	3.4	38
	(1.5)	(.80)	(.72)	(.86)
R^2	.82	.64	.75	.53
N	64	64	56	56

Note: t-statistics in parentheses

would exercise more thorough control over Blue Shield than hospitals do over Blue Cross. Finally, since physician insurance is less prevalent than hospital insurance in the United States today, there may be greater errors in the BMSR variable for Blue Shield (greater variation in the proportion insured across plan areas within a State). The loss of efficiency in estimation may cause these weaker results.

BLUE CROSS MARKET POWER AND HOSPITAL PRICES

Those who defend the existing market power of Blue Cross insurers argue that a strong Blue Cross plan can impose cost controls on the hospitals, through reimbursement policy. The idea is that for reimbursement policy to alter seriously the incentives of the hospitals, the local Blue Cross must be a large part of the market. If this cost control effect were the major result of Blue Cross market power, then strong Blue Cross plans should be associated with lower hospital prices.

On the other hand, there are two arguments that Blue Cross market power causes higher hospital prices. Clark Havighurst argues that a competitive insurance industry would be more likely to impose cost controls (largely in the form of claims review) than a monopoly insurer which is influenced by the providers (U.S. Congress, 1974, p. 1076). Indeed, in a recent paper, Goldberg and Greenberg indicate that the Blue Shield plan of Oregon was organized specifically to eliminate cost controls which had been employed by competitive commercial insurers. Although we know of no historical evidence, the incentives for the hospitals to use Blue Cross in the same way are clear enough.

The second argument is that Blue Cross plans use their market power to sell more complete insurance. This raises the demand for hospital care which, as shown by Feldstein (1971), results in an increased cost and price of hospital care.

We have competing theories or tendencies here, and we seek to determine whether more market power for Blue Cross tends to raise or lower hospital prices. To investigate this, a simple model determining hospital demand price was estimated. Determinants of demand price include quantity, income, urbanization, the price of insurance, and the Blue Cross market share. This represents a modification of the work in Frech (1974, 1976b) which included a variable for the average coinsurance rate, rather than the insurance price and Blue Cross market share. The 1974 regressions allowed one to trace the effect of Blue Cross market share on hospital price only through raising the completeness of insurance. By including Blue Cross market share directly, we can measure its effect, through both avenues of increasing insurance and cost controls to observe the net effect. In doing this, it is important to hold the price of insurance constant because low insurance prices will raise both Blue Cross market share and the average completeness of insurance, thus hospital prices. Failure to hold the price of insurance constant would lead to a specification bias, which would artificially raise the estimated coefficient on Blue Cross market share.

The regression is estimated by ordinary least squares on State data for 1969. States with no Blue Cross plan and the District of Columbia are excluded. The dependent variable is PHOS, the price of hospital care. This is a weighted average of charges for semi-private rooms. The independent variables are QHOS, quantity of hospital care (bed days per thousand population), PINS, price of hospital insurance (premium-benefit ration)[16] INC, per capita disposable income, and BCMSR, Blue Cross market share (proportion of insured population enrolled in Blue Cross).[17]

The results are shown in table 3, equation (1). One can see that Blue Cross market power tends to increase hospital prices. The estimate is that prices would be about $18.00 higher in a State with a virtual Blue Cross monopoly than in a State with no Blue Cross insurance. Since the average State has about a 40 percent Blue Cross penetration, prices are about $8.00 per day higher than in the absence of Blue Cross in 1969. More recent data would probably show a larger dollar difference because of generally higher hospital prices.

Two additional versions of this model were estimated to investigate whether certain biases may have contributed to this result. The first addresses the issue of whether high hospital prices could result from the discount that often accompanies use of cost reimbursement by Blue Cross plans. The concern is that prices are higher because hospitals increase charges on private patients to offset losses on cost reimbursed Blue Cross patients. Thus, part of the impact of BCMSR could be on pricing *structure* rather than average prices.

In order to deal with this problem, we interacted with BCMSR a dummy variable for whether Blue Cross reimbursement was on a charge basis (BCMSR · CHARGE). Inclusion of this variable should separate out from the BCMSR coefficient any impact of discounts on hospital charges. The results (table 3, equation (2)) strongly confirm those discussed above. The coefficient and t-statistic on BCMSR are virtually unchanged—they show the significant impact of Blue Cross market share on price. BCMSR · CHARGE has an expected negative sign, indicating that when cost reimbursement is used, charges to private patients are increased to compensate for the discount. This is perhaps the first evidence from a statistical model that cost reimbursement increases prices paid by other patients. It gives credence to the frequently expressed concern with this issue. It also is important in that it gives certain Blue Cross plans an additional competitive advantage over commercial insurers.

A second modification of the model deals with the dependent variable. In equation (3) we substituted cost per day for semiprivate room charges. There are two reasons for this. First, it is an alternative approach for dealing with the discount issue. If prices are higher because of a higher mark-up, this should not affect the cost variable. Second, the price variable is based on room charges only, and thus neglects prices of ancillary services. The cost variable has wider coverage. However, the cost variable confounds quantity charges (service intensity) with unit cost charges. This can be an advantage or a disadvantage depending on one's view of what the appropriate output unit should be for the analysis.

The results for this specification are quite similar to those for the others. The coefficient on BCMSR is slightly larger, but its standard error is also larger, leading us to have slightly less confidence in the result.

Thus, it seems clear that the net effect of Blue Cross market power is to raise hospital prices. There are two possible interpretations of this. One is that the more complete insurance induced by Blue Cross plans is more important than the cost control policies of Blue Cross plans. The other,

Table 3 Equations for Hospital Prices and Costs

Dependent Variable	**(1) PHOS**	**(2) PHOS**	**(3) CHOS**
Independent Variable			
BCMSR	18.2	17.9	19.5
	(2.2)	(2.2)	(1.5)
INC	.0135	.0124	.150
	(5.2)	(4.8)	(3.7)
QHOS	−.0112	−0106	−.0185
	(3.2)	(3.1)	(3.4)
PINS	−12.8	−5.69	−23.2
	(0.8)	(0.4)	(1.0)
URB	−8.11	−5.33	−8.6
	(0.9)	(0.6)	(0.6)
BCMR·CHARGE		−7.57	
		(2.0)	
CONSTANT	26.9	19.8	55.3
	(1.1)	(0.8)	(0.8)
R^2	.75	.78	.74
N	46	46	46

Note: t - statistics in parentheses.

following Havighurst, is that Blue Cross market power actually reduces insurer efforts at cost control. These results cannot separate between these interpretations, but they do indicate that more market power for Blue Cross leads to higher hospital prices.

PREMIUM TAX PREFERENCES FOR DOMESTIC COMMERCIAL INSURERS

Within the commercial segment of the health insurance market, regulation plays a role. While all States assess premium taxes on commercial insurers, some States exempt "domestic" insurers, or those with headquarters in the State, from all or part of the premium tax. This should lead to an increased market share for domestic insurers. However, the share of the "foreign" insurers need not fall to zero because (a) economies of scale may allow these firms to overcome their tax disadvantage (Blair, Jackson, and Vogel, 1975), and (b) many large purchasers of health insurance operate in many States, thus diluting any advantage that a domestic insurer has in a particular State.

We made some exploratory efforts to test the hypotheses that premium tax advantages lead to a greater market share for domestic insurers. Our difficulty was in not having data on small insurers. We dealt with this by examining the market share of the six largest and twelve largest national insurers[18] in each of a sample of States. A sample of ten States with no difference and ten States with large differences in premium taxes between domestic and foreign commercial insurers was selected.[19] The results are given in table 4.[20] For the six largest insurers, their market share was 58.8 percent and 54.0 percent in the no difference and large difference states, respectively. Calculating a t-statistic for the difference in means, we obtained a value of 1.0 (18df), which was not statistically significant at conventional confidence intervals. For the twelve largest companies, the market shares were 71.3 percent and 69.4 percent, but the t-statistic was only 0.5.[21]

While these results are in the direction hypothesized, they are quantitatively small and not statistically significant. Presumably, it is

Table 4 Market Share of Large Commercial Insurers

	No Difference in Premium Tax	Large Difference in Premium Tax	t-statistic
Top 6	58.8%	54.0%	1.0
Top 12	71.3%	69.4%	0.5

reasonable to ignore these tax biases within the commercial sector in modeling health insurance.

SUMMARY AND CONCLUSIONS

There are several findings of this work. First, Blue Cross and Blue Shield insurance is more complete than commercial insurance. Second, there is evidence that regulatory advantages of Blue Cross plans are used to raise market share and also to allow administrative costs to rise. The first seems related to the fact that more complete insurance raises demand for hospital care, while the latter would be expected for any nonprofit firm. The evidence for Blue Shield points in the same direction, but is weaker.

Third, the net effect of Blue Cross market power is to raise hospital prices. Thus, the ability of a strong Blue Cross plan to control costs through its reimbursement policy is either (a) not put to use, as Havighurst would argue, or (b) outweighted by the tendency of Blue Cross plans to encourage purchase of relatively complete insurance.

Fourth, the premium tax bias against foreign (out-of-State) insurers in some States reduces the market share of large national firms. However, the effect is quite small. Thus, treating the commercial sector as a competitive national market may be reasonable.

Policy recommendations deal with regulatory advantages, antitrust policy, and national health insurance. Clearly, the market power of the Blue plans leads to inefficiency. An obvious remedy is to remove differences in premium taxes. Another valuable remedy is to force the various Blue plans to compete by prohibiting market-sharing agreements. To eliminate the influence of medical care providers on the Blues, they could be required to convert into conventional stock insurers, with a prohibition against medical providers holding stock in the Blues. Short of this, the influence of medical suppliers could be reduced, as is already occurring under political pressure. This last will be less effective if individuals with an ideological interest in complete health insurance replace medical providers as controllers of the plans. This unfortunate outcome seems likely.

For national health insurance, the evidence presented here indicates that giving the Blues a significant role in national health insurance would lead to inefficiency in several ways. First, there is evidence from many sources (Frech 1976a, 1977; Vogel and Blair) that the Blues are less efficient than commercial firms at processing claims. This paper indicates that as their market power increases, the Blues' inefficiency increases. Secondly, if there is scope for private insurers to determine the type of benefits in national health insurance and/or to supply supplemental insurance, the Blues would tend to favor relatively complete first dollar coverage, which would undermine the cost-control features of the insurance plans. As a result, one can say that national health proponents who envision a role for private insurers are well-advised to ensure sufficient competition among health insurers.

NOTES

1. By complete, we mean policies with small (or no) deductibles and with no coinsurance, so that the patient pays only a small fraction, if any, of the cost of medical care.

2. Premium taxes are assessed by States on most types of insurance. The revenue is used to finance the insurance regulatory apparatus.

3. Since the loading charge (premiums minus benefits) on group policies is usually small (less than 10 percent of premiums), a 2 percent premium tax differential is a 20 percent advantage in net revenue.

4. All of the numbers in the following four paragraphs are from Andersen and Anderson (1970), chapter IV.

5. Market share is defined in terms of individuals insured. The remainder consisted of independent insurers (such as prepaid group practices) and Armed Forces insurance. Note that this market share data corresponds very closely with those reported by insurance companies (see table 1, above).

6. In our multivariate analysis of market share (below), we show that, when other variables are held constant, Blues have greater market shares in rural areas.

7. More specifically, these data are for admissions covered by one basic policy with some benefits received—469 admissions out of 991 surveyed admissions. Andersen and Anderson use the term "private insurers" for non-Blue insurance companies. Since Blue plans are also private, we prefer to label the non-Blue companies as "commercial insurers," reflecting the fact that States tend to recognize Blue plans as private organizations operating in the public interest.

8. The price of insurance is the loading charge (ratio of premiums to benefits).

9. See Frech (1974) for the complete model.

10. Frech's percentage of hospital expenditures paid by insurance is really a composite of both the number of people insured and the completeness of their insurance. However, it is inconceivable that the Blue Cross plans' market share influences the number of people insured, except in so far as they might offer insurance at a lower price. Since the price of insurance is included in the equation, this effect should not be a problem. Thus, we can attribute the entire effect of this variable to completeness of insurance.

11. Frech (1974) did estimate an equation relating Blue Cross market share (a function of regulatory variables) to whether Blue Cross plans offered a deductible option. The analysis was hampered by the necessity of using a binary dependent variable in a small data set and by little variation in the dependent variable. While the sign was in the expected direction, the standard error was large, so the results must be considered inconclusive.

12. See Frech and Ginsburg (1977) for a discussion of the assumptions necessary to obtain such a result.

13. See Blair, Ginsburg, and Vogel (1975) or an extensive discussion of data sources and editing.

14. A double-log formulation yielded results that were somewhat better (larger t-statistics for regulatory variables, higher R^2), but the constant elasticity constraint seemed inappropriate for the premium tax difference variable.

15. Variables for whether hospitals are reimbursed by cost or charge and the proportion of policies that are major medical policies were not included because they are endogenous. Experimentally including them did not alter the results of interest.

16. PINS may be a function of BMSR, biasing the coefficient on BCMSR downward (against our hypothesis). However, we feel that PINS is more reflective of the proportions of group and individual policies in an area than of BMSR. Exclusion of PINS from the equation raised the coefficient and t-statistic on BCMSR.

17. See Frech (1974) for more on the data and for results of two stage least squares estimation of the full model. That work indicated that the feedback influence of PHOS on BCMSR and QHOS was small, so that ordinary least squares estimation is preferred.

18. Relative size was based on group health insurance premiums in 1975. Data are from The National Underwriter, June 26, 1976, p. 15. The companies were Aetna, Travelers, Prudential, Metropolitan, Equitable, Connecticut General, Provident, John Hancock, Continental, Accidental, Mutual of Omaha, and Lincoln National, respectively.

19. The ten States with no difference in premium taxes are California, Colorado, Connecticut, Georgia, Maryland, Massachusetts, Minnesota, Missouri, New York, and Pennsylvania. The ten States with large differences (and their percentage differences) were Arkansas (2.5), Florida (2.0), Illinois (2.0), Kentucky (2.0), Michigan (2.0), Ohio (2.5), Oklahoma (4.0), Oregon (2.25), Texas (2.2), and Wisconsin (2.0). Where sampling was required, we chose the largest States.

20. We are grateful to David Robbins of Health Insurance Association of America for providing us with the market share data by State.

21. These concentration ratios are higher than those found in Vogel's unpublished work. We do not understand the reasons for this.

REFERENCES

A. Alchian and R. Kessel, "Competition, Monopoly, and the Pursuit of Money," in National Bureau of Economic Research, *Aspects of Labor Economics*, New York 1962, 157-175.

R. Andersen and O. W. Anderson, *A Decade of Health Services*, Chicago 1970.

_____ and J. Lion, *Two Decades of Health Services: Social Survey Trends in Use and Expenditure*, Cambridge, Mass., 1976.

R. Blair, P. Ginsburg, and R. Vogel, "Blue Cross - Blue Shield Administration Costs: A Study of Non-Profit Health Insurers," *Econ. Inq.*, June 1975, 55-70.

R. Blair, J. R. Jackson, and R. Vogel, "Economies of Scale in the Administration of Health Insurance," *Rev. Econ. Stat.*, May 1975, 185-9.

M. Feldstein, "Hospital Cost Inflation: A Study of Non-profit Price Dynamics," *Amer. Econ. Rev.*, Dec. 1971, 853-872.

_____, "Welfare Loss of Excess Health Insurance," *J. Polit. Econ.*, March/April 1973, 251-80.

H. E. Frech, III, *The Regulation of Health Insurance*, Ph.D. dissertation, University of California, Los Angeles, 1974.

_____, (1976a), "The Property Rights Theory of the Firm: Empirical Results from a Natural Experiment," *J. Polit. Econ.*, Feb. 1976, 143-52.

_____, (1976b), "Demand for Reimbursement Insurance: Comment," in Richard N. Rosett, ed., *The Role of Health Insurance in the Health Services Sector*, New York 1976, 156-60.

_____, "Mutual and Other Nonprofit Health Insurance Firms: Comparative Performance in a Natural Experiment," unpublished paper, 1977.

——— and P. Ginsburg, "Regulation and Competition Among Health Insurers," in preparation.

L. Goldberg and W. Greenberg, "The Effect of Physician-Controlled Health Insurance: U.S. v Oregon State Medical Society," *J. Health Politics, Policy, Law,* Spring 1977, 48-78.

H. Liebenstein, "Allocative Efficiency vs. X-Efficiency," *Amer. Econ. Rev.,* Sept. 1977, 392-415.

L. S. Reed and W. Carr, *The Benefit Structure of Private Health Insurance, 1968,* Research Report No. 32, Social Security Administration, Office of Research and Statistics. Washington 1970.

R. J. Vogel and R. D. Blair, "Health Insurance Administrative Costs," Staff Paper No. 21, DHEW Publication No. (SSA) 76-11856, Office of Research and Statistics, Social Security Administration, Washington 1976.

O. Williamson, *The Economics of Discretionary Behavior: Managerial Objectives in a Theory of the Firm,* Englewood Cliffs, N.J. 1964.

National Underwriter Co., *Argus Chart of Health Insurance,* Cincinnati (various years).

U.S. Congress, Senate Subcommittee on Antitrust and Monopoly of the Committee on the Judiciary, Hearings: *Competition in the Health Services Market,* Parts 1-3, 2d sess., 93d Cong., May 14, 15, 17, 29, 30; July 10, 1974, Washington 1974.

Comment

Howard Berman
Vice President, American Hospital Association*

The real issues that the authors raised are those of concept of public policy. They, I believe, understand this—for, at its "core," their paper is fundamentally an ideological presentation.

Given this basic understanding and perspective, I would like to address two matters.

First, I would like to clarify several of the paper's more troublesome errors. And second, I would like to comment- from the perspective of operational reality—on the issue which the Commission has asked Frech and Ginsburg to address: "The matter of competition among health insurers and prepayment."

ADMINISTRATIVE SLACK

The authors "use" an interesting word—when they talk of "administrative slack." The concept is never defined. However, they seem to use it interchangeably with the notion of inefficiency; both alleging that Blue Cross Plans are inefficient and implying that this is particularly the case relative to their commercial insurance competitors.

This is a peculiar contention, particularly when one realizes the authors have a serious limitation in their research design—making neither a direct performance comparison nor a comparison of the total cost of health services to the consumer. Nevertheless, their finding represents a serious misconception, unsupported by operational reality.

The authors weave several inferences together in trying to make their argument. They refer to operating costs, high salaries, and the benefit/premium rate. On each of these points, factual evidence is available which compels a different conclusion.

* Mr. Berman formerly was Vice President, Blue Cross Assn.

In 1975, the Government Accounting Office (GAO), at the request of the House Ways and Means Committee, conducted a comparative evaluation of the performance between the Division of Direct Reimbursement of the Social Security Administration and private intermediaries.

The private intermediaries compared were the Maryland and Chicago Blue Cross Plans and the Mutual of Omaha and Travelers insurance companies. These four private intermediaries were chosen because they had similar claims volumes and served similar types of providers. Also, since the analysis was focused on Medicare, the evaluation examined a uniform benefit. Thus, you have one of those interesting situations in which you are able to analyze almost like phenomena.

The GAO analysis (p. 266) showed that cost per bill processed, excluding audit, and using the Travelers weighting factor, was the lowest for the two Blue Cross Plans. Costs for the Maryland and Chicago Plans were $2.67 and $2.25, respectively; as compared to $3.50 for Travelers, and $3.18 for Mutual of Omaha. The Division of Direct Reimbursement costs, by the way, were $5.07.

These results are hardly indicative of either absolute or relative inefficiency.

Examining operating expenses as a percentage of premiums shows similar results.

Marjorie Smith Mueller and Pamela A. Piro report in the March 1976 *Social Security Bulletin* (p. 12) that Blue Cross Plans have the lowest ratio of operating expense as a proportion of premium income of all insurers. When operating expense per enrollee is examined, the same performance result is obtained.

Operating expenses for group and individual policies as a percentage of premium income—for both group and non-group policies—were 5.4 percent for Blue Cross Plans and 7.4 percent for Blue Cross and Blue Shield Plans versus 13.0 percent for group policies of insurance companies and 47 percent for insurance company individual policies.

On a per enrollee basis, costs were $6.21 for Blue Cross Plans and $13.41 for Blue Cross and Blue Shield Plans. This compares with $15.89 for insurance company group policies and $53.47 for individual policies.

These, again, are hardly the facts and the performance statistics which one would expect to associate with inefficiency. In fact, they clearly indicate, at the very least, relative efficiency.

HOSPITAL PRICES

With respect to hospital prices, the authors first suggest that Blue Cross Plan market power causes higher hospital prices. They then attempt to prove this point by showing that hospital prices increase as market share increases. They define hospital price as the hospital charge for semi-private rooms.

This, also, is a peculiar approach. Unfortunately, it is one which, by ignoring the complexity as well as the operational subtleties of the problem, results in an overly simple and unusable answer.

The price variable, hospital charges for semi-private rooms, which the authors use is in itself an unreliable measure. First, it does not reflect the total price paid for hospital care. Second, it is a price which is more a function of internal hospital management compromises than either the completeness of benefit coverage or routine service costs.

One could pursue this point—probably with some benefit. However, falling to the technical level clouds the examination of the fundamental policy issues.

To begin with, it is important to understand that Blue Cross Plans are not controlled by providers. In reality, Blue Cross Plan governing boards are composed in substantial majority of public, non-provider, non-physician representatives.

Second, the simple notion set out in the paper that the Plans' objective is to benefit providers by increasing the demand for care is specious. As representatives of their subscribers, Plans could not survive if they acted to benefit only the alleged needs of hospitals. This point is evidenced by plans which provide benefits which go considerably beyond hospital services, and the strained relationships with hospitals that have resulted from attempts to implement cost containment measures. Third, as a matter of philosophy, Blue Cross Plans have from the outset been committed to provision of service benefits and comprehensive coverage. This commitment is intrinsic to the principle of non-profit prepayment plans and is one of the factors which distinguishes Blue Cross Plans from commercial insurers. The authors refer to this commitment as a matter of ideology—and appear to gloss over its importance. Instead, they focus on trying to prove the "completeness" of coverage is greater for Blue Cross Plans than for others.

There is no question that this is the Blue Cross Plan goal. Plan success in reaching this goal is a clear reflection of the competitive market's preference for a service benefit product.

Let's thoroughly understand what the orientation of prepayment is. Its objective is to assure that financial barriers to needed health care are overcome. To the extent that people obtain needed care, health expenditures will obviously increase. Conversely, to the extent that needed care is foregone, health expenditures might be less—but other societal costs will increase.

To assure that only needed and appropriate care is obtained, Blue Cross Plans have pioneered a variety of new benefits and cost control mechanisms.

Plans across the country have been the leaders in utilization and claims review, health care facilities and services areawide planning, and prospective payment. The Blue Cross Plan track record in these areas is the standard that others have yet to achieve. This fact is a far cry from the opposite implication of the authors.

I should note that Blue Cross Plans have not undertaken all these activities only out of a sense of altruism. There are practical economic reasons why Blue Cross Plans must assure that only necessary and appropriate care is provided.

It does not take much analysis to understand that these measures are necessary if a service benefit providing first day, first dollar coverage—is to be competitive in the market with indemnity and large deductible programs.

This last point is related to a third area which, to my understanding, is really supposed to be the central issue of the paper the matter of competition among health insurers.

COMPETITION

The authors, in addressing this topic, make an interesting assumption. They seem to begin by arguing that the private insurance market is divided in half, with commercial health insurance making up about half the market and behaving in a somewhat competitive manner. They then argue that Blue Cross Plans make up the other half of the market and represent a monopoly segment. They also argue that commercial insurers survive only because Blue Cross is inefficient while, at the same time, Blue Cross leaves a segment of the market to the commercials.

There is an interesting set of inconsistencies here. We have already discussed the efficiency issue.

With respect to competition and market segment, the authors seem to wander between recognizing different market segments and presuming that that market falls into two "neat" categories. Why the market falls into these two segments is never addressed. One, however, is left with the feeling that it is due to some sort of external to the market phenomena.

At one point, the authors talk of "informed buyers." However, they never seem to give the informed purchasers credit for making rational decisions about either which product they wish to purchase or from whom they wish to purchase it.

The market obviously is not divided by predestination. Rather, it falls the way it does due to tough, head-to-head competition, with that "informed buyer" deciding which product he wants. Success in the marketplace is due neither to ideology nor to lack of competition but, rather, to offering a product which meets consumer preference.

This is illustrated clearly in the case of the Federal Employee Program where Blue Cross Plans are—under common ground rules; e.g., constant employer contribution, etc.—in explicit, direct competition with both commercial insurers and independent health carriers. In the 1976 Federal Employee Program enrollment period, Blue Cross Plans lost 107,000 contracts. In a follow-up survey of employees who opted for other benefits, the employees indicated that they were changing their demands for health coverage—that they wanted a different product. The loss of contracts indicated that, given the economy and other expenditure alternatives, some people were opting for lesser benefit coverage and a lower cost premium. From our perspective, this is a legitimate economic decision reflective of the workings of a competitive market. With respect to today's topic, it illustrates that there is competition—competition focused on market segments and product.

The private health benefit market can more appropriately be characterized not as two parts but, rather, as a whole, with stiff competition between Blue Cross Plans and others with respect to the type of product which will best meet the buyer's needs. If the buyer feels that access to care and service benefits are important and that he is getting value, he opts for the Blue Cross Plan product. If he wants lesser coverage, he opts for a different segment of the market.

The competition—at the level of the large groups—where the real informed buyers are, is not only "real" but "tough." If the authors do not believe it, let the next phase of their study focus on how the decisions are made by such purchasers as the steel, telephone, and auto industries.

Let us all understand, however, that the Blue Cross Plan/commercial insurer competition is focused at the product decision level. The difference in product offering and the resulting market decisions should not be confused with a lack of competition.

Blue Cross Plans generally limit their product line to comprehensive coverage. This limitation reflects the long-held belief that such coverage is in the best economic interest of the consumer, allowing for maximization of the benefits that can be received from available health dollars.

One other matter relative to competition should also be clarified. The authors contend that Plans "collude almost perfectly," agreeing to limit geographical market areas and the coverage—physician or hospital benefits—which they provide.

For the record, it should be noted that there are 70 Blue Cross Plans in the United States and Puerto Rico. Each is a separate corporation, locally chartered, managed, and controlled. Each is also closely monitored and rigorously regulated by State authority, usually the insurance commissioner. Thus, Blue Cross is not the monolith that the authors would have one believe.

Let me close with a final observation. I must confess that I had looked forward to this paper and the opportunity for a productive exchange which would have moved us all closer to workable solutions. I am disappointed that my comments had to focus on correcting misconceptions and errors of fact instead of reaching for those new frontiers.

If I had reviewed this paper as part of a journal refereeing process, I would have been substantially more blunt. My conclusion, and the conclusion that I leave with you, however, would have been the same. Simply, we deserve better work than the Frech/Ginsburg paper.

REFERENCES

M. S. Mueller and P. A. Piro, Private Health Insurance in 1974: A Review of Coverage, Enrollment, and Financial Experience," *Social Security Bulletin,* March 1976, 3-20.

U.S. House of Representatives, Committee on Ways and Means, Subcommittee on Health, *Performance of the Social Security Administration Compared with that of Private Fiscal Intermediaries in Dealing with Institutional Providers of Medicare Services,* Hearings, 94th Congress, 1st session, Washington, 1975.

TECHNICAL APPENDIX*

Page 167

"Blue Cross and Blue Shield Plans, organized by hospitals and physicians respectively and controlled by these providers. . . ."

COMMENT

Blue Cross Plans are not controlled by providers. A majority of Blue Cross Plan board members are public representatives.

A public member is defined as an individual who is not an employee of, nor has a financial interest in, a health care facility, nor is a member of a health profession which provides health care services. As of December 31, 1976, 67 percent of Blue Cross Plan Board Members were public representatives. Nationwise, over two-thirds of all the Blue Cross Plan, accounting for 90 percent of the Blue Cross membership, are controlled by public boards.

---

* The Appendix was written by William B. Elliott, Health Economics Center, Research and Development Division, Blue Cross Association.

Pages 168-169

"American health insurance is characterized by two major types of firms. First are the commercial health insurers, both profit-seeking and mutual, who make up about half of the private insurance market. . . ."

"The other half of the industry comprises the Blue Cross and Blue Shield Plans, organized by hospitals to provide hospital insurance and by physicians to provide physician services insurance respectively. . . ."

"Thus the health insurance industry as a whole, cannot be characterized as a competitive one, but as one with monopoly and competitive segments."

COMMENT

The authors have taken a peculiar approach to characterizing the health insurance market. They have apparently assumed an arbitrary division of the market between commerical insurance companies and Blue Cross and Blue Shield Plans. Further, they have stated that one segment, the commercials, is competitive, and that the other is not. This division does not seem to have any logical basis or at least none was demonstrated.

On the other hand, the authors argue that the market is dominated by "informed buyers," which infers that choices between the products offered would be made carefully. Purchasers can and do evaluate differences in products and determine their needs for the different offerings. The success of Blue Cross Plans would seem to indicate that they typically offer a superior product or a better price when matched against the commercial companies' offerings.

Page 169

"This means that from a national antitrust perspective, we can treat the entire Blue Cross/Blue Shield complex as one firm."

COMMENT

In both legal and operating reality, Blue Cross Plans are each independent corporations, locally chartered and controlled.

Page 169

"As is argued by Frech (1974, 1976b), the Blue Plans prefer more complete insurance. There are two reasons for this. First, more complete insurance raises the demand for medical care. The medical providers who control the Blue Cross Plan obtain higher revenues as a result."

COMMENT

There are several errors in this statement. First, as indicated earlier, medical providers do not control Blue Cross Plans.

Second, the Blue Cross Plans were created not as insurance companies but, rather, as non-profit prepayment mechanisms for assuring their members access to needed hospital services. As such, they could not survive in the market if they acted to serve the goals of providers—as opposed to the needs of their members. Evidence of their need to serve their members' needs and not just the goals of hospitals—is demonstrated by the fact that Blue Cross Plan benefits extend considerably beyond hospital care, tending increasingly toward health—as opposed to sickness—services.

The Plans believe that service benefits are desirable, so that high costs do not deter individuals from using needed medical services. It is felt that the appropriate decision criteria for medical treatment should not be an individual's ability to pay additional costs for coinsurance and deductible but the patient's need for appropriate treatment and its incumbent benefits. It is thought that these decision processes can be more appropriately controlled through correctly designed utilization and peer review procedures.

Page 169

"The mechanism by which more complete insurance is induced is through a special kind of discriminatory (in the economic theory sense) price—an all-or-nothing price. Consumers are confronted with an attractive price because of the regulatory advantage, but only complete insurance is offered."

COMMENT

The argument that Blue Cross Plans should not "discriminate (in the economic theory sense)" on ideological grounds is distasteful. The reasons for limiting offerings are clear enough. The Plans want to remove the financial barriers to the appropriate use of covered services and feel a "service benefit" is a key to that end. If the purchasers want to purchase a different type of insurance, it is available elsewhere.

The rationale is faulty. Using a similar logic, it follows that a Catholic obstetrician would be condemned for not performing abortions in a church-operated clinic when the procedure is readily available to patients elsewhere. The costs may be lower. There could be some subsidy effect from a nonprofit status. The authors seem to be implying that if there is a legal market, an individual or organization should become involved in it, regardless of ethical considerations, in order to keep the price down.

It might also be noted at this point that it is not demonstrated, nor even attempted to show, that a "regulatory advantage" is the sole or even a primary reason for Blue Cross attractiveness. The Plans seem to be more efficient in processing claims, judging from the GAO report provided to the U.S. House of Representatives, Committee on Ways and Means, Subcommittee on Health. The fact they are willing to operate as a not-for-profit corporation also reduces their administrative costs. By not producing profit they pass this savings on to the customer.

Page 170

"Consumers wind up demanding medical care that is not as valuable to them as what it costs to produce it."

COMMENT

There are a number of other non-monetary costs to treatment that are often overlooked by those advocating less complete coverage and higher out-of-pocket costs as a method to insure that the consumer is discriminating in the use of services.

The use of medical care and particularly hospital treatment is often disquieting, painful, and dangerous. It is the rare patient who uses more care than is thought to be medically necessary.

Page 170

"Thus, the social problem of monoply here is not the standard one of restriction of output but rather the inducement of an overexpansion of an aspect of output—completeness of health insurance."

COMMENT

The contention of monopoly is unproven. A monopoly does not exist. Moreover, the authors seem to indicate that the fact that a substantial segment of the market prefers a full service benefit is some subversion of competition. If the market prefers this level of benefits (coverage) and wishes to invest in it, then what exists is the market mechanism working as it should. It would seem that what the authors have difficulty with is that many individuals in the current market value health insurance differently than the authors believe they should.

Page 170

"Another link between Blue market power and medical care costs is through restrictions on cost control (claim review) activities. Lawrence Goldberg and Warren Greenberg have documented a case of Blue Shield using its market power to prevent commercial insurers from implementing an activist claims review process."

COMMENT

To be generous, this paragraph is misleading. The track record of Blue Cross Plans in cost containment activities far exceed the performance of their commercial insurance company counterparts. It appears that Frech and Ginsburg ". . . do not deal with this issue . . ." because, if they were to present the facts, they would find that the results are inconsistent with their hypothesis. It would seem that the model they have selected positing that the Blue Cross Plans were agents of the providers has limited their ability to deal with the facts of the case. The Plans have been active in a wide range of cost control efforts (B. Tresnowski, Larry Lewin). The reference to Lawrence Goldberg and Warren Greenberg is also somewhat misleading. The paper examines behavior during the formation of a Plan some thirty years ago. Conditions have obviously changed since then.

In fact, one of the major flaws with many of those efforts has been the presence of commercial insurers. Providers of service have been able to exploit the competition between the Blue Cross Plans and commercials and undercut cost control efforts. It would seem that competition to control administrative costs could discourage efforts to control the total costs of the system.

Many of the Plans' efforts at cost control are directed at systematic improvement and not merely controlling payments for covered services. The efforts by the Plans produce savings that are shared by other payers who bear none of the costs. Part of the problem with this paper, that is probably a function of availability of data, is that it does not deal with total costs for a region and how administrative and claims costs and consumer out-of-pocket costs interact. It is difficult to make an accurate analysis of the situation by measuring the difference between Plans when the types of populations covered and benefits offered vary widely. It is clear that differences exist, but the analysis does not explain why.

Page 170

"Some States also regulate Blue Cross and Blue Shield rates, but in terms of the overall premium rather than the benefit/premium rate. Regulations on benefit/premium ratios, overall premiums, and required reserves are expensive to enforce and often are not. We do not have precise knowledge of the extent to which they are enforced."

COMMENT

As a point of fact, most States regulate Plan rates and

operations—with strict enforcement. Again, the authors seem to select information deliberately and present it in a fashion to imply that the data supports their presumption without critically dealing with all the facets and complexities of the issues.

Page 171

"As shown in the results below, the regulatory advantages conferred on the Blue Cross Plans are used to "purchase" two items of value to (or goals of) those controlling and influencing the Plans. The first good purchased is administrative slack or inefficiency."

COMMENT

At the request of the House Ways and Means Committee, the General Accounting Office conducted an evaluation of a comparison of performance between various private intermediaries under Medicare. The Blue Cross Plans and two commercial insurance intermediaries were compared to the Division of Direct Reimbursement.

Using the Travelers' weighting factor for variations in claims complexity and excluding auditing expense, (p. 266) cost per bill processed by the Division of Direct Reimbursement averaged $5.07. This compared to $3.50 for Travelers and $3.18 for Mutual of Omaha. In contrast, the Blue Cross Plans' average in the case of Maryland was $2.67 and Chicago, $2.25. Thus, in comparing administration of similar benefits programs, Blue Cross Plans were able to perform at a significantly lower cost than their commerical counterparts.

In examining administrative cost as a percentage of premium revenue, the same results occur; i.e., Plans are able to perform at a significantly lesser cost. It should be noted that the "regulatory advantages" carry with them stringent obligations which go beyond the regulation applied to commercial health carriers; e.g., premium approval, board composition standards, investment standards, and so on.

It is not at all clear from their results that the regulatory advantages are used for the purposes described. What is shown is that there are variations in cost per enrollee between Plans. The analysis makes a comparison between Plans without attempting to account for variations in benefit offerings and complexity of coverage variations. For example, the proportion of supplemental insurance for Medicare varies widely between Plans, but there is no adjustment for this variation.

Page 172

"This second item of value purchased is more complete insurance. While all-or-nothing prices do induce some consumers to purchase insurance more complete than their optimum, others will still choose to purchase a policy with large deductibles, and will purchase such insurance from commercial insurers."

COMMENT

This sentence indicates that the market looks for different things. For that segment of the market which is interested in comprehensive full service benefits, the Blue Cross Plan product is quite competitive. For those who are interested in another form of coverage, they go to as indicated commercial insurers.

Blue Cross Plans do not use their not-for-profit status to induce more complete coverage. Rather, Plans attempt to assure that complete—or more complete coverage can be made available at a price competitive with the price quoted by commercial carriers for a different product.

Page 174

"Blue Cross Plans are offering a smaller loading charge than their competitors, and some buyers undoubtedly will find it attractive to buy a more complete policy in order to obtain the smaller loading charge—as in a quantity discount."

COMMENT

If the Blue Cross Plan price is more expensive in total than the commercial price, then the fact that one component of the total price—is cheaper, would not seem to be a sufficient motivator to attract one to buy a more expensive total package.

Page 177

"The dependent variable in equation (1) ENCOST is administrative costs net of premium taxes per enrollee."

COMMENT

Cost per enrollee is not a suitable variable to use as a measure of output. The output of a firm is typically measured, not by the number of customers, but by the number of services or items sold. This dependent variable was justified by inserting in the regression "output mix adjustment" variables; amount paid out in benefits (in millions of dollars), number of claims in millions, and number of enrollees. However, no adjustments were made for variation in benefit mixes and complexity due to exemptions and limited coverage. These are critical factors in the costs of administration. Blue Cross data indicates that these two additional dimensions vary systematically, with larger Plans offering a greater variety of benefits. Additional services raise costs.

Pages 177-180

COMMENT

The analysis as it is structured, obviously presumes that each Plan is dealing with a similar segment of a uniform population who are provided services by a uniform grouping of providers. An adjustment is made for numbers of claims but not claims complexity. The organization and behavior of the medical care industry varies widely between areas. No adjustments were made for many of these variations.

It is interesting to note that all output mix variables that were used turn out to have statistically insignificant "b" (regression) coefficients except the enrollee variable for Blue Shield's data. Although statistically insignificant, the benefit variable has a negative effect on administrative costs for Blue Cross data but a positive effect for Blue Shield's data. It is difficult to make anything out of these findings. It would probably have been more useful to run other regressions using different measures of administrative costs, such as costs per claims and benefit structure, to determine if there is some insight to be gained rather than using inadequate output mix adjustment variables.

These measurement problems certainly raise questions about the validity of any inferences that can be drawn from this analysis. The failure to account for variations is a serious problem.

The positive, statistically significant coefficients of DIFTAX and ENCOST in table 2 are also open to somewhat different interpretations than that offered in the paper. The positive association of DIFTAX and ENCOST is explicable on the grounds of the additional "public interest" restriction placed on the Plans. Any reputable economic theory of regulation suggests that when a State government requires additional non-remunerative tasks of a firm or industry, the government also compensates it partly for the cost. In this view, government requirements that Plans (or domestics in general) who take on additional costly business which increases ENCOST are balanced by a "grant" of higher "tariff protection" from foreign competition.

The authors are not particularly careful in their use of the results. They state that the tax "causes" higher Blue Cross costs. Regression analysis coannot be used to impute causality.

The paper did not mention that the "b" coefficients of number of enrollees in the Blue Shield regressions are negative and significant. These indicate economies of scale which contradict Blair, Jackson and Vogel's (1975) findings cited in the French and Ginsburg paper on page 220.

A serious drawback to the analysis presented here is that it does not attempt to determine if the Plans are dealing with similar populations and products. Based on other evidence it would seem that the products and clients vary widely. An analysis that does not adjust for these variations is suspect.

Page 180

"On the other hand, there are two arguments that Blue Cross market power causes higher hospital prices. Havighurst argues that a competitive insurance industry would more likely to impose cost controls (largely in the form of claims review) than a monopoly insurer which is influenced by the providers (U.S. Congress 1974, p. 1076). Indeed, in a recent paper, Goldberg and Greenberg (1977) indicate that the Blue Shield Plan of Oregon was organized specifically to eliminate cost controls which had been employed by competitive commercial insurers. Although we know of no historical evidence, the incentives for the hospitals to use Blue Cross in the same way are clear enough."

COMMENT

Blue Cross Plans have claims review at all levels in all Plans. Claims review is only one of several cost containment mechanisms used by Plans to contain the rate of increase in health cost. Plans historically have been pioneers in initiating cost containment efforts. The track record of Blue Cross Plans in this area is the standard which others have yet to achieve.

Page 181

"One can see that Blue Cross market power tends to increase hospital prices. The estimate is that prices would be about $18.00 higher in a State with a virtual Blue Cross monopoly than in a State with no Blue Cross insurance. Since the average State has about a 40 percent Blue Cross penetration, prices are about $8.00 per day higher than in the absence of Blue Cross in 1969."

COMMENT

There are a number of methodological shortcomings that led the authors to this conclusion. The first has to do with the dependent variable, State average charge for a semi-private hospital room. This price is influenced by a number of factors related more to reimbursement patterns than insurance coverage. First, charges for a semi-private room reflect only a portion of daily hospital costs and are subject to a wide variety of adjustments. Reflecting local conditions, the hospital administration can raise or lower the room rate without affecting the total price paid per day. The price of ancillary services can and are adjusted accordingly in order to generate the desired total revenue. Local competitive conditions and local reimbursement rules dominate this decision process. One of the primary factors is how the local Blue Cross Plan pays for services. Plans with larger market shares are more likely to reimburse hospitals on a cost basis. The room rate is a poor measure of the actual price paid or costs incurred.

In the regression equation in table 3, URBC (present urban population) has a negative and statistically insignificant "b" coefficient for "PHOS." This is unexpected because urban areas have higher room charges. One interpretation is that this anomaly results from the cross correlation between URBC and BCMSR. The paper has pointed out that Plans have higher market shares in urban areas (p. 217). If URBC has a negative and statistically significant "b" coefficient on hospital prices because of its cross correlation with BCMSR, then BCMSR's is not a reliable base for the paper's assertion "that Blue Cross Market power tends to increase hospital prices."

The models for both dependent variables are incomplete. They leave out at least one critical variable in determining price of care within a State—the effect of government programs. There are wide variations in State Medicaid programs. A generous program will increase demand and drive hospital prices up. There is a marked tendency for States with generous Medicaid programs to have a high Blue Cross market penetration. The zero-order correlation in 1976 between proportion of poor individuals covered by a State Medicaid program and Blue Cross market penetration is .57. This suggests at least two things about the demand for medical services. First, demand for hospitalization will be substantially higher. A more inclusive Medicaid program makes more dollars available by enfranchising many of the poor. Secondly, it is axiomatic that greater demand produces higher prices.

The relationship between Medicaid and Blue Cross Plan coverage strongly suggests that there are substantial differences between States in the evaluation of the utility of protection against loss due to illness. State legislatures. in designing Medicaid programs, chose more inclusive coverage, more eligibles, and higher payment levels, where more individuals and groups had chosen Blue Cross Plan service coverage. It seems very unlikely that the authors' "market advantage" notion forced the legislatures into more complete coverage than they wanted. Instead, the choice is far more likely to be a reflection of preference of the citizenry of the particular States to minimize barriers to access to medical care.

It is difficult to determine the direction of causality in Frech and Ginsburg's estimate on hospital prices. It certainly is not demonstrated that Blue Cross Plan market power raises hospital prices as stated. None of the analytic methods used can be used to impute causality as is done so liberally throughout the discussion sections. The direction could well be the other way; a higher price, for any other reason, may result in a higher fraction of the market choosing prepayment coverage. The environment from State to State also changes in ways not considered. The Medicaid program is only one such element. Variations in the practice of medicine is a key variable. Adjustments for these factors are likely to produce a much different outcome.

In response to one of our criticisms of the orginal paper, the authors have added an analysis examining cost reimbursement effects on the price structure of hospitals; unremarkably there is an effect. There are costs to the hospital associated with "charge paying" patients which justify the difference in rates paid. When a Plan pays charges, its subscribers may well be susidizing commercial and self-pay patients. Blue Cross Plan coverage minimizes a variety of costs for the hospital. Among others, there are savings from bad debt losses, collection costs, working capital, and bill processing expenses.

It should be noted that payment on a cost rather than charge basis is a cost control technique. Charges are almost invariably set higher than costs. Payment of only allowable costs reduces the surplus funds available to hospitals and acts to slow the rate of hospital cost increases.

When cost per hospital day is used as the dependent variable as we had suggested, the presumption that high Blue Cross Plan market penetration produces higher hospital costs is substantially less credible.

Page 183

"We made some exploratory efforts to test the hypothesis that premium tax advantages lead to a greater market share for domestic insurers. Our difficulty was in not having data on small insurers. We dealt with this by examining the market share of the six largest and twelve largest national insurers in each of a sample of States. A sample of ten States with no differences and ten States with large differences in premium taxes between domestic and foreign commercial insurers was selected."

COMMENT

This would seem to be a very strange test. For it to be valid, it is necessary at a minimum, that none of the commercial insurance firms be "domestic" with regard to the States in the high difference groups. To the extent that any is "domestic" (e.g., has local affiliates qualifying it for domestic treatment) the results may prove to be quite different.

The inference of the authors' hypothesis is that a decrease in the commercials' market share is due to Blue Cross Plan's premium tax advantage. However, as noted by the authors on page 232, the results of this test of the differences in market share for those firms are "quantitatively small and not statistically significant."

An ability to circumvent the "foreign" premium tax may serve to explain the results found. The tax barrier to competition may not be as "burdensome" as suggested.

Page 184

"Second, there is evidence that regulatory advantages of Blue Cross Plans are used to raise market share and also to allow administrative costs to rise."

COMMENT

It's important to move from the abstractions of models to reality. As shown earlier, Blue Cross' administrative costs are less than those of commercial insurers.

Page 184

"Third, the net effect of Blue Cross market power is to raise hospital prices."

COMMENT

The authors arrive at this through an incomplete analysis. It is equally likely that regional demand, and medical practice, vary in different parts of the country and that this dominates regional price variations. The presumption that Plans are operating in the same types of environments in each State is obviously unreasonable. Unfortunately, the model used takes very little of the variation into account.

Page 184

"Clearly, the market power of the Blue Cross Plans leads to inefficiency."

COMMENT

The evidence just doesn't support this.

Page 184

"This last will be less effective, if individuals with an ideological interest in complete health insurance replace medical providers as controllers of the Plans. This unfortunate outcome seems likely."

COMMENTS

It is interesting that Frech and Ginsburg feel that this particular outcome is unfortunate. They are merely substituting their own ideological preference.

Page 184

"There is evidence from many sources (Frech 1976a, 1977; Vogel and Blair, 1976) that the Blue Cross Plans are less efficient than commercial firms at processing claims."

COMMENT

The GAO study controlling for product mix is completely contrary to this. Two sources by one of the co-authors of the paper and a citation to Vogel and Blair hardly constitute "many sources."

REFERENCES

L. Goldberg and W. Greenberg, "The Effect of Physician-Controlled Health Insurance: *U.S. v. Oregon State Medical Society," Journal of Health Politics, Policy and Law,* Spring 1977, 48-78.

L. Lewin and Associates, Inc. Nationwide Survey of State Health Regulations, Health Resources Administration, Washington, D.C., 1974.

B. Tresnowski, Speech before the Council on Wage and Price Stability—Hearings on Health Care Costs, Chicago, Illinois, July 20, 1976.

U.S. House of Representatives, Committee on Ways and Means, Subcommittee on Health, *Performance of the Social Security Administration Compared with That of Private Fiscal Intermediaries in Dealing with Institutional Providers of Medicare Services,* Hearings, 94th Cong., 1st sess., Washington 1975.

Comment

David Robbins
Vice President and Director of Research and Statistics,
Health Insurance Association of America

I am pleased to be here this afternoon to participate in this important conference on competition in the health care sector. I am particularly pleased to have the opportunity to discuss the interesting paper delivered by Doctors H. E. Frech and Paul Ginsburg with respect to competition among health insurers. To be perfectly truthful, a good part of my pleasure comes from having reviewed the Frech/Ginsburg paper and finding myself in almost complete agreement with its conclusions. Actually, I believe most people in this room would also agree with the Frech/Ginsburg conclusion that competition among health insurers is basic to meeting the many diverse needs of the health care marketplace.

The history of health care delivery in this country has been one of rapid movement and change. The kinds and types of care that are being delivered today are far different from the care rendered just a few years ago, and the dynamic nature of the health care system will undoubtedly continue indefintiely. Inasmuch as the financing arrangments for prepaying health care have been able to operate in a free and competitive environment, they have been able to adjust their policies and practices to keep up with the continuing evolution of the health care system.

I need not trace for this audience the remarkable growth of private health insurance coverage to the point where today close to 9 out of every 10 persons below the age of 65 have some form of such coverage. What I would like to re-emphasize is that this coverage has evolved and continues to evolve in keeping with changes in the health care system. To mention just a few of such changes, we have seen the enormous growth of catastrophic health insurance coverage with very high or unlimited maximum benefits that today cover some 149 million Americans. We have witnessed the development of dental insurance, coverage for vision care, nervous and mental disorders, drug abuse, alcoholism, and care in the home. These developments would probably not have taken place in the absence of strong competition among Blue Cross/Blue Shield plans, insurance company plans, HMO's, and so forth.

In the brief time alloted to me, I would like to comment on four areas of the Frech/Ginsburg paper with which I find myself in disagreement. These are: the apparent omission of one of the major forces which has resulted in an unfair competitive advantage to my friends in the Blue Cross system; what appears to be a somewhat unsophisticated understanding of how insurance companies are regulated; the use of some very out of date statistics on the adequacy of private health insurance; and finally, some comments on what is or is not comprehensive health insurance coverage.

COMPETITION BETWEEN BLUE CROSS AND INSURANCE COMPANIES

The authors have quite properly called attention to several of the competitive advantages of the Blue Cross/Blue Shield system in that, in the very large majority of States, they are free from paying State premium taxes of the order of 2-3 percent of premiums. The Blues are also generally free from other kinds of corporation taxes paid by insurance companies such as real estate taxes and Federal income taxes. Although these taxes in themselves do provide a significant competitive advantage, the authors have apparently overlooked what is, in our judgment; the major reason why Blue Cross has had a greater market penetration in a number of key industrial States. I refer to what some impolite people label the "Blue Cross discount," but which I would choose to call the hospital price differential. As a number of people in this audience know, in the Northeastern States of New York, New Jersey, and Pennsylvania, and in Michigan, where the Blue Cross market penetration is upwards of 80 percent of the private health insurance in force, the Blue Cross enjoys a hospital price differential, in amounts varying between 14 and 30 percent. With some significant advantages, competition from insurance companies in those States has obviously been most limited. We, of course, regard these hospital price differentials as most unfair inasmuch as the practice of hospitals in the aforecited States, and in other States where the price differentials are much less, is to shift the cost of the differential to the patients who are required to pay charges—namely, patients insured by insurance companies or those who self-pay their hospital bills. In recent years, this particular problem has become even more acute with respect to such governmental programs as Medicaid and Medicare both of which have reimbursement arrangements with hospitals wherein patients under these governmental programs are called upon to pay even less than they would under Blue Cross arrangements and far less than under insurance company arrangements. We estimate, for example, that the private sector insured patients, both the Blues as well as ourselves, are subsidizing the hospital costs of these governmental programs to the tune of some $3 billion annually.

In States where the Blues receive a moderate hospital price differential, competition is greater, with each of us sharing the market evenly. For those States where hospital price differentials are minimal or non-existent, our studies indicate that insurance companies represent the bulk of the market. I would hasten to emphasize, however, that in no instance does any one insurance company have a majority of a given market. Our companies compete just as fiercely among each other as they do with our friends in the Blue Cross. Thus, one of our recent studies indicated that well over 90 percent of a given company's newly acquired group insurance business represented the transfer or "taking over" of a group case from a competitor.

REGULATION OF PRIVATE INSURANCE COMPANIES

The authors indicate that insurance regulation favors the Blue plans. There is a further implication on this and the following page that regulation of insurance companies not very extensive. I do not know in what depth the authors researched this question but I can assure you, based on my more than 20 years of dealing with State insurance departments on behalf of member companies, that quite the contrary is true. We are extensively regulated and this regulation has been refined over the years. Under the present system of State regulation of insurance companies, standards are established before a company can obtain and continue its license, including standards with respect to assets, reserves, and investments.

Each company must file annual financial statements, and be prepared for detailed periodic examinations by State insurance departments. These examinations cover not only a company's financial condition, but other facets of its operations that come under State statutory requirements. The results are a matter of public record, with State statutes providing for corrective measures in the event of financial weakness.

In addition, each company must file for approval both individual and group policy forms in every State; and in many States, the premium rates to be charged for such policies. If the forms are in any way unjust, unfair, inequitable, misleading, or contrary to law, they can be disapproved by the State insurance departments. For example, one basis for disapproval of individual policies would be proposed premiums that are unreasonable in relation to the benefits provided. Premium rates under group insurance must meet not only the competition between companies and among other types of plans, but also the review of management and labor.

Each State specifically provides under the State Fair Trade Practices

Act that rates for any health insurance coverage cannot be unfairly discriminatory.

All States have enacted the Uniform Individual Accident and Sickness Policy Provisions which were adopted in 1955 by the National Association of Insurance Commissioners. These provisions relate to incontestability, grace periods, proofs of loss, cancellations, uniform type size, claims procedure, and other provisions to protect the consumer.

Further guidelines for policy approval are contained in a Statement of Principles developed in 1948 by the National Association of Insurance Commissioners. This Statement calls in substance for keeping the number of policy forms within practical limits, the use of clear and direct language, properly worded insuring agreements, assurance of protection against substantial hazards, a clear definition of "Limited" policies, policy names or titles that are not misleading, and other points to protect the public and provide orderly growth of the business.

In addition, all State insurance departments are set up to handle inquiries and complaints from the public, thus constituting yet another approach to protection of the consumer interest.

COMPLETENESS OF INSURANCE COVERAGE

In their paper, the authors present an interesting mathematical analysis of marketplace performance between the Blue plans and private insurance companies which reaches the conclusion that the Blue Cross and Blue Shield have a preference for more complete insurance. I would like to highlight the fact, as the authors have done, that their entire analysis is based upon a review of 1963 statistics on the adequacy of coverage and, most particularly, on a study by Ronald Andersen and Odin Anderson which was based upon household surveys of samples of the United States population. There are far more current data available which the authors in our opinion, could have sought out before going through the mathematics which was employed. My association has conducted a number of more recent studies on the adequacy of private health insurance coverage. I will mention just two. In 1975, we published a study which indicated an enormous growth in catastrophic health insurance coverage during the preceding five years, including trends toward providing unlimited benefits for coverage of medical bills incurred whether or not hospitalized and toward out-of-pocket limits on the extent to which a family would have to pay for deductibles and coinsurance. I understand that the Blue Cross plans have likewise experienced an increase in catastrophic health insurance or major medical coverage. In 1969, my Association also conducted a study with respect to the adequacy of group health insurance coverage then in force and found that over 80 percent of the charges incurred by persons covered under group health insurance plans were reimbursed by their plans. What I am suggesting here is that a more thorough review of the recent literature and the use of studies such as the foregoing might well have led to different results than those reached by the authors.

COMPREHENSIVENESS OF COVERAGE

The authors have chosen to define completeness or comprehensiveness of coverage in terms of the presence or absence of deductibles or copayments. Inasmuch as Doctors Frech and Ginsburg have properly defined their term, I would not quarrel with it. I would strongly suggest, however, that there are many other possible definitions for what is or is not complete coverage or comprehensive coverage. For example, is a policy with no deductibles and copayment but which pays benefits only when a person is hospitalized more complete than a policy with a deductible and copayment but which pays benefits for both in and out-of-hospital expenses including the costs, which are considerable in many instances, of the iong-term out-of-hospital treatment of a cancer or heart disease victim. I am suggesting that emphasis of insurance companies on the sale of high limit major medical policies over the past 20 years—to the point where 92 million people have such coverage with us—is far more comprehensive in my mind than a policy which pays benefits only when hospitalized. The use of deductibles and copayments have a number of significant advantages beyond the pure administrative advantage of keeping down premium costs. We have evidence to the fact that deductibles and copayments are important cost containment devices in that they discourage unnecessary utilization of health care services. A major medical policy, which pays for out-of-hospital expenses, does not force people into a high-cost hospital for treatment in order to receive reimbursement for their health care expenditures.

Just as we have evidence to the effect that deductibles and copayments serve as cost containment devices, we have seen no evidence to the effect that these devices discourage the use of necessary care.

Incidentally, another policy provision which appears in our major medical policies, and I believe in those of the Blues, and which also serves to contain health care costs, consists of the coordination of benefits provision. Simply stated, coordination of benefits prevents the insured individual from being reimbursed for more than 100 percent of the costs of his care when covered by two or more group insurance contracts. It also serves to prevent patients from seeking unnecessary care. A study which we conducted several years ago indicated that claim costs have been reduced by approximately 5 percent because of the coordination of benefits device.

REFERENCE

R. Andersen and O. W. Anderson, *A Decade of Health Services*, Chicago 1970.

Part Three

Insurance, Competition, and Alternative Delivery Systems

The Structure of Health Insurance and the Erosion of Competition in the Medical Marketplace*

*Joseph P. Newhouse***
Senior Economist
Rand Corporation

The recent proposals for new legislation to "contain" hospital costs have focused attention on the operation of the medical marketplace. It has been alleged that hospitals are "obese" because of the dollars provided them through private and public health insurance plans. The prescribed diet for hospitals envisions a limit on hospital revenues that has analogies with price controls.

Economists usually treat price controls as being either ineffectual or as interfering with the workings of a competitive marketplace, thereby creating artificial shortages. For example, both rent controls and controls on natural gas prices have been portrayed in this light. From this point of view, controls on hospital revenues or prices make little sense.

The case for such controls seems largely built around two points: (1) The rate of increase in hospital prices has been unacceptably high. Price increases have in fact been substantial; data presented below show that hospital prices as conventionally measured have increased at three times the annual rate of

---

* This paper is a nontechnical version of a paper prepared under the Health Insurance Study grant from the Department of Health, Education, and Welfare. The technical paper is entitled "The Erosion of the Medical Marketplace" and is available through the Rand Corporation.

** The author owes a considerable debt to Lindy Friedlander and Sally Carson for careful data collection and computation. Rodney Smith and Charles Phelps were extremely helpful in pointing out an error in a preliminary draft; Will Manning, Bridger Mitchell, and David Salkever also gave me helpful comments. I am grateful to the Social Security Administration for providing me unpublished data on dental and drug insurance coverage.

The research on the technical version of the paper was performed pursuant to the Health Insurance Study grant from the U.S. Department of Health, Education, and Welfare, Washington, D.C. The opinions and conclusions expressed herein are solely those of the author and should not be construed as representing the opinions or policy of any agency of the United States Government.

[Ed. note: The "Comment" on this paper was unavailable].

the Consumer Price Index over the 1949-1974 period. (2) Widespread health insurance has "lowered consumer resistance" to substantial price increases.

The first point cannot lend much strength to a price control strategy, because rates of price increase can be very large in competitive markets if, for example, input (factor) prices are increasing rapidly or if the nature of the product is changing rapidly. If the market for hospital services were competitive, there is a presumption that consumers would be made worse off by precluding the price increases. Hence, the case for controls cannot rest solely on the first point, that increases have been large.

We thus come to the second point, the role of health insurance in affecting the amount of price competition, thereby inducing price increases. Health insurance in the United States is largely sold as basic health insurance or major medical health insurance (or both). Basic hospital policies typically pay for either the full cost of a stay up to a maximum number of days or dollars (service benefits) or a given number of dollars per day (indemnity benefits). The latter type of policy usually, although not always, covers the daily charge in practice. Major medical policies pay a stipulated fraction of the total cost (typically 80 percent) above a deductible which is usually on the order of $50 or $100 per person per year. For our purposes, it is sufficient to characterize health insurance as subsidizing each unit of purchase by a fraction denoted as I; thus, for each unit of purchase (day in hospital, visit to physician), the consumer pays an amount equal to 1-I times the price charged by the provider. If, for example, the consumer has full insurance, I equals one. This is exactly like major medical and service benefits. Indemnity benefits are somewhat different, but since in practice they often cover all expenses, the differences can be ignored for present purposes.

What is the effect of such insurance on the medical marketplace? The tale implicit in many discussions of medical prices can be told with the following diagram:

Figure 1

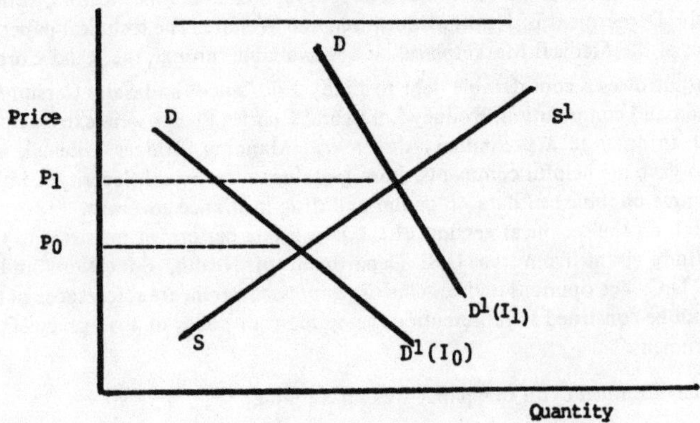

SS^1 is an industry supply curve; $DD^1(I_0)$ and $DD^1(I_1)$ are two market demand curves that are drawn for two levels of insurance coverage ($I_1 > I_0$). When insurance increases from I_0 to I_1, the demand curve rotates clockwise. The equilibrium price rises from P_0 to P_1. The important points of the tale, however, are that the market is assumed to be competitive, and that an equilibrium price exists. Because the market is assumed to be competitive, price controls are presumptively bad policy.

But is the market in fact competitive? Consider the implication of an equilibrium price. As insurance increases, prices will increase during an adjustment period, but at some point the effect of the increase in insurance will be fully registered, and price increases on account of the change in insurance should cease. Thus, *changes* in price are related to *changes* in insurance and not to *levels* of insurance. This distinction will form the basis of the empirical tests of competitiveness discussed below. Unfortunately, the empirical tests are complicated because any given change in insurance has a larger effect on price at higher levels of insurance. This can be seen by inspecting figure 1. If, for example, a given increase in insurance causes the demand curve to rotate from 10 o'clock to 11 o'clock, price will increase from P_0 to P_1. A further increase that causes the demand curve to rotate from 11 o'clock to 12 o'clock (i.e., become perfectly inelastic) will cause an even greater increase in price. Technically, there is an interaction between a change in insurance and the level of insurance, such that a given change in insurance has larger effects on price at higher levels of insurance. (This is proved in the technical version of the paper.)

The problem addressed in this paper is whether observed behavior in the medical market appears to be more consistent with a competitive model or an alternative model sketched below. To anticipate the conclusions, I find that there is some evidence that the competitive model does not predict well for hospital services, although for other medical services the predictions of the competitive model are consistent with the data. The findings thus provide some justification for revenue or price controls on hospitals, although an alternative remedy designed to enhance competition may well be preferable, as discussed in the concluding section.

Before sketching alternative models of the medical marketplace, some discussion of forces other than insurance that could cause prices to rise is warranted. Increases in income will cause demand for most goods to rise; if supply is less than perfectly elastic, prices will rise. Increases in income should increase the demand for medical services, and as a result, the empirical work seeks to control for the effect of changes in income on changes in price. Similarly, increases in the cost of inputs (factors) will cause product prices to rise. Medical care services use a wide variety of factors, and I have not attempted to develop a factor price index for each type of medical care service. Rather, as an approximation to changes in factor costs, I have used changes in the Gross National Product deflator to account for changes in factor costs.

Two other influences on medical prices are omitted from the empirical work below because of a difficulty in measuring them simply or meaningfully. The first is the supply of services. However, virtually any measure of the supply of medical inputs (e.g., short-term general hospital beds) shows steady increases over the past several years, so behavior of physical supplies cannot be used to explain price increases.

The second omitted influence is productivity. Medical care is a service industry, and service industries show a lower rate of productivity growth than other industries (Victor Fuchs). This would explain some of the relative price increase. But the price change that can be accounted for in this manner is the differential between the rate of productivity increase in medical care and the rest of the economy. Therefore, assuming productivity in medical care is not decreasing, an upper limit on the amount of price change that could be attributed to differential productivity change is the increase in productivity in the remainder of the economy. John Kendrick (table 3-2) estimates this to be around three percent annually in the 1948-66 period. Fuchs (table 15) estimated that the differential increase in productivity between all services and the rest of the economy was around two percent per year. We do not have an estimate of productivity change for medical care (as opposed to all services), but an estimate of productivity change for physician services concluded that over the 1955-65 period it was around three percent per year (Uwe Reinhardt, table 3-5). Thus, differential changes in productivity could explain perhaps a one to two percentage point increase in relative price each year. While this is nontrivial, there is a substantial portion of hospital price increases that remains to be explained (see the figures in table 1, below).

INSURANCE AND INDUCED TECHNOLOGICAL CHANGE

The simple supply and demand curves presented above assumed a given technology and a given product. As is well known, there has been considerable technological change in medical care. It is frequently stated that technological change in medical care has led to cost increases.[1] In fact, as Martin Feldstein (1971) several years ago pointed out, technological change could reduce cost as well as increase it. While this argument is correct in a general market, I shall argue that insurance (as presently structured) introduces a distortion so that technological change tends to increase the rate of medical care price and expenditure increases relative to a competitive market.[2]

A standard distinction in the literature on technological change is between product and process innovation. Product innovation leads to new products that enable new capabilities to be attained (e.g., the EMI Scanner, coronary care units); process innovations reduce the cost of existing products. In a competitive industry, process innovations will always be adopted; product innovations may or may not be adopted, depending upon whether sufficient demand exists for the product.

As the level of insurance increases, the rate of product innovation should rise; even if uninsured consumers were not willing to pay the entire cost of certain products, they may be willing to pay some fraction of the cost (with their insurance paying the rest). For a given rate of change in knowledge, therefore, there should be a greater rate of observed product innovation, the greater is the level of insurance. Moreover, it is reasonable to suppose that the rate of growth of knowledge is approximately constant from year to year.[3] The rate of adopted technological change in medical care is then a constant that depends upon the level of insurance. The higher the *level* of insurance, the higher the constant. It follows that the rate of expenditure growth will be higher with more insurance because some new medical care products will be bought each year that would not otherwise be bought.

Whether the rate of measured price increase (as opposed to expenditure increase) will be higher if the level of insurance is higher depends upon accounting conventions for unit price. Conceptually, a price index is for a given market basket and problems arise when new goods are introduced. In practice, medical care price indices are typically measured per visit, per admission, or per day in the hospital. Because product change will typically add to the products (services) that can be consumed during a visit, day, etc., the usual price indices will increase faster, the faster is product-enhancing technological change. Because the rate of change is a function of the level of insurance, the measured rate of price change will also be related to the *level* of insurance.

The thrust of the above argument is that insurance has induced too rapid technological change, and that this technological change has added to cost. It follows that there are too many resources devoted to product-enhancing technological change. Unfortunately, this argument is difficult to test, because it is difficult to distinguish between high levels of insurance causing too rapid technological change and high levels of insurance causing given changes in insurance to have larger effects on price (the interaction effect described above).

INSURANCE AND SEARCH BEHAVIOR

A different modification of the competitive model focuses upon the incentives facing the consumer (and/or the physician acting as an agent) to search for the lowest cost supplier of a given product. This modification attempts to make the introductory statement concerning the effect of insurance on lowering consumer resistance more formal.

A fundamental result of the competitive model is that inefficient firms are driven out of business. This result follows from the assumption that consumers maximize utility for a given level of income, but it assumes that the consumer benefits from locating a lower cost supplier of a similar product.

With complete insurance (I=1), the consumer does not receive any benefit from receiving services at a lower cost supplier. If he searches at all, it is because the "quality" (i.e., productivity) of service may vary among providers, and he is interested in the highest quality provider. Even though any single consumer is insured, a competitive *market* may continue to exist if completely (or nearly completely) insured consumers constitute a relatively small fraction of the market. In that case, there is a substantial number of uninsured (or nearly uninsured) consumers, and those consumers should be willing to arbitrage among alternative suppliers. It might be thought that some hospitals could specialize in insured patients and avoid the arbitrage; however, if insurance companies pay only the market rate, there is no advantage to specialization. It is interesting to consider the phrase "usual, customary, and reasonable" in this light. When insurance was a small factor in the market, insurers could observe a meaningful market rate, and define that rate as usual, customary, and reasonable. Insurance is, however, no longer a small factor in the market. At the present time, 92 percent of hospital expenditures are insured, and many of those expenditures that are not insured are for particular services that are not insured (such as maternity), or are for deductibles that are exceeded during the stay and so do not affect choice of hospital. In this context, a market rate cannot be observed (or has little meaning because the firms can essentially ignore the noninsured market in making pricing decisions). The phrase usual, customary, and reasonable then changes in meaning, so that for a given supplier it is defined relative to what other suppliers are charging the insurance company. If suppliers move their prices up together, say 15 percent per year, there is no check from insurers. Thus, if widespread, insurance operates to reduce the amount of price competition in the marketplace. It tends to convert the medical firm either into a monopolist facing a nearly perfectly inelastic demand curve, or a firm that competes on the basis of quality with little or no regard for price. In the former case, there is considerable scope for pursuit of goals that yield utility to the medical firm, but little to consumers; in the latter case, one would expect quality to be greater than consumers facing the true price would be willing to pay for.

Is there a way out through the effect of medical prices on demand for insurance? An increase in medical prices will cause insurance premiums to rise. Will consumers then buy less insurance, thereby reducing the rise in medical prices? The answer is theoretically ambiguous, and existing empirical studies of the question are both conflicting and far from definitive (Charles Phelps, H. E. Frech). However, the high rate of hospital insurance coverage despite persistently large price and premium increases is *prima facie* evidence that demand for insurance does not markedly decrease when medical care prices rise. Thus, in this model the usual link between the price the firm charges and its volume of business is weakened, and, in the limit, eliminated.

What governs prices in this world? Price changes are discretionary with the firm (hospital), a rather unsatisfactory outcome theoretically. One would expect that actual price changes would be large, because the firm could pursue its goals by raising prices. It is also possible that changes in factor prices would be much less closely related to change in product prices. But one must face up to the issue of why the firm does not adjust its price immediately to satisfy its goals; the answer may be that its goals evolve (satisfying behavior) or that there is some constraint on the rate of adjustment. Neither explanation is satisfactory from a theoretical point of view, and to the degree this model appears to receive empirical support, it is important to develop a theory of the firm that applies to these circumstances.[4]

To sum up, very high levels of insurance coverage structured like existing health insurance can erode price competition in the medical marketplace. It is reasonable to expect that such erosion will lead to continuing and large increases in price, although a model that is completely satisfactory from a theoretical perspective has not been presented. Nonetheless, this modified competitive model would predict that services that are nearly completely covered by insurance would show relatively large rates of price increase, while services that are not as well covered would not show such increases. It would also predict that the relationship between factor prices and product prices could be much looser for services where insurance is quite widespread than for services where insurance is a relatively minor influence.

SOME EMPIRICIAL RESULTS

Data were collected on the changes in price for four medical services: hospital services, physician services, dental services, and drugs. Table 1 shows descriptive statistics for the percentage change in the price of various medical services and the level of third-party payments for these services in the 1949-74 period. One measure of price change is the Consumer Price Index for the services. However, the Consumer Price Index for a semi-private hospital room is not entirely satisfactory as a measure of hospital

Table 1 Descriptive Statistics

Variable	Mean	Standard Deviation	Minimum	Maximum
Annual percentage change in expense per adjusted hospital admission, 1949-74	8.66	3.93	3.54	21.18
Annual percentage change in hospital semi-private room charge, 1949-74	8.10	3.85	3.41	19.76
Annual percentage change in physician fee index, 1949-74	4.09	1.99	1.47	9.12
Annual percentage change in dental fee index, 1949-74	3.59	1.77	0.49	7.63
Annual percentage change in drug price index, 1949-74	0.94	1.36	−1.55	3.53
Annual percentage change in overall Consumer Price Index, 1949-74	2.83	2.70	−0.97	10.97
Percentage of hospital expenditures reimbursed by third parties, 1949-74	82.3	6.7	62.7	92.2
Percentage of physician expenditures reimbursed by third parties, 1949-74	38.7	14.0	13.7	65.1
Percentage of dental expenditures reimbursed by third parties, 1949-74	3.3	4.9	0	14.7
Percentage of drug expenditures reimbursed by third parties, 1949-74	4.2	4.5	0.4	14.4

Source: See Sources of Data.

price, and so an additional hospital price variable is shown, the percentage change in expense per adjusted admission.[5] (The adjustment is designed to remove the effect of providing outpatient services on the costs of the hospital.) Expense per adjusted admission is a more comprehensive measure of unit price than the semi-private room charge, although the two measures are very similar in their first and second moments, as can be seen in table 1.

Sources of Data

Consumer Price Index: United States Department of Labor, Bureau of Labor Statistics, *Handbook of Labor Statistics, 1973;* Washington: Government Printing Office, 1973 (Bulletin 1790) gives values through 1972; United States Department of Health, Education, and Welfare, Social Security Administration, *Medical Care Expenditures, Prices, and Costs: Background Book;* Washington: GPO, 1975 (Publication Number (SSA) 75-11909), page 27, gives values for 1973 and 1974.

Expense per Adjusted Admission: United States Department of Health, Education, and Welfare, Social Security Administration, *op. cit.,* page 37, gives values for the adjusted measure from 1963 to 1973, and for the unadjusted measure from 1960 forward. *Hospitals, Guide Issue,* August 1, 1964, gives values of the unadjusted measure from 1960 and before. An adjusted measure was calculated from the unadjusted measure by multiplying the latter by 0.9, approximately the ratio of the two measures in the 1963-1966 period. The 1974 value is estimated from data in American Hospital Association, *Guide Issue to the Hospital Field,* 1975; the value of 878.95 equals the expense per unadjusted admission times the ratio of adjusted expense per day/unadjusted expense per day.

Third-Party Payments: Calculated at 100 (1-(Direct Payments/Total Expenditure)). Data on hospital and physician service coverage through 1973 are from United States Department of Health, Education, and Welfare, Social Security Administration, *Compendium of National Health Expenditures Data,* Washington: GPO, 1976, Table 12 (Publication Number (SSA) 76-11927). 1974 data (91.31 percent for hospital 65.075 percent for physician services) are unpublished estimates from the Social Security Administration. Data on dental and drug coverage are not available separately before 1970. For 1970 and forward data on these services are unpublished estimates made available by the Social Security Administration. Prior to 1970, two estimates were used that will bracket the true value. The first is the total of direct payment and private insurance payment; these values are again unpublished data provided by the Social Security Administration. This measure is probably quite accurate, but the resulting percentage third-party payment is somewhat understated. The second is to use the percentage of third-party payment observed in 1970 (9.96 percent for dental and 10.72 percent for drugs) for all previous years. This percentage almost surely overstates the true coverage in these years. The first method is used to derive the results presented, but the conclusions are not changed if the second method is used.

In the technical version of this paper, regression results are presented that attempt to explain variation in prices over time for these four services. In this paper, I will summarize verbally the results of that analysis. The competitive model, as well as the modified models discussed above, would predict that an increase in insurance would be accompanied by an increase in price. In general, the empirical results weakly supported this prediction.

There were two results that suggested a model that focused on reduced incentives for search behavior could well have some validity. The first such result had to do with distinguishing the effect of a higher level of insurance on incentives to search from an interaction with the change in insurance (meaning that a given change in insurance has a larger effect for more insured services). A variable measuring the level of insurance had a much larger effect on price changes for hospital services than would be predicted if the variable were only measuring an interaction between the level and change in insurance. The difference in size was on the order of three to ten times what might have been expected if only an interaction were being measured, and the difference was statistically significant. Such a finding is, however, entirely consistent with the model that focuses on reduced incentives to search for efficient suppliers. This model predicts that as complete insurance is approached, changes in the level of insurance could have substantial effects on the rate of price change because price competition is eroded. This very large effect of a variable measuring the extent of insurance coverage is not found for the other three services. Of course, an effect is not to be expected in the case of dental services or drugs, where the total coverage is small. Physician services are more interesting, because insurance coverage is substantially greater, although clearly much less than for hospital services. However, the results for physician services are much closer to those for dental services and drugs than they are for hospitals. The results for physician services are entirely consistent with a competitive model. But coverage for physician services is now beginning to approach the extent of coverage for hospital services. As this happens, these results suggest that price increase for physician services could markedly accelerate.

The second result that suggests a competitive market has been eroded for hospital services (but not for the other three services) has to do with factor prices. As mentioned above, the change in the Gross National Product deflator was used as a measure of change in factor prices. In the case of physician, drug, and dental services, this variable was related to changes in product prices. The relationship was statistically significant, and the size of the estimated effect was reasonable. However, in the case of hospital services, the estimated effect was statistically insignificant and actually had the "wrong" (negative) sign. Thus, while increases in factor prices are passed on with reasonable promptness in the other three sectors (this would be expected in a competitive market), there appears to be no consistent relationship in the case of hospitals. This need not mean that the price increases are not passed on, only that the hospital enjoys some discretion about whether and when they will be passed on.

An alternative explanation of this result is that the Gross National Product deflator is a suitable measure of factor costs for the other three industries but not in the case of hospitals. There is no obvious reason why this should be true; indeed, the industries draw to some degree on common factors (e.g., nurses). Moreover, hospitals use inflation in the general economy as an explanation of the rise in hospital prices (J. Alexander McMahon and David Drake), implying that a measure of prices that is economy-wide ought to be approximately correct for hospital services. I believe that the erosion of price competition is a much more plausible explanation of the lack of a relationship between changes in the Gross National Product deflator and changes in hospital prices than is the inapplicability of the GNP deflator for hospital services.

IMPLICATIONS AND CONCLUSIONS

I have argued that high levels of insurance can permit medical care prices and expenditures to increase at above-average rates independent of a change in demand that a change in insurance induces. Present insurance heavily subsidizes the marginal unit, and insurance premiums do not reflect choice of provider. Therefore, it is likely that the rate of technological change is higher than would be observed in the absence of such insurance and that price competition among firms is diminished (in the limit eliminated), thereby potentially giving the firm considerable discretion over its price. Both effects can serve to increase the rate of price and expenditure increase above what it would be without such insurance.

The empirical results, while not as firm as one would like, give support to this argument. If the argument is accepted, there are implications for both research and policy. For research, there are at least four implications. First, for those estimating models of the medical care sector, especially the hospital sector, the assumption of a competitive supply curve is a strong assumption. In particular, theories that seek to explain price rises from insurance as simply an increase in demand that presses against an inelastic supply curve may be missing an important part of the story. Second, estimates of welfare loss from insurance based upon the assumption of a competitive supply curve may be greatly understated (see, for example, the estimates of

Feldstein, 1973; and Emmett Keeler, Joseph Newhouse, and Charles Phelps, 1977; this comment also applies to John Marshall's (1974, 1976) critique of the other estimates).

Third, work is needed on theories of the medical firm (especially hospital) behavior. In particular, the nature of the constraints facing the firm needs attention.

Finally, the debate over demand-pull versus cost-push as an explanation of hospital cost inflation may have been largely beside the point. Cost-push theories have been tested by including in regressions of hospital cost a measure of the percentage of revenues derived from insurance that reimbursed cost (Mark Pauly and David Drake, Karen Davis), This variable has not been found to be associated with cost, and so cost-push theories have been rejected.[6] However, there is no reason to expect that the extent of cost reimbursement would be significantly related to cost; whether the hospital obtains reimbursement by quoting the insurance company a price ("charge"), which the insurance company pays, or by having its "costs" reimbursed should not be expected to affect costs. Thus, the existing tests do not really distinguish the two theories.

In fact, widespread insurance may make the distinction between the two theories moot. Insurance serves both to raise demand (demand-pull) and perhaps to grant the hospital an element of discretion (cost-push). One may argue that the hospital's discretion is arbitraged away by consumers and/or their physicians seeking the highest "quality" care (demand-pull). Either way, however, there is a substantial market failure. If the hospital has discretion, it can produce goods that provide it with utility, but may provide little or no utility to consumers; if its discretion is arbitraged away in the name of quality, resources that have little or no value to the consumer may be devoted to producing "quality." Moreover, it does not appear that the answer to the cost-push or demand-pull question has differential policy implications. Hence, resolution of the demand-pull versus cost-push issue would not seem to be of pressing importance.

For policy, the results are consistent with the view that hospital prices and expenditures could continue to increase at above-average rates for a very long period of time if present institutions are not changed. They are also consistent with the contention that additional insurance for other services could cause the rate of change of prices and expenditures for those services to increase. If these arguments are correct, three broad strategies may be pursued:

Do nothing: Proponents of doing nothing could argue that market failure has not yet been adequately demonstrated. They might also argue that the proposed cures are worse than the disease.

Regulate: This is the strategy currently being pursued; in its full-blown glory, it argues for public sector (or quasi-public sector such as health systems agencies) setting of budgets, at least for hospitals. More incremental interventions such as control of the entry of capital through certificate-of-need legislation are also consistent with this strategy. Proponents of this strategy argue that a market solution is either inappropriate (on equity grounds) or infeasible (on political grounds) in medical care.

A market-oriented strategy: There are two central thrusts that can be pursued as part of a market-related strategy. The first is appropriate only for nonhospital services (although the above results do not reject the standard model for nonhospital services). Insurance policies would be structured so that most individuals, most of the time, paid for their medical care services by including a substantial deductible in health insurance policies (which could be income related and need not apply to the poor). The tax subsidy to insurance would be ended. For hospital services, however, something else is needed. The desire to avoid large random losses leads to the public's desire to be insured, potentially creating the problems discussed in this paper. These problems would *not* arise, however, if the premium for the health insurance policy was related to the choice of provider and was higher for providers that imposed higher costs on their users. For in that case, inefficient providers (including those who introduced technological change at a rate consumers were unwilling to support) would lose business.

A health maintenance organization (HMO) is a device for relating choice of provider to the magnitude of the insurance premium, and if HMO's were more widespread, the amount of price competition could markedly increase.[7] HMO's are difficult to organize, however, and do not command a large market share. Fortunately, there are other ways to increase the amount of price competition. Several years ago, Vincent Taylor and I proposed rating hospital and possibly physician premiums on the basis of the unit price of the hospital (and physician) (Newhouse and Taylor); more recently, Paul Ellwood and Walter McClure have proposed rating physicians on the expenses they engender (Health Care Alliances). Both proposals should serve to strengthen price competition in medical care. There are questions of feasibility about both proposals; in addition, the Ellwood-McClure proposal could (but may not) introduce access difficulties for poor health risks.[8] In my view, both proposals deserve a trial.[9]

Thus, market-oriented solutions for hospital services may well be feasible. But when virtually the entire market is insured, health insurance as now structured does not appear to be consistent with the desirable properties of standard market forces.

NOTES

1. In the health services research literature, cost-enhancing technological change is often referred to as halfway technology.

2. Feldstein (1971) also reaches this conclusion, although his meaning is different from mine. His argument applies to a given state of knowledge and would not predict that the rate of price and expenditure increase would be related to the level of insurance. Put another way, if insurance were unchanging (but at a high level), Feldstein's model does not imply price increases, whereas mine does.

3. There is no evidence for medical care, but this appears to be the case in the aircraft industry. See Arthur Alexander and J. R. Nelson.

4. The possibility of discretionary behavior raises the issue of entry. Although nonprofit status, accreditation, and the like are barriers to entry, the important point is that price competition is unavailable to the entrant because consumers, by definition, are indifferent to the cost of the supplies. Hence, entry will not preserve price competition. In so far as entrants compete on the basis of quality, price and expenditure increases may be exacerbated.

5. The Consumer Price Index measure for hospital services was for many years based on the semi-private room charge. Room charges account for only around half of all hospital revenue, the remainder coming from charges for ancillary services such as laboratory, X-ray, and operating room, and these prices may have moved somewhat differently than room charges.

6. Davis finds the variable related to cost when data from across three years are pooled, but not related within year and also not when year dummies are included in the pool regression. She (correctly) infers that the extensiveness of cost-reimbursement is not the "true explanator."

7. Franklin Edwards has recently tested the hypothesis that the more competitive the environment for commercial banks, the less is the ability of a single bank to engage in expense-preference behavior. Edwards' test of expense-preference behavior is whether banks in more sheltered markets spend more on wages and salaries (add staff); he finds that they do. There is an obvious opportunity to test the same hypothesis for HMO's relative to the fee-for-service system, given that HMO's must compete on the basis of price, while firms within the fee-for-service system (especially hospitals) may not.

8. In particular, a provider who engenders expenses because he treats (on average) sickly patients must be distinguished from one who is simply inefficient, or providers will not wish to treat sickly patients. How well this can be done is an open issue.

9. One may reasonably ask why such schemes have not emerged. The answer may be that the fallacy of aggregation described above was not realized, or that medicine has colluded against them, or that legislation somehow precludes them, or that administrative costs render them impractical, or that there are unforeseen problems with them. A trial would settle most, if not all, of these issues.

REFERENCES

A. J. Alexander and J. R. Nelson, *Measuring Technological Change: Aircraft Turbine Engines,* Santa Monica, 1972.

K. Davis, "Theories of Hospital Inflation: Some Empirical Evidence," *J. Human Resources,* Spring 1973, 181-201.

P. Ellwood and W. McClure, "Health Delivery Reform," mimeo, 1976.

F. R. Edwards, "Managerial Objectives in Regulated Industries: Expense-Preference Behavior in Banking " *J. Polit. Econ.,* Feb. 1977, 147-162.

M. S. Feldstein, *The Rising Cost of Hospital Care,* Washington 1971.

______, "The Welfare Loss From Excess Health Insurance," *J. Polit. Econ.,* March/April 1973, 251-280.

H. E. Frech, "Comment on Paper by Charles E. Phelps," in *The Role of Health Insurance in the Health Services Sector,* ed. R. Rosett; New York 1976.

———, and P. B. Ginsburg, "Imposed Health Insurance in Monopolistic Markets: A Theoretical Analysis," *Econ. Inq.*, March 1975, 55-70.

V. R. Fuchs, *The Service Economy;* New York 1968.

E. B. Keeler, J. P. Newhouse, and C. E. Phelps, "Deductibles and Demand: The Theory of the Consumer Facing a Variable Price Schedule Under Uncertainty," *Econometrica*, April 1977, 641-655.

J. W. Kendrick, *Postwar Productivity Trends in the United States*, New York 1973.

J. A. McMahon and D. Drake, "Inflation and the Hospital," in *Health: A Victim or Cause of Inflation?*, M. Zubkoff, ed., New York 1976.

J. M. Marshall, "Moral Hazard," mimeo, Nov. 1974 (UCSB Working Paper in Economics, No. 18).

———, "Moral Hazard," *Amer. Econ. Rev.*, Dec. 1976, 880-890.

J. P. Newhouse and V. Taylor, "How Shall We Pay For Hospital Care?" *The Public Interest*, Spring 1971, 78-92.

M. V. Pauly and D. Drake, "The Effect of Third-Party Methods of Reimbursement on Hospital Performance," in *Empirical Studies in Health Economics*, H. Klarman, Baltimore 1970.

C. E. Phelps, "Demand for Reimbursement Insurance," in *The Role of Health Insurance in the Health Services Sector*, ed. R. Rosett; New York 1976.

———, and J. P. Newhouse, *Coinsurance and the Demand for Medical Services*, Santa Monica 1974.

U. E. Reinhardt, *Physician Productivity and the Demand for Health Manpower;* Cambridge, Mass., 1975.

The Emergence of Physician-Sponsored Health Insurance: A Historical Perspective

Lawrence G. Goldberg
Associate Professor, Graduate School of Business, New York University
and
Warren Greenberg, Ph.D.
Bureau of Economics, Federal Trade Commission*

Health care costs in the United States have risen considerably faster than the cost of living as a whole in recent years. In 1975, spending on health care rose at an annual rate of 12.6 percent compared to a 7.3 percent rise in the Consumer Price Index.[1] Whereas, in 1965, health care expenditures were 5.9 percent of gross national product, in 1975, they were 8.3 percent or more than $118 billion.[2] Many economists have suggested that increased coverage of health insurance is largely responsible for this rapid rise in health care costs. Between 1960 and 1975, third-party payments (both public and private) have grown from 44.6 percent to 67.4 percent of personal health expenditures and from 81.4 percent to 92.0 percent of hospital expenditures.[3] It has been convincingly demonstrated that this increased use of insurance has resulted in more services of a more expensive variety than consumers would elect to purchase in a market based on direct payment for services (Martin Feldstein, pp. 27, 28). Proposals to expand coverage of the population's health care expenses through a system of national health insurance have received serious consideration and are considered inevitable by many. National health insurance, however, if enacted, might increase demand even more than current insurance and compound the problems of rising costs.

Economic theory suggests, and experience indicates, that the injection of third-party payers into the marketplace need not result in uncontrolled costs. The costs of automobile accidents or of hospitalization are inputs into the service that insurers provide, and, as profit maximizers, insurance firms should have traditional incentives to minimize these costs.[4,5] In dental health

---

*The views expressed herein are those of the authors and are not necessarily those of the Bureau of Economics or the Federal Trade Commission. The authors wish to thank Professor Clark C. Havighurst for suggesting this case as an area for research and for comments on an early draft.

insurance, for example, many insurance companies actively monitor claims from dentists before authorizing payment for treatment expected to cost $100 or more. Under Aetna Life and Casualty's United Automobile Workers' benefits plan, several techniques are available for the investigation of questionable claims. Among them are (a) discussion with the attending dentist, (b) examination of dental X-rays, and (c) case review by Aetna's dental consultant when professional judgment is required.[6] That health insurance firms, by and large, however, exert little pressure to curtail these costs has been recognized.[7]

Are there imperfections in health insurance for physician services that cause health insurers to acquiesce to increased costs? Under circumstances different from the present, might one expect to find competition compelling insurance companies to review actively the procedures of hospitals and physicians in order to contain costs?

Experience in the State of Oregon in the 1930's and 1940's provides insight into the motivations and behavior of health care insurers. Prior to the creation in 1941 of the Oregon Physicians' Service (O.P.S.), the forerunner of the current Blue Shield system in Oregon, the State's health insurance industry consisted largely of private, for-profit hospital associations through which a patient was supplied physician and hospital care for a fixed fee under a closed and then open panel basis. Hospital association behavior was consistent with that of profit-maximizing firms since competition through cost-reducing measures was common. After the formation of O.P.S., however, the cost-reducing measures of the associations were gradually eliminated.

In 1948, the Justice Department brought an antitrust suit against Oregon Physicians' Service (O.P.S.), the Oregon State Medical Society, eight county medical societies, and eight physicians who were officers in these organizations, charging monopolization of the business of prepaid medical care and creation of territorial restrictions for doctor-sponsored prepaid medical plans. Although the Justice Department case was poorly organized and did not concentrate on the elimination of competition, the fact that the three largest hospital associations remained in the market after formation of O.P.S. critically damaged the Government's case. The Supreme Court affirmed the judgment of the trial judge ". . . That there was no conspiracy to restrain or monopolize this business." [8]

The first two sections of this paper describe the behavior of the hospital associations and the consequent emergence of O.P.S. The third section discusses the effects of O.P.S. on the health insurance industry in Oregon. The fourth section discusses the court decisions. Finally, the fifth section provides a brief analysis of the economic relationships in physician reimbursement. We conclude that, without O.P.S. or its equivalent in the marketplace, private insurers would have continued to play an active role in containing health care costs in the State of Oregon.

HOSPITAL ASSOCIATIONS

In the early part of the 20th century, a system of contract medicine developed in both Oregon and Washington State in response to hazardous working conditions in the lumber, railroad, and mining industries. These industries contracted for comprehensive medical and hospital care to be provided by "hospital associations" for a fixed fee divided between employer and employee.[9] Most of these "associations" were begun by physicians but were later managed by lay personnel. While some of them were financially strong enough to operate their own hospitals, others used the facilities of community hospitals. Originally designed to provide health care for employees injured on the job, the hospital associations gradually undertook insurance of all health care of employees and their dependents.

Many hospital associations began with closed panels of physicians and were similar to the health maintenance organizations (HMO's) of the present day. Like the HMO, the hospital association guaranteed a stated range of medical services and assumed the financial risk of health care delivery. Since many of the associations were profit-making firms, there were incentives to control the cost of medical care. Physicians worked either full- or part-time for the hospital associations as they do now for health maintenance organizations.[10]

In 1917, the private, for-profit hospital association movement in Oregon gained momentum when the so-called Hospital Association Act, permitting corporations to contract to provide medical and allied services without a medical license, was passed by the State legislature.[11] Previously, National Hospital Association, a physician-controlled association, was organized in 1913. In 1923, the physician-controlled Industrial Hospital Association was begun. Two smaller hospital associations, Weston and Pumphrey, entered in 1904 and 1926, respectively, but ceased operations in 1939 and 1940.[12,13] By December 1935, the for-profit hospital associations had disbursements of $843,727, or 60 percent of total hospital association disbursements in Oregon.[14,15]

The contract practice of medicine impairs a physician's ability to discriminate in the prices charged to his patients, and, therefore, in his ability to mazimize profits (Reuben Kessel). Because a physician is generally paid a fixed salary under contract medicine, he cannot charge different fees, based on patients' income, for the same services. In addition, as contract medicine began to evolve, it developed, according to the Oregon State Medical Society, "... commercial features which are in distinct contravention of established professional standards.[16] These features, compiled by the minority report of the Committee on the Costs of Medical Care and termed "unethical" by the American Medical Association, were:

(1) . . . solicitation of patients, either directly or indirectly;
(2) . . . competition and underbidding. . .;
(3) . . . compensation . . . inadequate to secure good medical service;
(4) . . . interference with reasonable competition in a community;
(5) . . . [impairment] of "free choice" of physicians.

Points (1) and (2) are typical components of a competitive market. Points (3) and (4) substitute the AMA's judgment for market forces. Point (5) reflects the AMA belief that third parties should not interfere with the patient's choice of physician.

Let us turn to the specific behavior of the hospital assocations in the State of Oregon in the 1930's. The basic policy of the hospital associations is presented in the following letter which the Industrial Hospital Association sent to physicians in November 1935:

> We solicit your cooperation in adhering to the following regulations:
>
> 1. All cases requiring major surgery, except in actual emergency, must be reported to the Association for authority before operation is performed.
> 2. It will be the policy of the Association to require consultation before authorizing major surgery.
> 3. No operation for hernia will be authorized until the same has been approved by the State Industrial Accident Commission or the Association has had the opportunity to make satisfactory investigation.
> 4. Hospital ticket or treatment order must be obtained in advance of giving treatments, except in the cases of actual emergencies. No bills will be paid without tickets being attached.[19]

Thus, the hospital associations in effect limited the doctor's freedom of action—a concept which has been traditionally considered an integral part of medical practice. Doctors were not accustomed to, and did not like, others, especially third parties, questioning their medical procedures. Because of the medical ignorance of most patients, doctors seldom have been questioned by their patients under the usual fee-for-service approach.

In addition, physicians' fees were scrutinized closely by the associations. Typically, when dealing with a patient, a physician can exercise some monopoly power. The patient is reluctant to search for the lowest priced physician, since he has neither sufficient knowledge nor information to be able to judge quality. Moreover, under the insured fee-for-service approach, the physician has little economic incentive to limit elective surgery, to limit hospital utilization, or to limit in-patient hospitalization stays. This is especially true if third-party insurance covers all of a physician's in-patient procedures. In Oregon, however, the introduction of the for-profit hospital association as an interested and informed third party seems to have resulted in upsetting the physicians' market position.

A sampling of letters, typical of those on the record in the Justice Department's case against O.P.S., illustrates how the private, for-profit hospital associations were able to restrain the physicians' market power as well as to alert the physicians to overutilization of facilities.

A letter written by the Industrial Hospital Association to a physician indicates that certain procedures would not be authorized without further investigation.

June 3, 1936

> In regard to the case of Ira Smith . . . we are assuming no responsibility for a hernia operation for any employee of a company outside of your district without having an opportunity to investigate the case before authorizing operation.[20]

Another letter from the National Hospital Association to a doctor questions the length of hospitalization for a patient.

December 28, 1938

> We have just learned that Mr. Kirk on whom you operated for appendicitis remained in the hospital until about December 19th. This seems rather a long period of hospitalization for a case of this kind, unless, of course, there were unusual complications. Will you, therefore, kindly furnish us a detailed report of Mr. Kirk's condition—including the operative finding.[21]

In the following two letters to physicians, the National Hospital Association indicated its close scrutiny of doctors' practices.

August 23, 1935

> . . . before authorizing this service (a cystoscopic examination and pyelogram) it will be necessary of course that we verify this man's eligibility to service at the expense of the Association. Also the

conditions as explained in your letter do not seem to be of sufficient severity to require the extensive examination for which authority is requested, and as experience has shown us these examinations sometimes result in stirring up inflammation rather than delaying it.

We hesitate granting authority unless it is absolutely necessary.[22]

July 15, 1939

On your bill for services rendered Oscar Homenyke you have charged for two X-rays of the chest. Will you kindly forward these films at your earliest convenience. . . . [23]

The hospital associations attempted to limit unnecessary surgery as indicated in the following letter from the National Hospital Association to a doctor:

January 3, 1968

We have your letter reporting further on the case of Harold Luhr employee of the Piggly-Wiggly Company. If this man is entitled to treatment at the expense of the Association and if he is suffering from acute attack of appendicitis necessitating an operation, the Association authorizes you to proceed. We, however, do not authorize appendicitis operations at our expense as a preventive for some future attack.[24]

The following exchange of letters between the National Hospital Association and a physician demonstrates how the hospital associations attempted to reduce doctor's fees and the doctor's opposition to these attempts. NHA to doctor:

September 30, 1939

We received a statement from you for care of Frank Robinson, an employee of the Smith Wood Products Company, whom you operated for a thyro-glossal cyst August 5. Your charge for care of this case seems to be out of proportion for services rendered when comparing it with other fees paid by the association for similar conditions. There is a charge for \$2.00 for examination of August 4, a charge for \$50.00 for operation on August 5, and an assistant's fee of \$7.50. Our understanding of the operation is that it would be considered a minor one. Therefore, an assistant's fee would not be in order, and the operative fee of $50.00, which also includes examination and diagnosis, is far in excess of what would ordinarily be paid.

Will you please review this account again and advise us if there was an error in presenting it.[25]

Reply by the doctor:

October 2, 1939

In reply to your letter of September 30, I do not feel that a fee of $50.00 for the removal of a thyro-glossal duct is excessive. This operation is certainly as difficult as the removal of a thyroid and certainly much more difficult than appendectomy. I am sure that if you will ask any of the doctors on your staff, who are in the habit of doing general surgery, that they will agree to this.[26]

In the next exchange of letters between the Industrial Hospital Association and a doctor, the doctor did agree to lower his fees.

IHA to doctor:

March 14, 1977

A fee of $150.00 which you have charged for the Winn case is undoubtedly in line with your private fees, but it is higher than any hospital association can expect to pay under their medical contracts.[27]

Reply by the doctor:

March 19, 1941

In answer to your letter regarding the fees in the above account, I wish to let you know that I will accept the mastoid fee of $75.00 for the operation and an additional fee of $6.00 for the X-rays taken.[28]

A final letter illustrates how deeply involved hospital associations became in the practice of medicine. The beginning of this letter from the National Hospital Association to a doctor stated that the organization would pay for shots of cold serum for the treatment of a cold but would not pay for preventive shots since this was not in the contract.

October 19, 1938

> Concerning the advisability of cold shots, we recently noticed an article in, *The Journal of the American Medical Association* dated September 24 which would indicate that cold shots, either orally or by injection, are of little or no value. Hope you read this article and if so, what is your opinion.[29]

It should be apparent from these letters that hospital associations were behaving in a manner similar to the way informed consumers might behave. Since in acting as proxies for consumers, the hospital associations did have to compete on the basis of quality as well as price, they would have to follow consumer desires or lose their insureds to competitors.[30]

The question arises as to why doctors continued to cooperate with the hospital associations even though the association policies interfered with the doctor-patient relationship. The answer seems to be that the hospital associations were serving a useful economic purpose for the doctors, guaranteeing payment for services by those struck with medical expenditures which they might not otherwise have been able to afford. This was especially true in the Depression when doctors found it more difficult than usual to collect from patients. In order to ignore the hospital associations, the doctors needed an alternative form of payment guarantee. This they began to develop in the 1930's and finally made effective in the 1940's.[31]

EMERGENCE OF O.P.S.

The reaction of organized medicine in Oregon to the practice of the for-profit hospital associations can be divided into two periods. In the first period (prior to 1941) the strategy consisted of (1) policy statements issued by the medical societies to warn physicians that contract medicine was unethical; (2) formation of alternative prepaid plans sponsored by the county medical bureaus; and (3) expulsion of "unethical" physicians from the county medical societies. In the second period, organized medicine began its own statewide insurance company, O.P.S., in order to eliminate the restraints of the hospital associations on health care cost and the accompanying interference with practice decisions.

In many ways the behavior of physicians was not unlike the behavior of other groups in society threatened with a reduction in income due to competition. It is well known that many regulatory agencies, for example, were established in order to circumvent the market by eliminating competition.[32]

In February 1936, the Council of the Oregon State Medical Society, cognizant of the growth of the hospital association, adopted a *Statement*

Concerning the Enforcement of the Principles of Medical Ethics. Essentially, the statement condemned commercial hospital associations for engaging in unethical practices such as the "... employment of paid lay solicitors, and advertising in newspapers and periodicals and pamphlets distributed to employers and employees.[33] In addition, the Council found it unprofessional for a physician to be employed by an association "... which permit [s] a direct profit from the fees ... to accrue to ... (the) individual employing him."[34]

Finally, the Council recommended "that the members of component societies engaged in unethical contract practice through association with [a] proprietary hospital association ... cease such activities,"[35] and that a "... copy of *The Principles* be supplied to every member of the component societies."[36]

Apparently prepaid hospital care was ethical only if it were in the hands of physicians.[37] For example, as early as 1931, a medical service bureau organized by physicians "... to provide prepaid medical, surgical, and hospital care to low-wage industrial and commercial groups ..." In Salem was readily approved by the Oregon State Medical Society.[38,39] In August 1938, the Oregon State Medical Society adopted a formal policy and program which encouraged local or component prepaid medical care plans.[40] In June 1939, the Oregon State Medical Society even attempted to encourage the Industrial Hospital Association, one of its chief competitors, to become an approved agency "... consistent with the policy and program of the Oregon State Medical Society and the *Principles of Medical Ethics.*"[41]

The policies of the Oregon State Medical Society seemed to be in consonance with the stance taken by the American Medical Association which first opposed contract medicine and then reluctantly accepted voluntary insurance, but only under the control of the local medical societies.

In 1932, the AMA based its opposition to voluntary health insurance on past experience with contract practice. "Wherever they are established there is solicitation of patients, destructive competition among professional groups, inferior medical service, loss of personal relationship of patient and physician, and demoralization of the profession."[42] Faced with the threat of nationwide compulsory health insurance in the depression-ridden 1930's, the AMA finally endorsed the voluntary health insurance concept, so long as it was under control of the medical profession.[43] In 1937, the AMA, in view of increasing physician support of voluntary insurance, accepted group hospitalization under the control of hospital and physician personnel.[44]

The actions of Oregon's medical societies were similar. In a direct step to limit physician participation in contract medicine, the Multnomah County Medical Society (the largest society in Oregon with more than 50 percent of

State society physicians) first attempted to expel physicians because of a "violation of the Principles of Medical Ethics in connection with contract practice."[45] Initially, the Multnomah Medical Society established the Multnomah Industrial Health Association in 1932 to eliminate the lay-owned commercial hospital associations as well as to provide a prepaid medical care plan (for those with incomes below $1,500 a year) to insure payment to physicians.[46] After only three years of operation, however, a county medical society report stated the plan ". . . resulted in a decreased income for that part of the profession within the Multnomah Industrial Health Association from patients who are able to pay customary fees and in the loss of some of these patients by doctors outside the Association."[47] Furthermore, the plan had "no appreciable effect" on commercial hospital associations.[48] In view of these "failures," the Society began to censure and expel physicians connected with commercial hospital associations for violation of medical ethics.[49] In addition, the Society required members of its own Multnomah Industrial Health Association to appear before the Board of Censors for unethical tactics.[50] Moreover, for some physicians, the mere threat of expulsion or censure was great enough to prompt resignation from the association, although the absence of an insurance-guaranteed payment undoubtedly hurt physicians.[51] By late 1939, the Oregon State Medical Society was urging all local societies to take "disciplinary action" against any of its members for unethical practice.

The results of the attack of Oregon State Medical Society on contract medicine in the 1930's were mixed. Though some physicians were willing to resign from them, the hospital associations still grew. In 1935, the five for-profit hospital associations had disbursed a total of $843,272, or sixty percent of all insurance company disbursements.

In 1940, the three remaining for-profit hospital associations disbursed $1,045,914, or 51 percent of all insurance company disbursements.[54] Apparently the hospital associations were still able to capture a significant market share since they provided broader and more complete coverage throughout the State than did the local county medical organizations which were confined to single geographic areas.[55] Furthermore, boycott and expulsion tactics of the kind practiced by the Multnomah County Medical Society were, in 1940, held in violation of the Sherman Act by the United States Court of Appeals for the District of Columbia.[56] The Court ruled the AMA had prevented practicing physicians' accepting employment from Group Health Association, Inc., a nonprofit corporation organized to provide prepaid medical and hospital benefits. The Supreme Court later affirmed the decision, and ruled that the fact that the defendants were physicians and medical organizations did not exempt them from the law ". . . if the purpose and effect of their conspiracy was such obstruction and restraint of Group Health."[57] If the growth of hospital associations was to be curtailed by the medical society in the State of Oregon a new strategy would have to be developed.

That new strategy, employed in the second period of opposition to the hospital associations, included the introduction by the State medical society of a statewide medical plan, the Oregon Physicians' Service, and a refusal by physicians to deal directly with hospital associations—a step which would destroy the ability of the private plans to control costs. Since subscribers could use the services of O.P.S. throughout the State, hospitalization in a county other than that of residence would not preclude collection of benefits. Moreover, only one plan need be promoted and sponsored by physicians.[58] In order to make the plan more attractive to doctors, stock in O.P.S. would be controlled by physicians who would not attempt to interfere with the doctor-patient relationship. With these advantages, only the most renegade physicians would not value membership.

In essence, the development of the Oregon Physicians' Service was instituted to eliminate the practices of insurers by creating, in effect, a vertically integrated structure and payment. The costs of monitoring physician behavior by the private insurers would become substantial, as shown below.

We have already shown that, despite physician opposition, associations were able to grow between 1935 and 1940. If a large portion of physicians chose not to cooperate with them, association growth could be curtailed. Given the desire of physicians for insured patients, physicians could be persuaded not to cooperate with the associations only if they could turn to their own physician-controlled health insurance as an alternative. It follows that the more patients enrolled in a physician-controlled insurance plan the less costly it is for physicians to reject hospital association insurance when cost-cutting occurs. Furthermore, for physicians who would not or could not understand the value of O.P.S., denial of O.P.S. membership could be a severe discipline.[59]

This strategy was implemented when the Oregon Physicians' Service was begun in December 1941 as a prepaid medical, surgical, and hospital plan. In addition, special services such as X-rays, physical therapy, and ambulance service were included.[60] By the mid-1940's, O.P.S. operated in 32 of Oregon's 36 counties, while cooperating fully with the county medical society plans of Clackamus, Coos, Lane, and Klamath Counties.[61] Each local society controlled the day-to-day activities of the O.P.S. in its district, although the State medical society seemed to control overall policy in matters such as territorial allocations, fees, and coverage.[62]

Like most present-day Blue Shield arrangements, O.P.S. paid cooperating physicians and hospitals on a service basis (claims paid directly to physicians) rather than an indemnity basis (claims paid directly to patients). A flat fee schedule was used to determine payment for each medical or surgical procedure. Physicians who were not "cooperating" had to incur the additional expense of billing patients directly. Membership and eligibility for stockholder status were open to any physician who was a member in good standing of the local medical society.[63]

The growth of O.P.S. was substantial between its formation and the date of the Justice Department complaint in 1948. In early 1942, O.P.S. had less than 5,000 subscribers, but by July 1943, it had 70,000, and by July 1948, nearly 100,000.[64] Disbursements by 1948 were nearly one-third of total health insurance disbursements.[65] This growth was undoubtedly the result of the medical profession's preference for O.P.S. The physicians finally had a statewide insurance plan which would cover their costs, but would not question their procedures. There were, in effect, no third-party controls on physician behavior. For example, a witness for the defense testified that O.P.S. never questioned the number of gastro-intestinal tests performed on a patient in a single year.

> A. Well, we never had to write in for authority on that. We go ahead and do the work and give them our reasons for doing it and it's always been satisfactory.[66]

This lack of third-party control was verified by the general manager of the Oregon Physicians' Service.

> Q. Well, does O.P.S. ever try to regulate doctors in the manner in which they treat patients who are subscribers to O.P.S.?
>
> A. No, we don't.[67]

Although it did not interfere with physicians' procedures, O.P.S. did not always pay whatever the physician billed. A letter from a member physician illustrates this point, and reveals some reasons for the founding of O.P.S.

> October 1, 1948
>
> I have refused to be on the panel of the O.P.S. because fees allowed for internists have been ridiculously small. The fee schedule makes it impossible for me to participate in your activities.
>
> . . . . . .
>
> Just why we should have cut-rate fees in order to fight hospital associations (it was the original purpose in organizing the O.P.S.) I cannot see, but I do wish you to bring this letter before the

attention of your board and see if some just method of compensation can be arrived at for internists.[68,69]

The great majority of the active membership in the Oregon State Medical Society became members of the O.P.S. By the middle of the first year of operation, 95 percent of the membership of the Society and 85 percent of all licensed practitioners in Oregon belonged to O.P.S.[70]

At the same time, the importance of the hospital associations began to diminish. By June 1944, the general manager of O.P.S. was able to boast that his plan was already larger than all of the commercial organizations combined.[71] In 1948, the three remaining for-profit hospital associations made approximately 24 percent of total health insurance disbursements, down from 51 percent of all disbursements at the end of 1940.[72] Moreover, during this period the level of health insurance disbursement increased nearly fivefold in Oregon.

The reasons for the relative decline in hospital association disbursements can be readily understood. One had to be a member "in good standing" of the county medical societies in order to be eligible for O.P.S. membership.[73] Although there were no outright expulsions from any society for cooperating with the hospital associations, it seems that non-cooperation with associations was at least an implicit requirement for membership and for a "good standing" rating. In addition, county medical societies inhibited the growth of the associations by their encouragement of physician refusal to accept "tickets" for medical work performed.

Tickets were provided to patients by the associations to be shown as evidence to the physician that the patient belonged to such an association. A cooperating physician would take the ticket and bill the association directly. If the physician refused to accept the ticket, the patient would be liable for payment to the physician. An association which would subsequently reimburse the patient for less than the physician's charge (after a determination that a physician's procedures were unwarranted or too costly) would find itself in disfavor with the patient.

A letter from a physician to the National Hospital Association is illustrative of a physician's refusal to accept tickets:

December 29, 1943

In answer to your letter of December 27, I wish to state that it is through no fault of the Association that I am not taking any more slips [tickets] by them, but I promised the Oregon Physicians' Service that when all the other doctors quit the National I would also. I am the last doctor to do so. . . .[74]

Another letter from a physician to a patient demonstrates the importance to the physician of O.P.S. membership:

> May 19, 1944
>
> Enclosed is the check which came in this morning to pay your bill. As I am on the list of the Oregon Physicians' Service, I am not allowed to sign a check of any other health association operating in the same district. . . .[75]

Further evidence that physicians were willing to go along with the county medical societies, even absent any viable threat of expulsion, is provided in the following letters to a patient and a lumber company:

> April 3, 1947
>
> This letter will serve as a means of establishing a diagnosis in your case with the National Hospital Association. Due to the fact that this hospital association is operated for a profit, members of the Medical Society are not allowed to make direct reports to them or to receive remuneration from them directly. . . .[76]

> April 3, 1947
>
> It is a rule of the Douglas County Medical Society that it's [sic] practicing physicians do not do any business with the National Hospital Association.
>
> However, the patient who is responsible to us for his own bill, is entitled to an itemized statement for his treatment. Such a statement is enclosed. . . .[77]

Finally, the major reason for the relative decline in hospital association disbursements was undoubedly the Oregon State Medical Society's support of its first statewide medical plan. For example, O.P.S. was even given permission to advertise in order to inform prospective patients about the "doctors' plan". . . .[78] Before O.P.S., only a threatened expulsion from a medical society could influence a physician to renounce the benefits of insurance of the associations; after its formation, the inducements to leave the private groups were far greater.

CONSEQUENCES OF O.P.S. ACTIVITIES

Faced with a rapidly declining market share, the for-profit hospital associations could either persist in their traditional cost-cutting procedures or abandon their aggressive tactics in anticipation of future doctor cooperation. Dr. Pitman, a witness on behalf of the defendants and former president of the Washington County Medical Society, indicated that the associations chose the latter approach:

> I started taking tickets again in March of 1948. By that time the hospital associations themselves had assumed the role of insurance companies. They no longer interfered with the relationships of the physician with the patient. They allowed the patient to choose any doctor in the community. They did not attempt to dictate to the physician what he should do for the patient. Their fee schedule had been adjusted upward so that it was comparable to the schedule of O.P.S., which is our own organization. It ran a little less, but they usually pay 100 percent, so it balanced out the same.[79]

In reply to a question about whether his experience with the hospital associations in 1948 was different from that in previous years, he stated:

> It is very much different yes. I think it was only the opposition of the doctors and the organization of competing hospital associations that has brought about the difference in the relationships.[80]

Thus, the refusal of physicians to "take tickets" forced the hospital associations to reimburse the patient directly rather than to pay the physician. This put the onus of controlling physician charges upon the patient and largely eliminated the ability of the hospital associations to control costs.

Three separate situations could arise in instances where physicians refuse to accept tickets. In the first situation, the insurance company agrees to pay the patient for the full amount of the physician's bill. The patient then pays the physician, although there can be a lapse of time before the patient is reimbursed by the insurance company. In the second instance, the physician bills the patient, but the insurance company pays only a portion of the bill. If the physician bills the patient for the remainder, the patient may be disillusioned with the insurance company for not paying the entire bill. In the third situation the physician bills the patient, but the insurance company pays only a portion of the bill, and agrees to defend the patient, if necessary, in a court of law. If litigation does occur, legal costs can be imposed on all three parties. Furthermore, insurance companies may not be able to assess properly their expected chance of winning in a legal action if patients' records are withheld from the insurance company by the physician.

Though their market shares decreased, the three for-profit hospital associations were able to continue in the market by changing their methods of operation.[81] The elimination of severe competitive pressures enabled the hospital associations to lead the "quiet life" under an O.P.S. umbrella. In addition, in the early 1950's, the commercial insurance companies entered the prepaid health insurance market in Oregon and by 1957 were able to secure more than half of total membership in all health plans.[82,83] We have found no evidence that these firms acted aggressively to control costs.

THE COURT DECISIONS

In our description of the Oregon case we have focused on the cost-reducing activities of the hospital associations as an important element of competition. Since creation of the Oregon Physicians' Service brought an end to this type of competition among hospital associations, we believe the mere existence of O.P.S. should have been the crucial issue for antitrust enforcement.

The Justice Department complaint charged the defendants with monopolization of prepaid medical care (the more important part of the charge), and agreements not to compete among themselves for the prepaid medical care business.[84] The Department further alleged that "prepaid medical care organizations other than those sponsored by the defendants have been prevented and hindered in entering into or expanding their business in Oregon."[85] The relief sought by the Government was consistent with its view of the case. There was no proposal to eliminate the physician control of O.P.S. Rather, the defendants were to be "... perpetually enjoined from further engaging in or carrying out said restraint and comspiracy, from doing any act in furtherance thereof, and from engaging in any similar conspiracy or course of conduct. . . ."[86]

The U.S. District Court for the State of Oregon ruled against the Justice Department in a misguided, irrelevant opinion.[87] Unconcerned that cost cutting by the hospital associations had ended, the Court was more disturbed by the "... trend and drift towards socialized medicine."[88] Apparently the Court was convinced that "... the purpose of the doctors in O.P.S.... was to save themselves and their profession from threatened socialization."[89]

In the main body of the opinion, the Court contrasted the events in Oregon prior to and subsequent to the formation of O.P.S. in December 1941. Prior to O.P.S., the Court acknowledged, some physicians would not cooperate with the associations, but subsequent to the formation of O.P.S. expulsions from medical societies ceased. Moreover, with the formation of O.P.S. a new competitor would be placed in competition with the privately owned insurance firms.[90] In any event, according to the Court, O.P.S. could not be a monopoly "since only 120,000 of 1,510,000 residents" in Oregon belonged to the organization.[91]

The Court also ruled against the Government's allegation that the State and local medical societies had agreed not to compete among themselves in any specific territory in Oregon. The Court's conclusion that "if the needs of the public are adequately taken care of in a particular county through the activities of local physicians, the profession's duty as to prepaid medical care in that particular county is fully discharged,"[92] ignores any benefits from competition among physicians.

In April 1952, the U.S. Supreme Court, in a 7-1 decision, upheld the District Court.[93] The Court seemed to be persuaded by the argument that, since any anticompetitive behavior by the Oregon State Medical Society and its members was abandoned with the establishment of O.P.S., relief that might be ordered would be unnecessary.

SUMMARY ANALYSIS AND CONCLUSIONS

The facts presented in this case, in contrast to the opinions and conclusions of the courts, reveal a great deal about the workings of the market for health care and the incentives facing the major participants. A careful analysis of the Oregon experience can lead to the development of an effective remedy for some of the current cost problems of the health care sector.

Before the development of O.P.S., the policy of the private hospital associations to reduce their payments to physicians was consistent with the effects in any competitive industry of individual firm efforts to reduce input costs in order to remain competitive. This active competition appeared to benefit consumers by reducing many medical procedures and thereby reducing premiums. By restraining demand for medical services, the associations were able to reduce prices charged by physicians.

It is not difficult to understand why doctors were so vehemently opposed to the practices of the hospital associations. Many physicians believe their profession is essentially different from any other profession or business because medicine deals directly with human life. The sentiment expressed by physicians and the medical societies that no one should make a profit from health appears throughout the case. However, it is essential to recognize the economic motives of physicians themselves.[94] Evidence of physician concern for their economic well-being is revealed in the letters and other materials presented in this case. In fact, the physicians appear to behave in the manner one would predict for any group which felt threatened economically and which also considered itself exempt from antitrust prosecution.

The intervention of an interested and informed third party into the doctor-patient relationship would remove much of the market power which lack of consumer information has conferred upon the physician. No longer could the doctor deal with an uninformed consumer; he must, instead, contend with an informed buyer.[95] As discussed earlier, the strong market position of the doctor has allowed him to discriminate in price among patients. With an informed third party either paying the full charge or backing the patient who refuses to pay that part of the charge not covered by insurance, the doctor could no longer absorb as much consumer surplus.

As we have seen, the reaction of health care providers to the practices of the hospital associations in Oregon may be divided into two periods. In the 1930's, the main weapon used was expulsion or threat of expulsion from county medical societies of doctors who worked for hospital associations or cooperated with them. The loss of medical society membership could have serious consequences for a doctor. He could lose his hospital privileges, his prestige in the eyes of his patients, and his access to the physician-controlled county medical service bureaus. After the AMA decision of 1940, the Oregon medical establishment had to end the practice of expulsion and find an alternative way to combat hospital associations. The methods used prior to 1940 had not been very successful in encouraging doctors to stop cooperating with the hospital associations, for, without an alternative system of health insurance, the typical physician found it too costly to discontinue the relationship, even though he disliked association interference in his affairs.

The formation of O.P.S. provided a viable alternative to the hospital associations. Several county medical bureaus were already in existence, but the formation of a statewide company greatly strengthened the attractiveness of the doctor-run plans since patients throughout the State could be treated. Now organized medicine in Oregon could effectively advocate the boycotting of hospital associations by doctors and could successfully urge patients to join O.P.S., which was physician controlled and thus would not check on physicians' charges and procedures. As O.P.S. grew, the physicians' need for hospital associations to guarantee payment became less urgent, and they could afford to refuse direct dealing with the hospital associations.

It is important to recognize that the refusal of doctors to deal directly with the hospital associations was the factor which made it impossible for the associations to serve as a cost-cutting instrument, even though the hospital associations still could reimburse the patient for expenditures. In this latter situation, if the hospital association felt that the patient was overcharged or that unnecessary procedures were performed, it would not fully reimburse the patient. Since the patient is interested in receiving guaranteed payment of his health care costs, the patient would likely blame the hospital association and change his health insurance coverage. In addition, after

1940, the hospital associations often found it impossible to obtain full records of procedures from doctors; thus they could no longer effectively restrict unnecessary procedures. Faced with this situation, one would expect the hospital associations to eliminate their cost-control procedures in order to survive in the market.

The question arises whether it is necessary for the dominant insurer to be controlled by physicians in order to eliminate cost cutting by the other insurers. Without a physician-controlled insurance company, one would expect the market to produce an array of private insurers offering a variety of price/quality packages to consumers. Those firms offering a high premium and mild physician surveillance package might be the ones physicians would be expected to endorse. If cost pressures become too intense, however, there is always the possibility that the private insurer would begin to interfere with the doctor-patient relationship.

The Oregon State Medical Society case illustrates that competitive cost cutting by private insurers can occur under certain circumstances. Doctors will be unhappy about such an arrangement, but this is not surprising. All suppliers of services would prefer to deal with acquiescent consumers rather than with knowledgeable buyers who have incentives to question charges. The case also shows that a strong doctor-controlled insurance company can compel private insurers to curtail cost-cutting procedures.

The experience in Oregon suggests that competition among insurers was most effective in health insurance in the absence of physician control of the carriers. The existence of a competitive insurance market was an effective force in restraining rather than adding to health costs.

NOTES

1. Council of Economic Advisers (p. 124, table 34 and p. 71, table 12).

2. Council of Economic Advisers (p. 118, table 35).

3. Council of Economic Advisers (p. 118, table 35).

4. Apparently, auto insurers attempt to minimize automobile accident costs. Allstate, the largest stock company auto insurer, has led a nationwide campaign to require air bags on automobiles. In addition, many insurers examine the extent of accident damage before authorization for repair is given.

5. The problem of "moral hazard," increased usage due to a reduction in marginal cost in insured services may be more common in health than in accident insurance. However, coinsurance, deductibles, and vigilant insurance companies can serve to reduce "moral hazard" in medical services. See section I, below.

6. Aetna Dental Claim Procedures provided by Aetna to one of the authors, December 23, 1976.

7. Data from Blue Shield suggest that only 0.04 percent of benefit claims paid to physicians are disallowed because of questionable patterns of practice. Though it is difficult to suggest a hypothetical standard to which these savings may be compared, they appear negligible relative

to the cost-cutting procedures of the hospital associations in Oregon in the 1930's which are described below. See Ohio Medical Indemnity. See also *The National Underwriter and The New York Times.*

8. *United States vs. Oregon State Medical Society*, 343 U.S. 326, 337 (1952), affirming 95 F. Supp. 103 (D. Or. 1950).

9. See Louis S. Reed, (pp. 136, 137) and George A. Shipman, Robert J. Lampman and S. Frank Miyamato (pp. 7-9) for an early history of the hospital associations.

10. For a description of the health maintenance organization concept, see Clark Havighurst.

11. Record at 2168, *United States vs. Oregon State Medical Society,* 343 U.S. 326 (1952).

12. See T. H. Hammond (pp. 1, 2).

13. In addition to the for-profit hospital associations, two physician-sponsored contract practice associations, Eugene Hospital and Clinic and Hillside Hospital Corp., also were in the market. Finally, three medical service bureaus, approved by the Oregon State Medical Society, in which physicians practiced solely on a fee-for-service basis, sold prepaid insurance. These medical service bureaus were merged into the O.P.S. in the early 1940's. Hammond (pp. 2,3).

14. R.4810.

15. Market shares are calculated here on a disbursement rather than a revenue-received basis. There appears to be no significant difference between the two measures, however.

16. See *Statement of Principles and Procedures for the Control of Contract Practice,* adopted by the House of Delegates of the Oregon State Medical Society, October 10, 1936. R.2798.

17. Committee on the Costs of Medical Care (pp. 156, 157). See also Elton Rayack (p. 152).

18. Due to consumer demand for free choice of physicians and to opposition of organized medicine to the closed panel, the associations gradually allowed free choice of physicians while maintaining only a few physicians on their own staffs.

19. R. 6832 - 33.

20. R. 6836.

21. R. 6874.

22. R. 6931.

23. R. 6882.

24. R. 6959, 6960.

25. R. 6887.

26. R. 6887, 6888.

27. R. 7025.

28. R. 7026.

29. R. 7048.

30. Consumer desires should also dictate that competition among insurance companies would not result in excessive emphasis on cost control at the expense of desired technological change.

31. In a similar manner, the King County Medical Society in Washington State began to develop a physician-controlled prepaid insurance plan after boycotting the private contract practice plans. See Shipman, Lampman, Miyamoto (pp. 22-25); and *Group Health Cooperative of Puget Sound vs. King County Medical Society,* 39 Wash. 2nd 586, 237 P. 2d, 737, 1951.

32. See George Stigler.

33. R. 3691.

34. R. 361.

35. R. 3696.

36. R. 3695.

37. The Oregon State Medical Society disapproved of the C. H. Weston Hospital Association in September 1940, for the stated reason that ". . . it is not owned and controlled by physicians who are members of their local society and the Oregon State Medical Society." R. 3148.

38. R. 5193.

39, As in most other States in which physicians developed their own medical plans, the initial emphasis was on insurance for low-wage groups only. By insuring only low-income groups, physicians were able to receive payment from those most likely to default yet charge their more affluent patients what the market would bear. See Kessel (pp. 32-42) for a review of the development of physician-sponsored plans and the conflicts with private prepaid plans in Oklahoma, California, Washington, and Illinois. See, also, Hyde, and Wolff, and Herman Somers and Anne Somers.

40. R. 120. By 1940 five medical service bureaus, all of which operated as distinct organizations under the guidance and approval of the Oregon State Medical Society, were formed. According to the *Report of the Oregon Insurance Commissioner,* the five bureaus had 35 percent of the total "hospital association" market. ("Hospital associations" as summarized in the Report of the Insurance commissioner apparently included prepaid medical service bureaus.) See *Report of the Insurance Commissioner,* R. 4818 and R. 5189-5193, for a brief description of the medical service bureaus.

41. R. 5503. There is no evidence that Industrial Hospital Association ever accepted the offer.

42. *Journal of American Medical Association,* December 3, 1932, 1951, quoted in Elton Rayak, (p. 155).

43. Rayak (pp. 164-166).

44. Rayak (pp. 172-175).

45. See the letter from the Multnomah County Medical Society to Dr. Steagall Sept. 17, 1936. R. 4460-61.

46. See R. 2558, 2564.

47. R. 2569.

48. R. 2570.

49. See R. 5512, 5616, 5709 and Defendants' Opening Statement, R. 334-3.

50. See R. 6072 (letter from Oregon State Medical Society, dated April 21, 1938, to physician inquiring about ethical standards of Association). One aspect of medical ethics appears to be a prohibition against solicitation of patients (see R. 5512). Apparently, the initial lack of success of the Association forced it to engage in these commercial tactics.

51. See R. 4208, 4434, 3601 (resignation letters dated December 3, 1937, June 7, 1938, and November 29, 1938, from physicians to the Prudential, Pumphrey, and Industrial Hospital Associations.).

52. R. 2166-67 (letter from Oregon State Medical Society to Jackson County Medical Society, December 11, 1939).

53. In Washington State, physicians also tried the legislative approach in attempts to reduce competition. Helgerson reports that after a meeting of the Washington State Medical Association in 1942 on "medical economics," within "several months, a host of bills was prepared by State legislators for the 1932-33 meeting of Washington's State legislature." See Steven D. Helgerson.

54. See State of Oregon, *Report of Insurance Commissioner,* 1936 (R. 4810) and 1941 (R. 3829).

55. See letter from Industrial Hospital Association to Southern Oregon Credit Bureau, Jan. 28, 1939, R. 3575.

56. *United States vs American Medical Association,* 110, F.2d 703 (D.C. Cir. 1940); aff'd., 317 U.S. 519 (1943).

57. 317 U.S. at 528.

58. Cf. the differences in medical service bureau plans, R. 2326.

59. Cf. with Kessel (pp. 31-32). Kessel suggests that expulsion from the county medical society is the "most formidable sanction" to control unethical physician behavior such as price cutting (p. 31). Expulsion from the medical society can mean denial of hospital privileges for physicians. Kessel did not consider, however, the effect that denial of insurance plan membership would have on physician behavior.

60. R. 2060.

61. R. 2332.

62. R. 3518-3522.

63. See "Memorandum of Understanding" between O.P.S. and Cooperating Physicians of Jackson County, Oregon, August 24, 1942, R. 3470-71.

64. R. 2397.

65. R. 4866.

66. R. 1215.

67. R. 1661.

68. R. 3538-39.

69. It has been suggested to us that O.P.S. paid low fees to physicians in order to offer attractive low-priced premiums to subscribers—a form of predatory pricing. However, we found nothing in the record to indicate this directly, nor were we able to compare unambiguously the health benefit premium package of the hospital associations with O.P.S. See below (letter from Dr. Pitman).

70. R. 3520.

71. R. 4371.

72. R. 4866, 4829.

73. See letters from physicians to patients, R. 2121, 2127, and 2157. See also R. 5340, *Pretrial Stipulation of Facts.*

74. R. 2154.

75. R. 2157.

76. R. 2121.

77. R. 2121.

78. R. 6592.

79. R. 1580.

80. R. 1580.

81. Two of the five associations, Pumphrey and Weston, went out of business by the end of 1940, before the emergence of O.P.S. See R. 4818, 4829. (*Reports of the Insurance Commissioner of Oregon* for December 31, 1939, and December 31, 1940.)

82. Hammond (p. 9).

83. In 1974, Blue Shield covered only 16 percent of Oregon's population. See *Blue Cross/Blue Shield Fact Book,* 1975 (p. 17).

84. U.S. Department of Justice, *Complaint*, Oct. 18, 1948, Sections 32(a) and (i), R. 6-7.

85. U.S. Department of Justice, *Complaint*, Oct 18, 1948, Section 35 (a), R. 8.

86. U.S. Department of Justice, *Prayer*, Section 3, R. 9-10.

87. *U.S. vs. Oregon State Medical Society*, 95 F. Supp. 103 (D. Ore. 1950); *aff'd* 343 U.S. 326 (1952).

88. 95 F. Supp., p. 109. The Court quoted from an editorial in a bar association publication. Editorial, *Oregon State Bar Bull.*, Aug. 1950, p. 2.

89. 95 F. Supp. p. 109. The Court further warned in a self-protective mood that "the trend and drift towards socialized medicine should be all the lawyer needs to recognize that socialized law is but the next step for those dedicated to the socialized-police state." (95 F. Supp. p. 109).

90. 95 F. Supp., p. 116.

91. 95 F. Supp., p. 107.

92. 95 F. Supp., p. 107.

93. *United States vs. Oregon State Medical Society*, 343 U.S. 326 (1952).

94. The situation in Oregon can be viewed as an attempt by physicians to decrease the elasticity of the demand for health care by eliminating the price conscious element of the market, the hospital association.

95. Michael Darby and Edi Karni have used the term credence goods to describe goods which "cannot be evaluated in normal use" such as the removal of an appendix or the replacement of a television tube.

REFERENCES

M. Darby and E. Karni, "Free Competition and Optimal Amount of Fraud," *J. Law Econ.* Apr. 1973, 67-88.

M. S. Feldstein, *The Rising Cost of Hospital Care*, Washington, D.C., 1971.

T. H. Hammond, "Corporate and Organizational History of the Oregon Physicians' Service and Other Hospital Associations in Oregon," speech before the Oregon Physicians' Service Annual Statewide Staff Meeting, Feb. 27, 1958.

C. C. Havighurst, "Health Maintenance Organizations and the Market for Health Services," *Law and Contemporary Problems*, Autumn 1970, 716-795.

S. D. Helgerson, "The Founding of a Medical Service Bureau in King County, Washington - 1933," *Western J. Medicine*, Jan. 1976, 67-69.

D. R. Hyde and Wolff, "The American Medical Association; Power, Purpose and Politics in Organized Medicine," *Yale Law J.*, May 1954, 937-1022.

R. A. Kessel, "Price Discrimination in Medicine," *J. Law Econ.*, Oct. 1958, 20-53.

E. Rayack, *Professional Power and American Medicine*, Cleveland, Ohio, 1967.

L. S. Reed, *Blue Cross and Medical Service Plans*, Washington, D.C., 1947.

G. A. Shipman, R. J. Lampman, and S. F. Miyamato, *Medical Service Corporation in the State of Washington*, Cambridge, Mass., 1962.

H. M. Somers and A. R. Somers, *Doctors, Patients and Health Insurance: The Organization and Financing of Medical Care*, Washington, D.C., 1961.

G. J. Stigler, "The Theory of Economic Regulation," *Bell J. Econ.*, Spring 1971, 3-21.

Aetna Dental Claim Procedures, Dec. 23, 1976.

American Medical Assn. Journal, Dec. 3, 1932.

Blue Cross/Blue Shield Fact Book, 1975.

Committee on the Costs of Medical Care, *Medical Care for the American People,* Washington, D.C., 1970 reprint.

Council of Economic Advisors, *Economic Report of the President,* Washington, D.C. 1976.

Group Health Cooperative of Puget Sound vs. King County Medical Soc'y, 39 Wash. 2nd 586, 237 P. 2nd 737 (1951).

Industrial Hospital Association letter to Southern Oregon Credit Bureau, Jan. 28, 1939.

Multnomah County Medical Society letter to Dr. Steagall, Sept. 17, 1936.

National Underwriter, Jan. 22, 1972.

New York Times, Aug. 4, 1975.

Ohio Medical Indemnity, Inc., *Cost Containment Reports - Second Quarter 1975,* July 9, 1975.

Oregon Physicians' Service, "Memorandum of Understanding" to Cooperating Physicians of Jackson County, Oregon, Aug. 24, 1942.

Oregon State Bar Bulletin, editorial, Aug. 1950.

Oregon State Medical Society letter to Jackson County Medical Society, Dec. 11, 1939.

Oregon State Medical Society House of Delegates, *Statement of Principles and Procedures for the Control of Contract Practice,* Oct. 10, 1936.

State of Oregon, *Report of the Insurance Commissioner,* 1936, 1939, and 1940.

United States vs. American Medical Association, 110 F.2d 703 (D.C. Cir. 1940) aff'd 317 U.S. 519 (1943).

United States vs. Oregon State Medical Society, 95 F. Supp. 103 (D Ore. 1950), aff'd 343 U.S. 326 (1952).

Competition of Alternative Delivery Systems

*Alain C. Enthoven**
Marriner S. Eccles Professor of Public and Private Management,
Graduate School of Business, Stanford University

Competition serves consumers well in the production of many goods and services. It is the basic regulator of our economy, and an important factor in our high standard of living. It forces producers to offer better products at lower prices, and to offer a diversity of products that matches the diversity of consumer tastes. It has stimulated many desirable innovations. However, competition is not strong in all sectors, and even where it is strong, it does not always produce the best results. So while competition is usually desirable, increasing competition may not guarantee better performance for the consumer. A challenge for public policy analysis is to sort out exactly how competition works in particular industries and how it can be enhanced to the benefit of the consumer.

Economists have identified a number of conditions that must be satisfied for competition to produce optimum results. The economist's model of the competitive economy is made up of profit-maximizing firms that produce goods and services, and utility-maximizing consumers who pay for them out of their own incomes. Within the framework set by market prices, firms control the cost and quality of their products, and their quest for maximum profits leads them to minimize the costs of what they produce. Because consumers pay for what they consume out of their own incomes, they are cost conscious, and the prices they pay reflect their marginal valuations of the goods and services they buy. The health services economy in the United States today does not fit this model at all well. Think of one of its main products as being the treatment of a serious illness. In the predominant economy of independent fee-for-service physicians and community hospitals, neither the physician nor the hospital has complete control over the

* I wish to acknowledge gratefully valuable criticisms and suggestions on an earlier draft received from Scott Fleming, Harold Luft, and Arthur Weissman. However, the views expressed in the paper, and any remaining errors, are mine, not necessarily theirs.

cost and quality of this product. Each controls some aspects of it, and each responds to its own incentives. Not being profit-maximizing firms facing given market prices, neither has an economic incentive to minimize the cost of production. The insured consumer pays at most a small fraction of the cost of this product, so he is not cost conscious. Moreover, the natural barriers to competitive economic behavior in this market are large. It would be very costly for a consumer to attempt to shop around for a less costly product, even if he had the motivation. There is little competition among physicians. There is some competition among hospitals, but that is not to attract consumers by offering a better product at a lower price. There is competition among third-party payers, but in most cases they have little if any control over the price of medical care services. While competition forces them to hold down administrative costs, which is good, it also leads many of them to experience rating, which has socially undesirable aspects.

Sorting out the actual and potential effects of competition in health services is particularly complex, and it certainly cannot be assumed that any action that increases apparent competition will necessarily make things better for consumers. For example, increasing the number of surgeons in a community already well supplied with them may serve only to increase the amount of surgery with no discernible net benefit in terms of health status, to increase the amount surgeons charge per operation as they seek to protect their target incomes, to reduce their workloads and proficiency, and to increase per capita spending for medical care. Increasing the number of hospital beds in an area already well supplied may only increase the amount of hospitalization with no discernible net benefit in terms of health status, increase the number of empty beds, increase the daily costs passed on to the third-party intermediaries, and increase per capita spending for medical care. Increasing the number of third-party intermediaries in an area may merely assure that none of them has any bargaining power over physicians and hospitals for controlling costs.

The main purpose of this paper is to explore how different market structures affect competition, and how the market for medical care services might be restructured with alternatives to the dominant system of fee-for-service physicians, cost-reimbursed hospitals, and third-party intermediaries, so that the competition might yield more of the benefits that it yields in other markets.

SOME CHARACTERISTICS OF MEDICAL CARE DELIVERY SYSTEMS

Modern medical care in the United States is, for the most part, provided by systems of physicians, hospitals, laboratories, and other agencies, and most is paid for through financial intermediaries. These elements are interdependent; the behavior of each is strongly influenced by the structure and behavior of the others. The product the consumer receives is their joint product. A system may be more or less formally organized. For example, care may be provided by the very loose organization of individual physicians on fee-for-service and community hospitals, financed through third parties, or it may be provided by a tightly organized hospital-based prepaid group practice plan, or by any of a large variety of intermediate possibilities.

Competition between systems takes place in many dimensions, not just in cost and "quality" measured in one dimension. Medical care is not a standard product. Its many dimensions include the following:

1. **Perceived quality of care:** If one is really sick or injured, will one's providers of care bring about the best possible outcome? Or a good outcome? What do they consider to be good outcomes? Do they have good quality control? What are the attitudes of the personnel? Do they emphasize caring as well as care? Or are they impersonal and unconcerned?

2. **Basic value judgments about priorities:** In cases in which any course of treatment has a low or uncertain net marginal value in terms of health status, different physicians will have different value judgments as to what to do. If in doubt, is it better to intervene or not? For example, different physicians respond differently to the information that clinical trials do not support the effectiveness of a given procedure. Or, in a given circumstance, one may use more diagnostic tests than another. Different providers offer, and different consumers prefer, a more or less technological style of care. For example, an increasing number of mothers in northern California, including educated middle-class women, prefer to have their deliveries at home to avoid the costly high technology style of care (including routine fetal monitoring) offered in some of the leading hospitals. Different physicians and consumers see more or less value in checkups, screening, health education, and other forms of preventive care.

3. **Accessibility and convenience:** Different provider systems offer different travel times and distances, waiting times for appointments, and waiting times in doctors' offices. Some provide good access to physicians on nights and weekends; others provide none. Different systems ration access by different mixes of money cost, in the form of cost-sharing, and time cost in the form of waiting. Some systems require the consumer to keep detailed records and to understand complex cost-sharing provisions; others do the bookkeeping for him.

4. **Cost:** Different systems offer different total expected costs for a family's medical care. And different systems divide the costs differently among premiums, cost-sharing, and costs not covered at all. Thus, a family may be able to trade acceptance of a higher degree of risk for a lower monthly premium.

From a public policy point of view, the most important differences in cost are differences in the total per capita costs for comprehensive health care services for similar populations. Such variations can be quite substantial. They are not necessarily related to variations in the quality of care, or to the neglect of necessary care. The explanation for such variations is very complex and very imperfectly understood at this time. Among the many contributing factors are these:

(a) *Utilization:* J. P. Bunker, Paul Lembke, John Wennberg, and others have noted wide variations in the per capita consumption of certain health care services among similar populations without any apparent difference in medical need or health status. Clifton Gaus *et al.* found a large and significant difference in hospital and surgical utilization rates between Medicaid beneficiaries served by group practice health maintenance organizations (HMO's) and control groups served by fee-for-service physicians, with no significant difference between the study groups and their controls in terms of health status perceived, number of chronic conditions, or disability days per month. Various studies have noted similar differences between Federal employees and their families cared for by group practice HMO's and those cared for under fee-for-service.[1] Although these studies generally have not attempted to measure differences in health status, the beneficiaries have a free choice among plans, and apparently the ones choosing the group practice HMO's have not found themselves at a disadvantage in terms of needed health services.

(b) *Physician judgments:* There are significant variations in the judgments of different physicians as to how best to treat various conditions. These differences may or may not be influenced by differences in fees and costs, yet they have very different cost implications.

Since these variations are usually not related to significant differences in morbidity or mortality, the differences in their consequences, if any, must be in the general area of "quality of life" where there is a great deal of room for differing value judgments. So it is not a question of whether or not patients under one system or another will or will not have access to, e.g., coronary artery bypass graft surgery or computed tomography; it is a question of differences in marginal judgments about the indications for such procedures.

(c) *Resources:* There are differences in the amount of resources used to do the same number of procedures. One community or system might have several heart surgeries or CT-scanners to do a given number of procedures that another system does with one. Because average unit costs of heart surgery or computed tomography decline substantially with volume, the system that concentrates all the procedures at one or fewer facilities can have much lower unit costs.

(d) *Consumers* may be more or less educated as to how to use the health care system, and as to personal health practices.

So there is not a simple trade-off between cost and quality.

5. **Referral patterns and choice of physician:** To which specialist and hospitals will one be referred under what conditions? The choice of family doctor will have implications for referrals. Does the primary physician rely extensively or only a little on specialists? How is the consumer's choice of physician constrained or enhanced?

Moreover, different providers have different preferences. Some physicians prefer the freer entrepreneurial lifestyle of the fee-for-service solo practitioner. Others prefer the stability and freedom from managerial duties and financial concerns offered by an organized system. Since a physician is more likely to perform well in an environment that he prefers, these preferences should be respected and the physician should be free to choose—provided that his income is related to the value of his services within a financial framework that reflects his contribution to consumer satisfaction and responsible use of resources.

Public policy should recognize that there is good and legitimate reason for considerable variation in systems and styles of care. The variation is not simply a matter of cost versus quality. Quality comes in many different flavors, and it is a matter of physician and patient judgment, for the most part not reducible to numerical measures. There is plenty of room for product differentiation to suit the needs and tastes of different people. There is not a single pattern of care that is best for all people. Elderly people who prefer a program that emphasizes low-cost home care rather than high-cost technological care should be allowed to exercise that choice on a financial basis equal to that of people with the opposite preference. Time-poor money-rich professional people ought to be able to trade money for convenience while time-rich money-poor people do the opposite. The poor should not be required to take out their share of society's assistance in the form of extremely costly medical technology if they feel it would be better for their health and well-being to spend less on medical care (by choosing a less costly system) and more on food and housing.[2]

Thus, I believe it is likely that several competing organized systems, each emphasizing a different mix of characteristics and designing its program for a different market segment, can increase consumer satisfaction considerably over what would be the case if there were a single uniform plan. This principle has important implications for Medicare and for the design of a rational National Health Insurance program. Moreover, I believe that people are likely to be able to do a much better job of exercising an informed intelligent choice from among competing organized systems of care than they can picking their way through the occasional episodes of care provided by the fragmented fee-for-service, cost-reimbursed, third-party financed system because the costs and characteristics of the organized system can be better defined and predicted.

THE SIGNIFICANCE OF ORGANIZED SYSTEMS

In the system of (a) independent physicians on fee-for-service, (b) community hospitals paid essentially on a cost-reimbursement basis, and (c) patients well insured by third-party intermediaries, none of the actors on the scene has enough control over enough parameters to be able to offer, for example, a significantly less technological or more cost-effective alternative to the costly standard of care that predominates in our country. Each actor must respond within the limits and incentives offered by the economic framework in which he finds himself.

The ability of the individual fee-for-service doctor to offer his insured patients a less costly style of care—in exchange for lower cost to the patients—is very limited. As an individual, he has no influence over his patients' insurance premiums. He has some choice over where he has hospital privileges, and where he admits his patients, but he has little or no incentive to direct his patient to a less costly hospital. In most cases, at the margin (i.e., after the deductible), practically all the hospital bill will be paid by a third party, in which case there would be no way to pass the savings on to the patient. (This may not be the case for patients insured on a specified indemnity basis—so much per hospital day, etc. If the hospital exceeded the indemnity limit, the patients would realize the savings from choice of a hospital with lower charges.) On the contrary, the physician is likely to be rewarded for using more costly technology. The individual physician has very limited, if any, ability to induce the hospital to reduce cost. Given the financing arrangments, such a reduction would offer no direct benefit to him or his patient.

The typical community hospital operates in an environment of competition for doctors who bring in patients and cost reimbursement by third parties. Hospitals compete for doctors in a variety of ways including amenities, quality and convenience of facilities, freedom from controls, residency programs, and expensive equipment which allows the doctors to do costly procedures, for which they are well paid, and which build prestige. The general effect of this is to increase total costs. And, for the most part, the hospital can pass on the increased costs to third parties. Suppose that a hospital administrator sincerely believed that many people in his community would be better off with a less costly style of care. Suppose he were able to do such things as institute tighter controls on use of surgery and laboratory and avoid buying certain costly diagnostic equipment by referring patients to other hospitals. The first thing he would experience would be a loss in revenue, and since typically marginal costs are below average costs, a loss in net revenue. For each dollar he cut from cost, he would lose about a dollar in reimbursement from Medicare and Medicaid.[3] The next thing he would experience is a loss in physician staff as doctors took their patients to the hospitals offering the better equipment, looser controls, etc. So he would be punished for his efforts. And, assuming that their hospital insurance premiums are rated over a wider area, there would be no way that he could return much of the savings to the citizens in his community, so that there would not be many grateful citizens at his going-away dinner.

Under the arrangements that prevail today, most third parties appear to have few alternatives to paying the bills, provided the charges bear a reasonable relationship to costs, and the services provided are not clearly unnecessary. Most third parties have no serious leverage over the cost-generating behavior of the hospitals or doctors. Most third-party payment plans assure the patient of free choice of doctor and hospital, so they cannot direct patients to less costly doctors and hospitals, thereby creating pressures for cost reduction. Operating in the present framework, about all they can do is argue over extreme cases. (However, this could be changed if third parties were to form alliances with provider groups—to use Paul Ellwood's term—and to offer plans with a limited choice of doctor and hospital.)

While the fee-for-service, third-party payment system offers the patient a completely free choice among doctors and hospitals in his community (subject, of course, to their capacity and availability), it does not offer him the alternative of keeping the savings he would generate by choosing a less costly style of care. The premiums and charges he must pay reflect the cost-generating behavior of the doctors and hospitals in his community and the experience of his insured group. Moreover, his choice of doctors and hospitals is limited to those who work within the framework of incentives provided by fee-for-service and cost reimbursement. If he would prefer, for example, a system that used half as much hospitalization per capita in exchange for more home care or better access to ambulatory care, at an equal per capita cost, the fee-for-service, third-party payment system would not be able to offer it to him.

In contrast to the world of independent physicians, hospitals, and third-party intermediaries, an organized system financed on a capitation basis, such as a hospital-based prepaid group practice, can exert substantial influence over the variables enumerated above, and within the limits set by competition, standards of medical care, Government regulations, etc., can design its program to appeal to one or another segment of the market. It can make conscious policy choices and control trade-offs among the variables. For example, an organized system financed on a capitation basis, serving a defined population might de-emphasize hospitalization and apply the savings to improved access to ambulatory care. It might allocate more resources to convenient access and to a more personal style of care, at the expense of less use of specialty care. It might emphasize caring and home care at the expense of less high technology care. It might achieve savings from more efficient operations (e.g., higher occupancy rates) and apply them to broadening its benefits in areas such as preventive care and mental health. Thus, capitation-financed organized systems are not merely a device for financing the same bundle of services as that offered by fee-for-service, cost-reimbursed third-party financed medicine; and they are not merely an incentive scheme for lowering cost or utilization. Rather, they are a framework within which providers can offer very different product mixes, emphasizing different values, depending on the tastes of the consumers served.

Of course, the fact that a system is organized does not assure that it is in a position to control all of these variables. Between the large hospital-based prepaid group practice (PGP) serving a defined population on a capitation basis and the world of independent fee-for-service physicians, community hospitals, and third parties, there are many intermediate possibilities. And the specific details of their arrangements can make a great deal of difference. For example, a PGP that is largely dependent on one community hospital may have little control over hospital per diem costs. It may have to pay a share of the costs of expensive equipment whether or not its physicians consider the benefits to be worth the costs. Its degree of control may be limited to control over the utilization by its own members. The PGP's market power will be enhanced by its size (relative to the hospital's market), and by availability of other less costly hospitals. A Medical Care Foundation (or Individual Practice Association) may have more or less influence over the practice patterns of its member physicians depending on what percentage of the physicians' incomes depend on the Foundation. "Organization" is a matter of degree.

COMPETITION BETWEEN ORGANIZED SYSTEMS AND THE FEE-FOR-SERVICE SECTOR

What is the likely impact on the fee-for-service of the entry of a capitation-financed organized system? A natural response is to think that the organized system will put pressure on the fee-for-service sector, forcing it to lower its costs and improve its services. But this assumes that the fee-for-service sector can be managed and can operate on the basis of rational economic incentives. The actual response may be considerably more complex. Perhaps the most impressive thing about the market structure of the medical services industry is the very great variety of organizational forms, and the importance of the particular versus the general. Automobiles or electronics or life insurance or higher education are each produced by one organizational form or a small number of different ones. But when it comes to the delivery of medical care services, there is almost infinite variablility. For example, investigation of the impact of the HMO is inhibited by a lack of uniformity among these organizations. The Health Maintenance Organization Act speaks of two forms of HMO: the group practice and the individual practice association. But, legal definition aside, there are many forms of each. Though both are group practices, what differentiates Kaiser Foundation Health Plan from the Health Insurance Plan of Greater New York may be as important as what they have in common. The Kaiser program owns and operates its own hospitals, and its physicians share in the financial risk of hospital costs. With one exception, HIP does not own its own hospitals and does not itself provide hospitalization coverage, so its physicians bear no financial responsibility for many of the costly decisions they make (Lawrence Goldberg and Warren Greenberg, p. 64).

At the level of market structures, consider the differences among, say Hawaii, northern California, and Minneapolis. The Hawaii market for medical insurance is dominated by the Hawaii Medical Service Association (HMSA) which insures about 64 percent of the non-military (and dependents) population of the State. Kaiser membership is about 16 percent of the non-military population of Oahu. HMSA was started under employer sponsorship with a serious interest in controlling costs. (By contrast, Blue Cross and Blue Shield were started under hospital and physician sponsorship, respectively.) The HMSA board includes representatives of business, labor, government and consumers, as well as hospitals and the medical profession (Goldberg and Greenberg, p. 99). HMSA promotes utilization control, and their hospital days per 1,000 are low and similar to Kaiser's.[4] Most of the patients of a non-Kaiser doctor or hospital are likely to be covered by HMSA, which gives HMSA substantial power to influence charges, fees, and utilization. Competition between the two is very strong. The Hawaii market structure reflects some of the unique features of the history of the State: the dominance of the "Big Five" employers and the entrepreneurship of Henry Kaiser.

In northern California, on the other hand, Blue Cross of Northern California covers about 23 percent of the population in its territory; Kaiser covers about 16 percent.[5] Blue Shield competes with Blue Cross across the board; its statewide membership is roughly 1.2 million, or 5 percent of the population. The rest of the population is covered by many commercial carriers, government programs, etc., or not at all. Blue Cross or Northern California's market share is much smaller than HMSA's and it is not in a position to apply nearly as much influence over hospital charges, physician fees, and utilization. Blue Cross has worked with physician groups to create HMO's but none of the efforts is numerically significant. There are several foundations for medical care in operation in northern California, but their percentage of the population is small, they are not at risk for hospital costs, and their ability to reduce costs significantly is still in doubt (Gaus, et al.).

Goldberg and Greenberg report that Blue Cross, merged with Blue Shield, covers about 25 percent of the population of the Minneapolis-St. Paul market. There are numerous commercial insurers, but none has as much as 5 percent of the population. "In 1976 there were seven HMO's within the Minneapolis-St. Paul Standard Metropolitan Statistical Area (SMSA) with a total of 133,347 enrollees representing nearly 7 percent of the population of the SMSA" (Goldberg and Greenberg, p. 37). The largest HMO, Group Health Plan, Inc., with about 90,000 members, is not large enough to obtain important economies of scale in many specialized services, and does not own its own hospital. With about 4.5 percent market share, it cannot have a large competitive impact. The others are small, in the start-up phase, and below what is generally considered to be the break-even size. So Minneapolis has neither an 'HMSA" nor a "Kaiser Northern California." The competitive impact of the HMO's is reflected in Goldberg and Greenberg's finding that "Blue Cross/Blue Shield has not made any changes, however, in either their traditional insurance coverage or their attempts to control cost in response to HMO development" (p. 41). However, Paul Ellwood reports that total membership in the seven HMO's grew by about 40 percent in 1976, so a discernible competitive impact may not be long in coming.

It seems likely that the economic impact of, for example, a 16 percent HMO market penetration will be very different if the leading third-party carrier has 64 percent of the market, as in Hawaii, than if it has 23 percent as in northern California. In the former case, the third-party carrier has more power to respond with tighter cost controls, and more incentive to do so because a substantial part of the HMO's membership gains must be its losses.

One thing that seems clear is that there is not a single textbook model of competition that fits many different local markets the way the economists' models of industrial competition fit many industries. The market imperfections are too strong and the particular factors in each situation are too important. This makes it, in my opinion, almost impossible to sustain simple generalizations about the competitive impact of HMO's. Rather, there are many models of competition. To illustrate, let me describe, elaborate, and comment on three hypothetical cases. I offer them merely as vehicles for discussion in the hope of developing useful insights. They are not exact empirical descriptions and they do not exhaust all the possibilities.

Model I: Desirable Competitive Response by the Fee-for-Service Sector.

In this model, Blue Cross (and other third-party carriers) will respond to the competitive pressure of HMO's by strengthening their utilization review procedures in order to reduce utilization and per capita costs. This is the model implied by the Goldberg and Greenberg study. They relate three measures of Blue Cross hospital utilization to HMO market share, by State, while controlling for such variables as per capita income, climate, physician and hospital bed to population ratios, and percent of unionization of the State's work force. Using multiple regression on cross-section data by States, they find that (a) hospital days per 1,000 for nonmaternity cases for Federal employees and their families enrolled in Blue Cross, (b) length of stay for maternity care for Federal employees enrolled in Blue Cross, and (c) hospital days per 1,000 for Blue Cross non-Federal group enrollees, all have a statistically significant negative relationship to HMO market share. These results support the hypothesis that Blue Cross does respond to HMO market share. These results support the hypothesis that Blue Cross does respond to HMO competition by tightening its controls on hospital utilization.

Of course, as Goldberg and Greenberg observe, there are other dimensions besides cost controls in which the fee-for-service sector might make desirable competitive responses to the entry of HMO's into a market. For one, HMO entry has put employers and third-party intermediaries under competitive pressure to introduce insurance plans with more comprehensive benefits and reduced consumer cost-sharing. For another, HMO entry may put pressure on fee-for-service physicians to offer better service and to make their services more accessible. Third, the presence of Kaiser has been an important factor in the creation of Medical Care Foundations in California. The Foundations enable fee-for-service physicians to participate in plans offering comprehensive benefits on a prepaid capitation basis. While hospital utilization is a key indicator of cost control, it is not the only measure of competitive response.

While the Goldberg-Greenberg results are very interesting and desereve to be treated with respect, they are not completely persuasive. I do not doubt the proposition that, given time and fewer barriers to competitive entry, HMO's could have the favorable competitive impact they hypothesize. But they have not really shown that HMO's have had the desired effect so far. First, on the empirical side, the results are dominated by the three west coast States and Hawaii. Using Goldberg-Greenberg's measure of penetration, only these States and the District of Columbia have HMO enrollees equal to more than 5 percent of insured persons. And the D.C. data point is confounded by the overlap with the Virginia and Maryland suburbs.[6] When the four western States are omitted, the relationship between HMO share and Blue Cross utilization is not longer statistically significant. [7] Of course, the western States are a part of the United States and deserve to be included in the study. But the possibility remains too strong that other factors account for the generally lower utilization on the west coast. Second, neither Goldberg-Greenberg nor my own limited investigations have been able to identify the specific mechanisms that would account for the strength of the hypothesized competitive response. For example, most of the specific Blue Cross competitive responses mentioned in their description of northern California involve very few people. The Blue Cross Model Utilization Review System (MURS) to which they refer works on the principle of retroactive denial of claims for services is considered to be unnecessary. While Blue Cross only denies .2 percent of claims, its management feels that its deterrent effect is much greater. However, the threat of retroactive denial must be a comparatively weak form of utilization control. By the time the claim is presented, the expenses have already been incurred. If the claim is denied, the hospital and the doctor have recourse to the individual beneficiary. If the patient is a member of an important group, Blue Cross must feel under some pressure to pay the claim. Moreover, in many cases, in effect, because of experience rating or because the insured group's contract with Blue Cross is for claims administration, making the payment will be at the expense of the insured group and not Blue Cross. There are much stronger forms of utilization control such as pre-admission certification and mandatory second opinions for elective surgery, but, with small exceptions, these are not in effect in Blue Cross of Northern California. In some cases, Blue Cross uses Foundations for Medical Care to review admissions, but the Foundations have not yet proved to be very effective at cost control.[8] This argument would not be very persuasive if the Goldberg-Greenberg empirical evidence were much stronger. But when the empirical association really depends on four States in one region, I think it is reasonable to seek a believable "micro-economic" counterpart for the aggregate statistical results.

However, this is not to say that a potentially desirable competitive impact is not there. But there are also some perverse responses by the fee-for-service sector that work to offset the desirable responses. This brings us to Model II.

Model II: Perverse Response by the Fee-for-Service Sector.

Consider a hypothetical community served by 4.5 beds and 1.7 physicians per 1,000 population, with all the physicians on fee-for-service and all the hospitals on cost reimbursement by third-party intermediaries. Now suppose that a group practice HMO enters the market, grows rapidly, and cares for its members with 1.5 beds and 1 physician per 1,000 population. Suppose it buys existing hospital beds and hires doctors already in the community at the same annual cost per bed and doctor as in the fee-for-service sector. The HMO would enjoy a large advantage in per capita cost. Suppose the HMO grew to serve 20 percent of the population, while the total number of doctors and beds in the community remained unchanged. Then the 80 percent of the population cared for by the fee-for-service sector would be served by 5.25 beds and 1.88 physicians per 1,000. (If the HMO built its own hospitals and brought in its own doctors from outside, the population in the fee-for-service sector would be served by even more beds and physicians.) Thus, as the HMO grew in market share, its relative advantage in per capita costs would increase.

How does the fee-for-service sector respond? Does it cut costs to remain competitive? We should not assume that it is tightly organized like a single firm, or that it exhibits normal competitive economic responses. If we were talking about a normal competitive market such as, for example, the market for gasoline or convenience foods, some doctors and hospitals would experience a loss of revenue, would not be able to cover incurred or opportunity costs, and would leave the market. Along the way, doctors and hospitals would cut fees, charges, and costs to retain their customers. But various studies have shown that doctors and hospitals do not respond that way.

First, studies by Martin Feldstein and Uwe Reinhardt show that doctors respond to lower demand for their services by raising fees (to maintain their target incomes) and working less. Reinhardt has found that doctors in areas of comparatively low doctor-population ratio work longer hours, see more patients, use more auxiliaries, and *charge less.* Second, Victor Fuchs and Marcia Kramer found that doctors exercise power to increase the demand for their services, independently of the increased amount demanded attributable to reduced fees, so that a larger doctor-population ratio will mean more doctoring for the same health conditions. This is not an unmixed blessing. More doctors per capita may mean improved accessibility and better care; it may also mean greater per capita costs with no resulting improvement in health status. Third, since the hospitals are financed primarily through cost reimbursement, they face no pressure to cut back on the number of beds. On the contrary, they may merely allocate the same fixed costs over a smaller number of patients. In fact, if a hospital shut down a wing, it would no longer get its debt-service reimbursed by Medicare and Medicaid, so it has a strong incentive not to reduce capacity. Even if the reduced volume of business caused the community hospital to realize operating losses, as a not-for-profit institution it would not have the incentive that a for-profit firm would have to go out of business rather than accept continuing losses, as long as it had the resources to continue in business. Moreover, a hospital in our hypothetical over-bedded community would find it hard to redeploy its existing physical capital. There are not many good alternative uses for hospital buildings. And its legal structure would prevent it from redeploying its cash flow into some other business in need of capital.

Moreover, Goldberg and Greenberg found some evidence that Blue Cross plans have responded to the comprehensive coverage offered by HMO's by increasing their insurance coverage. This would have the effect of reducing consumer cost-sharing and, by inducing greater utilization of services, increasing per capita spending. Whether or not, on net balance, this would be a desirable response would depend on one's view of the value of the additional services, and the alleviation of individual hardship, in relation to the cost.

These factors suggest that those remaining with the fee-for-service sector would experience an increase in per capita cost, as a result of the competitive entry of the HMO. This should temper our optimism about what an HMO can do to reform the fee-for-service sector.

But this process is unstable; it cannot go on forever. As it continued, the per capita cost advantage of the HMO would increase until it became overwhelming, and consumers would leave the fee-for-service sector rather than pay the higher costs. However, this response by consumers is attenuated by a group of Government-created and other barriers to competition; because of them, those who stay with the fee-for-service sector do not have to pay all of the extra costs.

First, because it is based on cost reimbursement, Medicare pays more on behalf of people who choose more costly systems of care. For example, a recent study compared the Incurred Reimbursable Per Capita Cost to Medicare of members of six Group Practice Prepayment Plans (GPPP) with

Table 1

Group Practice Prepayment Plan	Year	Difference between GPPP Reimbursable Cost and AAPCC as % of AAPCC
Detroit Community	1969	35.2
Health Assoc.	1970	27.3
Hotel Union Family	1969	15.0
Medical Fund of NYC(a)	1970	8.0
Group Health Coop of	1969	38.1
Puget Sound	1970	43.2
Kaiser Southern Calif.	1969	23.9
	1970	20.3
Kaiser Northern Calif.	1969	27.1
	1970	28.0
Kaiser Oregon	1969	36.4
	1970	39.3

(a) This is the only non-hospital based plan of the group.

Source: Steven Goss.

the Adjusted Average Per Capita Cost (AAPCC) of similar beneficiaries living in the same areas—primarily on fee-for-service. In all cases, the GPPP's received less than the AAPCC from Medicare by the percentages shown in table. 1.[9]

In other words, for example, in 1970, Medicare paid $202.43 on behalf of a typical beneficiary cared for by Group Health Cooperative of Puget Sound, but paid $365.50, or 76 percent more, on behalf of similar beneficiaries in the same area who got their care from the fee-for-service sector. With that kind of a subsidy, the fee-for-service sector will be able to hold out for a long time. Moreover, the subsidy becomes greater as the cost differential widens. Medicaid, also based on cost reimbursement, suffers from the same defect. In both cases, there is no way that the alternative system can pass along to the beneficiary the financial savings it achieves through greater cost effectiveness. This is, of course, very important because, for example, Medicare and Medicaid account for about a third of the Nation's spending on hospital care.[10] It is easy to understand how someone who would prefer to join a GPPP for, say, a 20 percent saving would choose the comparative freedom of the fee-for-service sector if the alternatives cost him the same.

Second, many employees got their health benefits paid for through a single employer-furnished health plan, and do not see themselves as having a choice. In many cases, they probably do not even know how much the employer is paying on their behalf. They do not need to if there is nothing they can do about it. If they do have a choice, in some cases the employer may pay more on behalf of those who choose the more costly plan. The HMO Act should have the desirable impact of opening up many employee groups to competition by HMO's.

The tax laws provide a reason for the employer to pay all of the premiums, and to offer a generous health benefits plan, for the employer's contribution is not taxable income to the employee. Moreover, within limits, part of the employee contributions are tax deductible. These provisions of the tax laws were enacted for a commendable purpose; i.e., to encourage the spread of voluntary health insurance and broad coverage. But they do have the undesirable side effect of providing an extra tax subsidy to those who choose a more costly system for delivery of health care services.

These barriers to competition could be eliminated, if for example, the Federal Government were to put a limit on the amount of employer and employee premium contributions that were not treated as taxable income, and if the Medicare law were changed to allow each beneficiary to elect to have his Adjusted Average Per Capita Cost (the average per capita cost to the Medicare Program of people in a given age-sex category) paid as a fixed prospective capitation payment to the HMO of his choice. (The limit on the tax exemption of premium contributions should be related to the actuarial status or predicated health care costs of the taxpayer and his family.) If this were done, those Medicare beneficiaries who chose a delivery system offering comprehensive care for a lower per capita cost would be able to benefit from the savings through reduced cost-sharing, catastrophic coverage not provided by Medicare, or improved benefits.

Another similar market imperfection arises from the fact that many people are insured through groups whose rates are set on the basis of the experience of members in many communities besides their own. Thus, the premiums they pay do not reflect the per capita cost in their own community. This is true, for example, of Medicare, the Blue Cross-Blue Shield and Aetna plans in the Federal Employees Health Benefits program whose rates are set on a Government-wide basis, some insurance plans for companies with multiple locations, the indemnity and Blue Cross options in the public employees plan for the State of California, etc. Thus, if per capita health services costs increase in our hypothetical community relative to costs in the rest of the country, the increase is not likely to be reflected in the insurance premiums of many of the citizens of that community. Rather, the citizens in areas with high per capita costs will be subsidized by citizens in areas with low per capita costs. And the subsidy widens with the cost differential. In the long run, this kind of ratemaking should invite competition in the low-cost areas. But this market imperfection might be eliminated more quickly by a pro-competitive regulatory framework in which insurers were required to set rates based on the costs in individual market areas (such as Health Service Areas or groups of contiguous areas).

The potential competitive impact of HMO's may also be attenuated by other factors. First, the HMO must compete for doctors and for members. As the fee-for-service doctors charge more and work less—according to the hypothesized Model II response—the HMO will have to offer its doctors better pay. As service improves for the consumers served by the fee-for-service sector (because of its higher doctor-population ratio) the HMO will be inhibited from making further economies at the cost of convenience or accessibility for members. The fee-for-service sector sets the community standards of care (e.g., appropriate number of diagnostic tests for a particular condition) which may be very costly in relation to their benefits at the margin. But the HMO will be required to adhere to them to attract members and to limit its vulnerability to malpractice claims. Moreover, if the HMO is dependent on community beds, it may be forced to bear part of the cost of the over-bedding. Also, as its cost advantage increases, it may become less able or willing to resist the wage demands of its workers. Competitive wage levels will be set by the fee-for-service sector. So the Model II (i.e., perverse) response by the fee-for-service sector will generate some upward pressures on HMO costs.

Second, the financial incentives for an HMO to grow will be much weaker than those of a for-profit industrial company that could see greater economies of scale and experience and improved profit margins in a greater market share. Most HMO's are non-profit entities. Not-for-profit status will leave the HMO with weak financial incentives to press its cost advantage and grow as fast as it can. Moreover, medical care is, for the most part, a local business. Few economies of scale carry over from one market area to another. A physician-owned, for-profit HMO would presumably be run in the interests of the proprietors—which might not include growth. Some HMO's are consumer cooperatives, run by and for the members. In some cases, the members, acting in their own shortrun best interest, have been reluctant to vote dues high enough to generate the capital required for expansion. (Thus, a legislative requirement that a substantial part of the policymaking body of the HMO will be members of the organization may have the growth-inhibiting effect of making the HMO more of a club for existing members than an outward-reaching community service organization.) The HMO's that have sustained the greatest growth have been not-for-profit entities with a community service orientation; i.e., with the philosophy that potential members not yet enrolled ought to have the opportunity to join. HMO's may have reasons other than profit for continuing to grow and gain in market share, such as realizing economies of scale in costly specialized services, maintaining a favorable age composition of membership, providing opportunities for personal advancement for its employees, or carrying out its public service mission and meeting the demand for membership.

The not-for-profit HMO has no powerful incentive to *minimize* its per capita costs; it may find its competitive optimum by controlling its costs and keeping them 20-30 percent below those of its fee-for-service competition. In that case, as the per capita costs in the fee-for-service sector rise, the HMO will have no incentive to further reduce its relative costs. It may settle into an equilibrium with premiums about equal to those of Blue Cross and other third parties, and an overall 25 percent advantage in per capita cost. In this *Model II Equilibrium,* we would see the trend in per capita costs in the community being set by the fee-for-service sector, and going up at about the same rate as if there were no HMO. Some support for this idea is provided by an interesting study of 8 market areas over a 10-year period by John D. Valiante, comparing HMO premiums and Blue Cross-Blue Shield rates offered to Federal employees, Valiante found "HMO premiums more than $10 above or less than $5 below the applicable Blues rate appeared to be unsupportable over the long run. . . . Higher rates appeared to have the effect of reducing market share, and lower rates apparently failed to recover the cost of serving beneficiaries (or were for other reasons not sustainable over time)." The "Valiante corridor" is what Model II would predict.

Of course, there are important elements of unrealism in Model II's perverse response. First, the large HMO's have grown steadily over many years. Thus, there has been plenty of time for their presence to affect physician location and hospital construction decisions in the fee-for-service sector. Second, most of the large western HMO's have continued to grow in market share in response to consumer demand. Third, the equilibrium between the fee-for-service sector and the HMO in Model II could be broken by competition between HMO's. Many HMO's have been created by physicians, hospitals, and third-party intermediaries as a competitive response to existing HMO's (Goldberg and Greenberg). The main point of Model II is to caution against unrealistic expectations as to what one HMO can do in reducing per capita costs in the fee-for-service sector, and to illustrate some of the complexities and conflicting tendencies in the response of the fee-for-service sector to HMO competition. HMO's do a good job of controlling their own per capita costs, and they give us some useful yardsticks to help evaluate the fee-for-service sector's performance. But we should not necessarily expect them, through competitive impact, to bring the fee-for-service sector's per capita costs under control. The point is not that Model II is right and Model I is wrong, or vice versa. Both reflect important elements of reality.

Model III: Competition Among Organized Systems

The Model II Equilibrium could be broken if two or more organized systems were competing against each other as well as against the fee-for-service sector. In that case, each HMO would have to make significant efforts to cost reduction in order to maintain its position relative to the other(s). (Cost reduction does not necessarily mean premium reduction; it could mean more benefits per dollar.) As the HMO's compete with each other, they would grow stronger, relative to the fee-for-service sector because of improved efficiency, economies of scale, and possible Model II responses by the fee-for service sector. Competition between HMO's would supply the incentive to continue reducing costs that is missing in Model II. Thus in a Model III situation, one would expect to see lower premiums and greater market penetration by HMO's than in a Model II situation.

Unfortunately, today we have few examples of competing organized systems with substantial market positions. Probably the best example is Hawaii where there is strong competition between HMSA and Kaiser. HMSA is not an HMO, although it does operate an HMO with about 22,000 members. However, the market positions of Kaiser and HMSA go a long way toward dividing Oahu into two competiting groups of providers—Kaiser and non-Kaiser—with the latter getting most of their financing through HMSA. Thus, HMSA has some of the attributes of what Paul Ellwood and Water McClure have called a "Health Care Alliance." As such, third-party intermediaries are associated with specific groups of providers with whom they can cooperate to reduce costs and pass the savings on to consumers in the form of reduced premiums of subscribers to less costly provider groups. I believe that this combination rather than the mere fact of Kaiser's market share explains HMSA's very low hospitalization rate.[11] Southern California is moving toward a Model III situation. Kaiser there now has about 1.3 million members; Ross-Loos, a physician-owned plan, has about 160,000;[12] Family Health Program has roughly 115,000, and other HMO's have about 250,000 members. But the total HMO market share is only around 12 percent of the total population[13] (though much higher in some areas), and none of the smaller HMO's begins to approach the size, geographic coverage, and reputation of Kaiser. And there are areas such as Washington, D.C., and Minneapolis-St. Paul in which new HMO's are growing rapidly and, in the foreseeable future, may be able to offer significant competition to larger established HMO's.[14]

Model III might be a natural sequel to Model II as providers and third-party intermediaries perceive themselves increasingly vulnerable to HMO competition and start their own HMO's in self-defense. Certainly, encouragement of Model III market structures would be a desirable goal of public policy.

SUGGESTIONS FOR PUBLIC POLICY

It should be clear that there is no simple solution that will cut through the many market imperfections in the health care sector and restructure it along competitive economic lines. Whatever change does come in the health care delivery system is bound to come slowly. One important objective should be to avoid a national health insurance scheme or a regulatory scheme that will freeze the delivery system in its present costly and non-competitive state. This would be the result, for example, of extending Medicare to everyone.

The creation of organized systems that can compete effectively requires a certain amount of aggregation of consumer buying power in a market area, so that someone can negotiate for economies in the hospitals and for fees and utilization controls with the doctors. If there are too many third-party intermediaries, then none of them will represent a large enough percentage of hospitals' or physicians' business to be able to influence the providers' behavior. It is not at all clear that preserving atomistic competition among third-party intermediaries is in the best interests of consumers. For example, if the Federal Government were to break up HMSA into several smaller "competing" units, each of which reimbursed the fees and costs of all providers, on the mistaken theory that more units mean more competition, the result would be to destroy competition, not to enhance it. Thus, the

Federal Government should not prevent the aggregation of buying power into units large enough to form viable competing organized systems.

Perhaps the most important suggestion for public policy to come out of this analysis is that the Federal Government ought to find ways to put HMO's and other competing systems on an equal footing with respect to the (actuarially adjusted) per capita cost supported by tax dollars, and eliminate the subsidy of more costly systems of care through Medicare, Medicaid, and the tax laws. It is quite understandable how the subsidies came about. In part, the Federal Government wanted to help people to obtain better insurance coverage because so many people were so poorly covered. Moreover, those who spent more on health care were assumed to need more. However, recent research, such as the study by Mildred Corbin and Aaron Krute, and others, suggests that there are at least two reasons why some people spend more on health care services than others: greater need, and because they choose a more costly system of care for the same need (because of preference, income, or subsidy). While people should be free to choose the more costly system of care if they prefer it, there is no good reason for that choice to be subsidized with tax dollars once the level of care has reached a standard that is judged to be adequate. We need, then, to distinguish need from preference for a more costly system and subsidize according to need. As mentioned earlier, this could be done in the Medicare program, for example, by setting the Government's contribution in real terms (i.e., adjusted for inflation and regional price levels) at this year's Adjusted Average Per Capita Cost for each actuarial group, or at some percentage of it, and then allowing each beneficiary to assign it as a fixed prospective per capita payment to the HMO of his choice. In view of the large subsidies to the fee-for-service sector in the Medicare program, and the fact that many beneficiaries choose HMO's nontheless, it seems likely that the impact of such a change would be large.

The Federal Government has taken a number of steps over the years intended to help prepaid group practice plans and other HMO's. Perhaps the most important was including them as an option in the Federal Employees Health Benefits Program. Prepaid Group Practice plans have done well in this market in which they were allowed to compete on an equal footing with service benefit and indemnity plans. The list also includes Section 226 of the Social Security Amendments of 1972, providing for payments to Health Maintenance Organizations, the HMO Act of 1973, with its mandatory dual choice provision, and the HMO Amendments of 1976. However, as pointed out, by various persons and by the passage of the 1976 Amendments,[15] the 1973 HMO Act and its administration actually created impediments to HMO progress. As of February 1977, only 28 HMO's had qualified under the HMO Act, and the list did not include any of the large leading HMO's in whose image the new HMO's were meant to be created.[16] Those in the Congress and HEW who believe that HMO's are a valid alternative to fee-for-service deserving of an opportunity to compete on equal terms should continue to work to eliminate the "Factors that Impede Progress In Implementing the HMO Act of 1973."[17]

The unfortunate Prepaid Health Plan experience in southern California showed that some regulation is needed to prevent fraud, underservice, attempts to profit by weeding out poor risks, insolvency, and other abuses. But there now appears to be a danger that the pendulum has swung too far, that the regulation is too detailed, and that it is inhibiting HMO growth. The law and regulations should focus on the essentials, and not try to control HMO's in every detail. For example, the HMO Act specified two types of HMO's, Group Practices and Individual Practice Associations, and it defines them in greater detail. The problem is that there may be many other satisfactory ways of organizing services; it is surely too soon to tell. And a detailed law specifying the forms inevitably inhibits competition and innovation.

All this might be summarized by saying there is much the Government could do to bring about a fair market test between the fee-for-service sector and alternative delivery systems. That idea is not new.[18] But it still is untried.

NOTES

1. For example, see George Monsma, Jr., in Herbert Klarman and Donald Riedel *et al.*

2. I am referring here to choice of a system offering comprehensive benefits at a lower total cost, not to a system offering lower premiums at the cost of greater financial risk.

3. I assume charges are set about equal to average costs which exceed marginal costs. In the "immediate run" before charges are adjusted to the lower volume, there would be a loss in net revenue from third parties paying charges. When the hospital increased charges to reflect the lower volume, then again total revenue would be about equal to total cost. Medicare and other third parties reimbursing on a retrospective cost basis would pay higher unit costs right away.

4. The respective age compositions of the memberships are not published, so a reliable age-adjusted comparison is not available.

5. Blue Cross of Northern California's territory includes all of California from the San Jose area north to the Oregon border. This includes large areas in which Kaiser has no facilities and which are outside its service area. Kaiser Northern California Region defines its service area as 16 counties around San Francisco Bay and Sacramento, and its membership exceeds 20 percent of the population in those counties.

6. In the regression analysis, they use an HMO penetration in D.C. of 16.1 percent of insureds, apparently using the population of the District as the denominator. In a table on page 68, they report a penetration of 4.2 percent of total population, using the total population of the SMSA as the denominator. Since the Washington-based HMO's have many suburban members, use of the SMSA as the market area seems more appropriate.

7. Personal communication from Warren Greenberg, March 8, 1977. Morover, the least-squares regression technique, because it finds the line that minimizes the squared deviations, gives observations far from the sample means (i.e., the western States with large HMO market

shares) a much larger weight in determination of the regression coefficients than the other observations with HMO market shares close to the mean.

8. This should not be interpreted as a criticism of Blue Cross of Northern California. Its management is very concerned about costs. The problem lies in the nature of its contracts with members which gives them freedom to choose providers, and therefore leaves Blue Cross with little market power over providers, and with the Blue Cross market share which does not give them strong bargaining power over hospitals. Moreover, this is not to imply that Foundations could not be very effective at cost control if they and the rest of the fee-for-service sector were under sufficient competitive pressure.

9. Steven Goss. The Goss analysis uses the same data as the Corbin and Krute study, referred to below, but adjusts the costs for final settlements. The same point with slightly different numbers can be made with the Corbin and Krute study.

10. Marjorie Mueller and Robert Gibson.

11. HMSA had a group enrollee hospital utilization rate of 390 days per 1,000 in 1975, including retirees in groups, but not individuals 65 and over. Kaiser Hawaii Region had 357 days per 1,000 for members under 65 and 438 days per 1,000 overall. Because the HMSA and Kaiser numbers have not been normalized for age-sex composition, they cannot be compared accurately. However, these data do imply that both groups have low and similar hospital utilization rates.

12. Goldberg and Greenberg, p. 86.

13. Goldberg and Greenberg, p. 85.

14. The Valiante study referred to earlier presents some intriguing data. Of eight market areas examined, four offer Federal employees a choice of two competing organized systems, while in the other four they are offered no choice. He finds (p.4) that "In markets with competing HMOs, total HMO market share is larger and HMO prices have increased less rapidly than Blue Cross premiums than in markets with only one HMO." Unfortunately, the fit of the generalization to the data is not very good. And there are special circumstances in each market that would permit one to explain away the result. The "competing HMO" markets are New York, Seattle, Honolulu, and Los Angeles. Goldberg and Greenberg (p. 62) observe that "In many ways GHI (Group Health Inc. of New York) operates like a traditional Blue Shield plan." Honolulu and Los Angeles were discussed in this paper. The "single HMO" markets are Washington, D.C., Boston, Denver, and St. Paul. Harvard Community Health Plan in Boston and Kaiser in Denver have low market shares because they are so new. The slow growth of Group Health Association in Washington, D.C., and Group Health of St. Paul may be related to their consumer cooperative form of organization in which consumer members are reluctant to vote premiums adequate for capital generation. Valiante expresses many of these qualifications. But we are left without a good empirical test of the potentialities of Model III.

15. Alain Enthoven, Paul Starr.

16. *Group Health News,* March 1977.

17. Comptroller General of the United States.

18. See Institute of Medicine, National Academy of Sciences.

REFERENCES

J. P. Bunker, "Surgical Manpower: A Comparison of Operations and Surgeons in the United States, England, and Wales," *New England J. Med.,* Jan. 1970, 135-144.

M. Corbin and A. Krute, "Some Aspects of Medicare Experience with Group Practice Prepayment Plans," *Soc. Sec. Bull.,* Mar. 1975, 3-11.

P. Ellwood, Jr., *Twin Cities HMO Development*, Interstudy, Apr. 1977.

——— and W. McClure, *Health Delivery Reform*, Interstudy, Nov. 1976.

A. C. Enthoven, "Prepaid Group Practice and National Health Policy: Keynote Address 1976 Group Health Institute," *Proceedings of 26th Annual Group Health Institute*, Washington, D.C. 1976.

M. S. Feldstein, "The Rising Price of Physicians' Services," *Rev. Econ. Stat.*, May 1970, 121-133.

V. R. Fuchs and M. J. Kramer, *Determinants of Expenditures for Physicians' Services in the United States, 1948-68*, National Bureau of Economic Research Occasional Paper 17, 1973.

C. R. Gaus, B. S. Cooper, and C. G. Hirschman, "Contrast in HMO and Fee-for-Service Performance," *Soc. Sec. Bull.*, May 1976, 3-14.

R. M. Gibson and M. S. Mueller, "National Health Expenditures, Fiscal Year 1975," *Soc. Sec. Bull.*, Feb. 1976, 3-20.

S. Goss, "A Retrospective Application of the Health Maintenance Organization Risk Sharing Savings Formula for Six Group Practice Prepayment Plans for 1969 and 1970," U.S. Dept. of Health, Education, and Welfare, SSA, Actuarial Note No. 88, Department of Health, Education, and Welfare, Publication SSA 76-11500 (11-75).

P. Lembke, "Measuring the Quality of Medical Care Through Vital Statistics Based on Hospital Service Areas: A Comparative Study of Appendectomy Rates," *Amer. J. Pub. Health*, Mar. 1952, 276-286.

G. N. Monsma Jr., "Marginal Revenue and the Demand for Physicians' Services," in *Empirical Studies in Health Economics*, H. E. Klarman (ed.), Baltimore 1970.

U. E. Reinhardt, *Physician Productivity and the Demand for Health Manpower*, Cambridge, Mass., 1974.

D. C. Riedel et al., *Federal Employees Health Benefits Program Utilization Study*, Department of Health, Education, and Welfare Publication (HRA) 75-3125.

P. Starr, "The Underlivered Health System," *The Public Interest*, Winter 1976, 66-85.

J. D. Valiante, *Analysis of HMO Markets*, Washington, D.C. 1976.

J. E. Wennberg, Testimony and Statement in *Getting Ready for National Health Insurance: Unnecessary Surgery*, Hearings Before the Subcommittee on Oversight and Investigations of the Committee on Interstate and Foreign Commerce, U.S. House of Representatives, 94th Cong., Serial No. 94-37, July 15, 1975.

Comptroller General of the United States, *Factors that Impede Progress in Implementing the Health Maintenance Organization Act of 1973*, Washington, D.C. Sept. 3, 1976.

Institute of Medicine, National Academy of Sciences, *HMOs: Toward A Fair Market Test*, Washington 1974.

U.S. Federal Trade Commission, Bureau of Economics, *The Health Maintenance Organization and Its Effects on Competition*, July 1977 (staff report prepared by Lawrence G. Goldberg and Warren Greenberg).

Comment

Stuart O. Schweitzer
Associate Professor, UCLA School of Public Health and
USC Human Resources Research Center

While chairman of the President's Council of Economic Advisers, Walter Heller once remarked that it was terribly difficult being the Nation's chief economist; for, while people willingly delegated authority to their physicians or attorneys, in a sense we were a Nation of 200 million economists and everybody had suggestions for improving the work of the Council.

This flow of ideas is undoubtedly a healthy process. Economists have never asserted monopoly control over economic wisdom, and ours is probably one of the professions most free to engage in self-criticism. Many professions with which we are familiar are well known for a reluctance to apply peer review. There is little doubt that our profession is much the stronger for this free exercise in self-examination. More often, however, this process of self-examination begins to resemble self-immolation, as institutionalists are pitted aginst theoreticians, Keynesians against neo-classicists, and so forth. As the fires of debate rage, others are encouraged to feed them or at least fan the flames. We have been treated to a display of these pyrotechnics at this conference.

It is instructive every once in awhile to review some of the principles by which economic analyses can be judged and interpreted. Analyses of the health sector are particularly vulnerable to criticism, for example, on the grounds that initial assumptions are improper. A variant of this argument is that the data used to test a hypothesis were faulty or dated. As we all know, a hypothesis can never be proved; it can only be disproved, by showing it to be inconsistent with observations of the actual world. While our inability to prove such theories as monopoly power, demand creation, etc., would appear to weaken the value of economic analysis, it means that our own conclusions, and those of individuals with whom we compete in the free market of ideas, must hinge upon the question of which theories or models appear to be consistent with the data. When our findings are ambiguous, we must be frank in admitting so and, if the question is worth asking, resume devising a better test which will help us make a "differential diagnosis."

When the debate is elevated to this level, questions of underlying market behavior can be addressed without our being mired in side issues of definitions of variables, limitations of data, or theoretical specifications of a model. The question which must remain central is whether or not a hypothesis is consistent with our observations, or whether a counter thesis can explain this same (or improved) data better.

This conference addresses a question with which economists have dealt for at least 200 years and, in a more refined way, for at least 50 years following Pigou. This is the "Theory of the Second Best," which in one form tells us that a market that is in many respects noncompetitive will not necessarily be made to operate more efficiently if one of its noncompetitive characteristics is made to conform to the model of perfect competition. The example of the locomotive belching sparks and setting fire to wheat fields through which it passes is illustrative of the problem of dis-economies, and we realize that a solution imposing compensatory payments upon the railroad may not actually be in society's best interst.

The health care market is notoriously noncompetitive because of conditions affecting both consumers and producers. Some of these conditions are self-imposed by society (wittingly or unwittingly) while others may be technologically determined and are inevitable. The list of these characteristics is long and has already been enumerated in one form or another by most of us participating in this conference.

What is more difficult, however, than enumerating the list of health system characteristics which diverge from the model of perfect competition is defining the appropriate approach to remedy any of them. This, I would suggest, is the issue the papers we have been hearing should be addressing.

But I am concerned that we have not yet justified the remedies we are posing in terms of general welfare. If consumers are allowed to see advertisements pertaining to physician services but remain ignorant of factors determining quality of health care, will they be better off? The "Second Surgical Opinion" programs, such as the two in New York State, seem to ask more questions than they answer. Are two conflicting opinions of more value to a patient than the first opinion alone was? And what is the probability that the second opinion will be more correct than the first?

With these programs, and a myriad of others, we seem to be applying partial solutions to systemic defects under the assumption that a step in the right direction is better than standing still. This is not necessarily true.

From the perspective of "Competition in Health Care," let us address the Lawrence Goldberg-Warren Greenberg and Alain Enthoven papers on the structure of health insurance.

I was struck by the degree to which the two papers are related to one another, though each has a totally different starting point.

The Goldberg-Greenberg paper is a look at a fascinating sequence of events, whereby physician-sponsored hospital insurance in Oregon first failed and then succeeded in supplanting hospital-sponsored insurance. For our purposes, the most interesting aspect of this rivalry is the difference in the way the two types of plans acted as purchasers of health care. The case is carefully drawn that prior to the 1940's, health insurance in Oregon was organized in such a way as to act as an informed consumer representing patients. Anecdotal evidence is presented illustrating the extent to which the intermediary actively intervened to question either the propriety of a service or its charge. We wish we could see some evidence of the impact of this intervention, either in rates of service utilization (including surgery), charges, or expenditures. We often despair of our inability to trace these indices with today's data, and so it is clear that we are hardly able to do so for a period of time 40 years back. We have already seen the emergence of "econometric historians." Now we need "health-econometric historians"!

Having personally observed health insurance only in the 1960's and 1970's, being taken back in time to see how independent insurance once functioned is extremely enlightening.

From comments provided at an earlier session, there is some hope that private insurance may once again take on the responsibility of monitoring and questioning the care subscribers purchase through it.

The Enthoven paper carries on from where the Goldberg-Greenberg paper leaves off, as three alternative models of insurance competition are described.

Basic to the argument is that consumers have a number of elements defining their utility for insurance, including comprehensiveness (which was discussed at this conference), convenience, and the medical sophistication to be covered. Given this complexity of consumer preferences, it naturally follows that no single insurance "package" can maximize a community's social welfare.

The discussion of the dis-incentives facing individual providers as they contemplate containing costs is well done and plausible. The spectre of the lonely going-away dinner for the cost-conscious hospital administrator is compelling. Perhaps Health Care Financing Administration employees would be invited!

Enthoven presents three scenarios of competition between the fee-for-service sector and HMO's, each with a different degree of active participation or intervention in the market. The author asserts that private insurance will not be terribly willing to intervene on behalf of the consumers when HMO's succeed in making a substantial penetration of the insurance market. This is contrary to some recent findings of Lawrence Goldberg and Warren Greenberg in another paper. The Enthoven criticism of this second Goldberg-Greenberg paper is not compelling, however.

A second scenario would have the HMO sector widen its competitive advantage over the fee-for-service sector as its ability to utilize services more efficiently draws subscribers from the already over-capitalized fee-for-service sector, thereby exacerbating its problems and widening cost differentials.

One of the few stabilizing forces under this scheme is the Government, which is hypothesized to continue to pay full costs of fee-for-service care to its "subscribers" — the poor and the elderly.

Thus we have a perverse sort of two-class medical care system. The Government patients enjoy the fee-for-service sector services, while everybody else receives care through HMO's.

But soon the HMO begins to cease competing and acts as the fee-for-service sector, and so the price-competitive edge ceases to widen. In the event of multiple HMO's within a community, a sort of rigor mortis of the single HMO described in Scenario II relaxes, with clear advantages to consumers as efficiency incentives are reinstituted together with wide consumer choice. The spectre of Prepaid Health Plans being diffused nationally is enough to scare any Californian, however, underlining the responsibility of public authorities to regulate the newly formed HMO's.

The basic problem in evaluating the Enthoven scenarios is the paucity of empirical evidence which would either confirm or refute their plausibility. The author honestly describes the differences he has with the Goldberg and Greenberg, for instance, in interpretation of the same data.

The HMO movement has been at a plateau for many years. Only recently have we seen a resurgence in growth—not so much in membership as in numbers, and hence access to this mode of delivery. The dual choice feature of the HMO Act will encourage the membership growth. But until the newly reborn HMO movement has had time to mature, we will have to rely on thoughtful and carefully drawn theoretical expositions, such as the papers we have heard, to provide predictions as to the impact of these developments on the broader issue of Competition in Health Care.

REFERENCES

U.S. Federal Trade Commission, Bureau of Economics, *The Health Maintenance Organization and Its Effects on Competition,* July 1977, (staff report prepared by Lawrence G. Goldberg and Warren Greenberg).

Part Four

Competition and Regulation

The Role of Competition in Cost Containment*

Clark C. Havighurst
Professor of Law, Duke University

I propose to discuss health care cost containment as a service that, from most indications, has been undersupplied by the private sector and is therefore being demanded from government. The nature of the apparent "market failure" has not been analyzed as fully as it might have been, and I propose to present certain hypotheses concerning it as a means of provoking more attention to the possibilities for improving the private sector's performance. In attempting to establish why cost-containment services have not been forthcoming as a natural byproduct of market incentives and competition, I shall look for explanations on both the demand side and the supply side of the market.

Some of the causes that I identify to explain the private sector's inaction on health care costs seem subject to elimination by measures that are less than radical, and it seems to me that these steps should be taken even though considerable uncertainty necessarily remains as to precisely what would happen as a consequence. Some unpredictability attends any policy proposal, but market-oriented proposals always seem the most vulnerable to rejection on this score, probably because they concentrate more on means than on ends and rely ultimately upon consumer choice to dictate outcomes. Regulatory proposals, on the other hand, ostensibly allow governmental mechanisms to determine the outcome and therefore seem the safer bet as long as one has reasonable faith in government's ability to act wisely and effectively. Charles L. Schultze has recently suggested some further reasons why market-oriented proposals usually get short shrift in the political process.[1] His argument, like my own, is that they are frequently preferable and deserve a fairer hearing.

---

* Work on this paper was supported in part under Grant No. HS 01539 from the National Center for Health Services Research, U.S. Department of Health, Education, and Welfare.

The greater portion of this paper is an examination of how antitrust principles might be used to expand the private sector's opportunities for containing health care costs. I expect that there are many people who, though they could not agree with optimistic forecasts about what a more competitive market could ultimately achieve, could nevertheless support an effort to use the antitrust laws aggressively to challenge organized medicine's excessive influence over the mechanisms for financing and delivering health services. I would hope that we could agree on the desirability of this step even if we cannot immediately resolve the question of what else we must do. It is at least possible that such a step would permit some interesting things to happen.

SUPPLY AND DEMAND IN THE MARKET FOR COST-CONTAINMENT SERVICES

Health-Care Cost Containment as a Service

Control of health-care costs does not just happen. Because people need to insure (or to be protected by government) against unpredictable expenditures, cost containment must be worked at. The phenomenon known among economists as "moral hazard"—that is, the tendency of insurance to induce people to spend more on covered services (or less on prevention) than they would otherwise spend—appears to operate with particular force in medical care for a variety of reasons: the open-ended and subjective nature of disease; the desire for reassurance and comfort; the uncertainty necessarily involved, coupled with the desire to take no chances; and the related impulses called variously the "technological imperative,"[2] the "quality imperative,"[3] and the "livesaving imperative."[4] Moreover, the medical profession seems to have attached ethical importance to the removal of immediate cost considerations from clinical decisionmaking, thus adding what might be called a professional "ethical hazard" to the moral hazard of inappropriate consumer behavior under third-party payment.[5] The thesis here is that, while cost containment is undeniably difficult in the face of these powerful forces, it is not impossible, and that some more satisfying explanation than the complexity of the task must be found for the lack of innovation in cost containment by insurers and other third parties.

My attempt to show specific deficiencies in the private sector's performance can only be suggestive. Although I cannot show conclusively that certain promising cost-control ideas would work, neither can anyone establish that they would not—precisely because the necessary experimentation has not occurred. Indeed, the failure to experiment can itself be seen as evidence of inadequate incentive, inadequate opportunity, or inadequate competitiveness, matters to be explored below. Even more suggestive is the fact that similar techniques have been used with success in settings so closely analogous to the health insurance setting (e.g., prepaid dental plans) that a heavy burden rests on the private actors to provide an innocent explanation for the nonuse of comparable techniques in medical insurance programs.[6] Finally, I shall try to show enough evidence of the existence of distorted incentives and trade restraints to suggest that the problem lies primarily in the suppression of market forces and not in administrative or technological considerations. I shall then explore at some length the antitrust remedies for what I identify as the most immediate problem—the power of organized medicine to limit the scope of cost-containment initiatives.

The Illogic of Comprehensiveness in Health Insurance

Health insurers and other bulk purchasers of health care could do a wide variety of things to respond to consumers' desire to spend no more on health services than is necessary to get the quality, quantity, and style of service that they desire to pay for. The most crucial thing that can be done is to sell the consumer less insurance coverage, thereby leaving him to his own resources for much of the care that he requires. As a result of paying less for health insurance coverage, the insured will have more resources in hand to meet uninsured expenses. More important, he will also have an incentive to purchase only what he needs. As long as the insured is protected against unpredictable, big-ticket items, he should find less comprehensive coverage attractive since it permits him not only to escape some of the loading and administrative costs of the insurance plan but also to minimize the burden of the "moral hazard"—that is, the necessity for contribution to a fund upon which others may draw with wide discretion. It is widely recognized that self-insurance can be a wise policy as long as one is protected against the most serious risks. Although proponents of less extensive coverage and more self-insurance usually advocate across-the-board use of larger deductibles and co-payment requirements,[7] the argument here is that appropriate departures from comprehensiveness can take other forms as well, including greater selectivity in the coverage of particular services or particular diagnoses.

Economic theory suggests that optimal insurance coverage for an individual is a function of four things: the degree of risk, the individual's aversion to risk, the elasticity of demand for the insured services, and the administrative costs of the insurance plan.[8] If one focuses on the elasticity of demand, not for medical care in general, but for specific medical services,[9] the logic of less than comprehensive health insurance coverage begins to emerge. The elasticity of demand for a service—that is, the responsiveness of demand to price changes—is an index of the importance attached to the service by consumers and physicians and therefore of both the medical need for it and the value of insuring against that need. To illustrate, where demand is "inelastic," as in figure 1, a price reduction from p_1 (equal to 100 percent of cost) to p_2 (equal to 20 percent of p_1 due to insurance covering 80 percent of the cost) increases the quantity of the service rendered only from q_1 to q_2 and yields a "welfare" loss (deduced from some patients' unwillingness to pay as much as the full price, p_1) equal to the area of the shaded triangle. In contrast, where demand is "elastic," as in figure 2, the same insurance causes a much greater welfare loss as societal resources are employed to provide services that are valued at less than their cost. Other things being equal, insurance would be more sensible from the consumer's standpoint, and more socially efficient, for those essential services whose demand approximates that shown in figure 1.[10]

It should be obvious that defining covered medical services with greater particularity would allow more discriminating judgments to be made about whether or not to insure. For example, the overall demand for hysterectomies may look like figure 2, making insurance inappropriate, but, in a few cases with certain medical indications, the need for the service would be so clear that demand would not be significantly affected by price. If insurance coverage could be readily restricted to such medically necessary services, it would be appropriate for many people to purchase only this limited coverage. The administrative costs which obviously limit the

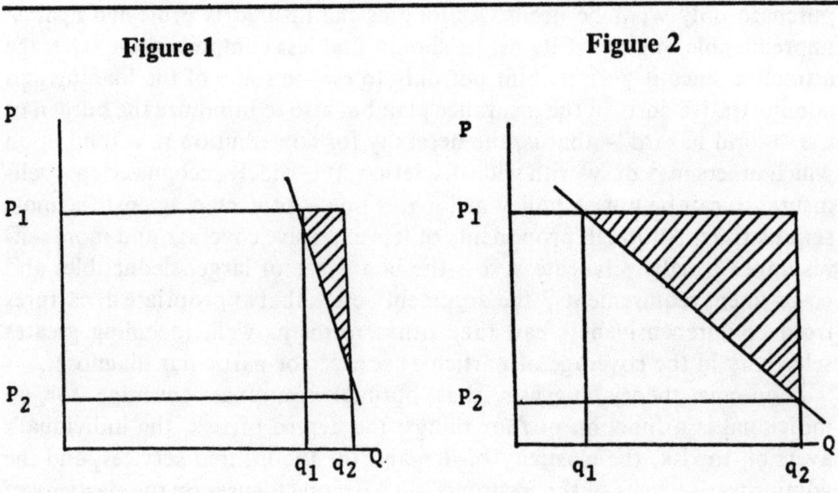

feasibility of minute specification of coverage do not invalidate the basic point that highly selective coverage could well make very good sense. By the same token, comprehensiveness in health insurance coverage is highly questionable.

Designing and Administering Coverage Limits

Despite the foregoing demonstration that rational consumers with correct incentives and a range of options would elect insurance coverage that was less than comprehensive, the trend has been toward increasingly comprehensive coverage with little private effort to contain the increased costs that this trend entails. Before identifying the factors that reduce the demand for and the supply of limited coverage and cost-contâinment services, it may be helpful to suggest some measures that might be taken by insurers and other parties to minimize or overcome the cost-escalating tendencies of insurance. The thesis is that, under normal market conditions, anyone who could supply health-care cost containment, either directly or by inducing providers to exercise restraint, would succeed in the competitive race and that, consequently, the neglect of many promising cost-containment opportunities results from causes other than consumer preference. The missed opportunities are, in effect, the measure of the marked failure—or, more accurately, the failure of governmental policy—that has occurred.

In a normal and unrestrained market for health services, competition among health insurers should lead to the development of benefit packages that are carefully designed to meet customer groups' particular expectations and needs. Employment groups are sufficiently homogeneous that a good deal of common ground probably exists as to the coverage required. It seems probable that a set of basic benefits could be designed to assure that high-priority needs are met and that low-priority items are excluded.[11] Exclusions would reflect a judgment that the "moral hazard" is particularly great with respect to the excluded procedures, not that they are valueless or medically unjustifiable.[12] Although, by hypothesis, the benefit from the excluded treatment or procedure is frequently not worth its cost, the patient who, with professional advice, values the treatment or procedure at more than its cost, is free to buy it.

Intelligent design of benefit packages might not be confined to totally excluding certain procedures but might include varying the copayment requirement (to, say, 50 percent) so as to limit the impact of the moral hazard but also to provide some financial protection. For example, a questionable procedure such as coronary by-pass surgery might be covered in this way. Another technique might be to pay a fixed amount based on the estimated cost of the lower-cost mode of treatment, allowing the patient to supplement that amount if the more costly treatment were desired.[13] As to care totally or partially excluded from coverage, a consumer-oriented plan might stand by to lend the insured the money to pay for the service, thereby reaffirming that the exclusion was not intended to deny the possible legitimacy of the treatment but simply to reflect the subscribers' collective judgment that such care should be provided at personal expense, if at all, in order that benefits and costs would be appropriately weighed.

Explicit coverage limitations can only go so far, however, in the direction of excluding from coverage all care that is apt not to be worth its cost. An insurer or other health plan might therefore seek to limit coverage further by adopting a utilization review mechanism similar to the PSRO program adopted by the Federal Government for the purpose of limiting Medicare and Medicaid coverage.[14] I summarized some of the numerous possibilities in a recent paper as follows:

> Utilization review procedures which insurers might introduce are simply another way of imposing coverage limitations [similar to the foregoing]. But, because advance specification of limits on hospital stays and use of ancillary services is practically impossible, a case-by-case review is needed to give effect to the plan's policy, which may be liberal or stringent in accordance with the premium charged and the attendant necessity for cost control. It would seem reasonable to require participating physicians to obtain advance approval of some hospital admissions and some costly procedures so that only medically necessary care would be paid for. Obviously the procedures for making such reviews would be of considerable importance, but one cannot reasonably object to the principle of allowing consumers to bind themselves in advance to accept the plan's determinations on the scope of coverage. The surgical second-opinion plans currently being experimented with have so far shrunk from applying this principle so as to make the second opinion or other review binding with respect to the plan's obligation to pay.[15]

A proper conceptualization of second-opinion plans would be as a mechanism for distinguishing truly essential care, such as that demanded as in figure 1 above, from care that, while desirable, is not without substitutes and is not so clearly worth its cost in every case that it should be paid for by insurance rather than out of pocket. To extend the earlier example, an insurance plan could specify the medical indications for a covered hysterectomy and require a second examination to verify their presence.[16]

The ability of a third-party payer to impose such controls depends in large measure on whether it can be perceived, not as a profit-hungry corporation, but as the reasonable executor of the wishes of the plan subscribers, who, having entered into a mutual bargain about the extent of coverage, rely on the plan administrators to enforce that bargain fairly and consistently. Procedures are thus extremely important, and plans will be under some pressure to come up with systems that do not expose patients to unfair decisions or apparent hardship. Retroactive denials of payment would seem particularly objectionable but could be avoided by a mechanism for advance determination of coverage. Dental insurance plans provide for pre-treatment review and allow patients to know their financial situation before proceeding with treatment.[17] Such procedures would seem potentially adaptable to many medical treatment situations. Indeed, the anticipated complexity of coverage provisions would make some arrangement for predetermination of benefits essential.

The cost of administering cost-containment measures would undoubtedly be another important limiting factor. Unlike the case with such public regulatory efforts as PSRO's, there is some guarantee that private cost containment measures will not be undertaken or will be discarded if they are not cost-effective from the consumer's standpoint, and this is as it should be. By the same token, there is an ever-present incentive to discover and adopt cost-effective measures. There is a real possibility, nevertheless, that many of the foregoing cost-containment ideas would not work well enough to justify the costs of claims review under circumstances where providers and patients sought actively to evade the restrictions so carefully developed.[18] But these problems would be avoided if there were some direct understanding with the participating physicians that they would follow prescribed procedures. Contractual arrangements between plan and providers could spell out obligations on both sides and would facilitate simplified claims review and some reliance on the providers themselves to apply the rules. Thus, health plans might well be led into some kind of "closed-panel" arrangements by the high administrative costs involved in trying to control independent private practitioners by indirect means.

Closed-Panel Arrangements

The organization of effective closed panels of physicians may well be the most valuable cost-containment service that the private sector can render. The possibilities are numerous and range through a wide spectrum, with health maintenance organizations (HMO's) of the prepaid group practice variety at one end and traditional free-choice health insurance at the other. HMO's have great promise[19] but are difficult to organize because, although Federal assistance is available for plans meeting certain requirements, most fledgling HMO's cannot be assured—in the short run at least, given patient loyalties—of enrollment sufficient to support a plan of the ambitious dimensions and high cost compelled by the Federal requirements. Some health insurers have already been deeply involved in HMO development, with widely variable results. In the case of Blue Cross, involvement in HMO's seems to have had a distinct monopolistic aspect, although more public-spirited purposes were also undoubtedly in evidence.[20] Nevertheless, it should be possible, even without impugning Blue Cross's motives, to use the antitrust laws eventually to restore appropriate competition between HMO's and Blue Cross by breaking up their anticompetitive joint ventures once they have served their admittedly useful purpose and are no longer needed to sustain the HMO in the marketplace.[21]

The HMO concept has been elastic enough to include prepaid plans which do not integrate physicians into a group practice but rely on so-called "individual practice associations" of practitioners (IPA's) to serve plan subscribers on a fee-for-service basis, much as traditional Blue Shield plans have done. IPA's have customarily been formed by or with the blessing and support of local medical socieities, although, as a practical matter, they might also be organized independently by an insurer, employer, or union seeking to solve some of the administrative problems of cost containment. Subsequent discussion suggests that antitrust principles could well exclude medical societies from a role in HMO or IPA development,[22] leaving insurers and others to organize competing and possibly overlapping panels.

A new and promising entrant into the discussion of "alternative delivery systems" is the so-called "health care alliance" (HCA), [23] recently conceived by Dr. Paul Ellwood, who also popularized the HMO concept. As Ellwood visualizes them, HCA's would include hospitals as well as doctors in a closed-end plan serving subscribers on a fee-for-service basis, with bills paid by the insurer. Ellwood believes that a multispecialty group practice would provide an ideal nucleus for an HCA, but an insurer-organized IPA with limited physician participation could also serve. Under the HCA model, subscribers pay premiums based on the participating providers' cost experience, an arrangement permitting providers and consumers to divide the savings from any efficiencies achieved. (Under present arrangements using communitywide experience, efficient providers are not rewarded, and patients have no incentive to select them.) In addition to the cost savings that flow from greater selectivity, both in coverage and in provider participation, and from closer control over providers, closed-panel mechanisms would facilitate quality-assurance activities as well as competition for identification in the consumer's mind as a reputable and reliable alternative.

Another cost-containment technique that leads logically to the closed-panel model is the establishment by the insurer of a fee schedule or the negotiation of fees or charges with individual physicians or hospitals.[24] Providers not accepting the plan's limits could be excluded altogether from seeing subscribers at plan expense, or the patient might be allowed to pay the difference. If these providers also resisted the plan's other cost-containment efforts, a larger copayment might be required to reflect the higher cost and discourage their use. Again, it is important to observe the wide range of possibilities.

As indicated, the striking thing is that so many promising ideas for private-sector actions to contain health-care costs seem not to have received a market test. A brief look at the demand and supply sides of the market will suggest some explanations and some possible remedies.

Consumer Demand for Cost Containment

It is arguable that the limited scope of private-sector cost-containment efforts, particularly on the part of health insurers, is traceable simply to a preference on the part of consumers for comprehensive coverage and for unquestioning payment of claims. Plans having cost-containment features may simply be unmarketable. Indeed, insurers report that employers and unions alike seem to prefer increasingly comprehensive coverage and claims administration that keeps the rank and file happy. Moreover, many companies that purchase large amounts of coverage have expressed a preference for other approaches to cost control. For example, the broadly representative Washington Business Group on Health appears to emphasize governmentally fostered collective controls, particularly health planning and PSRO efforts, over privately initiated competitive ventures.[25] Unions, on the other hand, are lined up behind major national health insurance proposals that would probably destroy the private sector's incentive, as well as its opportunity, to develop solutions of its own.

Of course, it may be simply that these interests lack confidence in the private sector's capability because they regard as immutable the trade restraints and other influences that currently prevent or inhibit significant change. In other words, purchasers' observed political behavior may not be a guide to their potential behavior in a market offering real alternatives. The widespread support voiced by both unions and business groups for the general notion of "alternative delivery systems" suggests that new configurations would receive a fair hearing.

It remains possible that the dynamics of labor-management relations and internal union politics might make union leaders and company personnel directors less than completely satisfactory representatives of the individual worker's interests, with the result that private-sector choices would not fully reflect the consumer's desire to economize. One hears it said, for example, that choices made between more take-home pay and more health benefits frequently reflect the union leadership's desire to provide some immediate in-kind benefits (such as come with shallow insurance coverage) which the rank and file can regard as a prize specially won by the union's efforts. Even though there may be some problems here, I find it hard to think that they would be insurmountable if health insurers had a reasonable chance to show what cost-containment services they could in fact deliver. Once a few employment groups had discovered that take-home pay could be increased significantly with only a small marginal reduction in the value of the health benefits package, the word would get around, and health benefits would begin to be looked at with increasing skepticism.

Although insurers frequently allege that active cost containment is resisted by employers because they are reluctant to appear to economize at the expense of employee health benefits, this "image" problem can be easily overcome. For example, Mobil Oil Corporation has offered its employees a year-end rebate of savings achieved in health insurance premiums, thereby legitimizing the company's cost-containment efforts. Similarly, an employer should be able to reduce health insurance benefits by expressly coupling it with an increase in take-home pay equal to the saving on premiums. The ideal approach to the problem would be to offer the individual employee a set of options that allow him to make the economizing choices himself and to profit from them personally. The employer's cost would be the same, except for the small administrative cost of offering the options, but the employees would derive a net benefit from the opportunity to economize and put the employer's contribution to a better use. There would thus seem to be a variety of ways in which employers could simultaneously cut back their health plans, increase their employees' overall welfare at essentially no cost to themselves, and maintain their beneficient image.

The really serious problem on the demand side of the market is the tax law's favorable treatment of health insurance as an employee fringe benefit. All consumers' demand for health insurance is heavily influenced by the tax benefits to be derived by paying health bills through an insurance plan rather than directly. The primary advantage is that dollars contributed to a group insurance plan for an employee's benefit are taxed to him as income neither at the time they are paid in nor at the time they are paid out on his behalf. Both State and Federal income taxes and FICA taxes are thus avoided, allowing the individual to purchase substantially more services for the same money by the insurance route. Management, union, and employee all perceive the greater efficiency of money spent in this way and the limited return from any economizing effort. Thus, the tax law has arranged things so that a penny saved on the purchase of health insurance is much less than a penny earned. The demand for cost-containment services has thus been greatly diluted by government's once well-meaning but now quite troublesome attempt to encourage fringe benefit programs. It is possible to believe that, by increasing demand for health insurance and decreasing demand for cost containment, the tax law is the primary cause of the problem of health-care costs.[26]

It is highly important for Congress to consider the desirability of switching to a system of limited tax credits as the vehicle for subsidizing the purchase of private health insurance.[27] A credit against taxes due could be given for 100 percent (or some lesser percentage, perhaps variable with income) of health insurance premiums paid by either the employer or the employee—up to some fixed amount. Among other things, this could mean that higher-bracket taxpayers would no longer be subsidized at a higher rate than lower-bracket taxpayers. More importantly, however, it would put an upper limit on the subsidy enjoyed by everyone, meaning that beyond some point additional insurance would, like most other things, be paid for with after-tax dollars. The incentive to economize in the purchase of health insurance would therefore be restored and, with it, the incentive for health insurers to offer only essential coverage and to supply cost-containment services. Although changing the tax law in this regard has long seemed politically impossible, the suggested switch to the use of credits fits well into the current tax reform movement and should be treated as a matter of the greatest urgency.

Changing the tax law to strengthen economizing instincts may nevertheless not be an essential prerequisite to getting us off the dime in private cost containment. Things may be so badly distorted already that even the poor return available on cost-containment efforts—owing to tax law's treatment of any economies achieved as taxable income—will frequently seem attractive because of the low value of some of the services that would be dispensed with. Employers and unions are increasingly aware that marginal health-care costs are not justified by the marginal benefits and have shown some signs of responding to cost-containment opportunities.[28] Although, as it stands, the law guarantees a permanently excessive allocation of society's resources to the health sector, some consumer demand for cost-containment services exists and could be exploited by careful design and marketing if it were not for certain problems that lie on the supply side of the market.

The Supply of Cost-Containment Services

Restrictions on the supply of cost-containment services include legal as well as nonlegal influences. While the legal restrictions seem not to be prohibitive in most States, they could be minimized still further by governmental efforts aimed at improving the private sector's ability to act. It is particularly important that ambiguous legal questions be resolved so as not to preclude responsible cost-containment measures. As to nonlegal obstacles, some of them would yield significantly to initiatives by health systems agencies and others, while the antitrust laws are available to deal with the most serious restraints.

Some types of closed-panel arrangements have been inhibited by restrictions on the corporate practice of medicine. The nature of this restriction varies from State to State, but in general it serves to exclude profitmaking enterprises controlled by lay interests from hiring physicians and selling their services.[29] The rule is broader than this in many places, however, and has precluded even nonprofit HMO's from operating in some States. The corporate practice rule has prevented many organizational innovations that could have imposed direct controls on physicians with potential benefits in the form of cost containment. Moreover, experience with restrictions on the corporate practice of such professions as pharmacy and optometry suggests that consumers are in fact deprived of the benefits of price competition by such restrictions.[30] It is of course argued that too intense competition would have undully detrimental effects on the quality of services, and, although this argument has been overstated, one cannot deny its force or hope to overcome its basic premise. Nor is it necessary to do so, since the corporate practice rule does not preclude all cost-containment ventures, although it may require tailoring them to meet certain concerns about preserving the doctor-patient relationship. It is an important insight that effective cost containment can be achieved without infringing on this valued relation. The corporate practice rule, if applied with reasonable appreciation of the competing interests at stake, can supply a useful guarantee against abuses, assuring that doctors and patients remain free to contract with each other for services without outside interference—though perhaps at the patient's rather than the insurer's expense.

Closely related to the corporate practice rule are provisions in a significant number of State statutes governing dental and medical service plans of the Delta (dental) or Blue Shield (medical) variety that purport to assure noninterference in the provider's diagnosis and treatment. An extreme reading of such provisions would restrict the plans to simply checking eligibility and paying bills, on the theory that any limitation on the resources available for financing care will necessarily influence, or "interfere" with, clinical decisions. I am not aware of any case law construing these provisions in the States, but a similar provision in the Medicare law has already created some difficulty in the Federal courts in litigation initiated by the AMA against utilization review regulations promulgated by the Department of Health, Education and Welfare.[31] In issuing a preliminary injunction against enforcement of the regulations, the courts appeared to conclude that any limitation on the coverage of the Medicare or Medicaid programs would be invalid if it might somehow influence doctors' clinical decisions.[32] One can perhaps attribute this result to the courts' vigilance in protecting Medicare and Medicaid beneficiaries against possible excessive cost-containment measures.[33] Under this view, private plans would be readily distinguishable, since consumers exercise some choice and can be presumed, in the absence of fraud or overreaching, to have looked out for their own interests.

Moreover, private plan beneficiaries are more likely than Medicare or Medicaid clients to have other resources available to pay for services which are desired but which, for whatever reason, are excluded from coverage. Again it would appear that legal restrictions on insurers and other health plans, if properly understood, should not prevent effective cost-containment measures taking the form of coverage limitations.

Another potential obstacle to insurer-initiated cost containment is a somewhat obscure provision in most State insurance laws that could conceivably be read to guarantee each insured absolute "free choice" of a physician or hospital, precluding the organization of closed-panel plans or HCA's except under special provisions in State or Federal law for HMO's, IPA's, or Blue Shield-type service plans. The provision permitting payment of claims on an insured's behalf directly to a medical care provider includes, in nearly all States, a statement such as "the policy may not require that the service be rendered by a particular hospital or person."[34] In the only case I have found construing this statutory language, the Indiana Supreme Court characterized it as:

> statutory language of differentiation, by which policy designs that would permit the insurer to direct the destiny of the cure through the specific designation of the person or facilities, is prohibited. The phrase "may not require that the service be rendered by a particular hospital or person" distinguishes accident and sickness policy standards from the standards of the Workmen's Compensation Laws, which expressly permit and authorize an employer to select for the treatment of his employee, specific physicians, hospitals, nurses, or spiritual healers. Therefore . . . [the statute serves] to prohibit this selective and discretionary designation of personnel for the treatment of the ill, rather than to affirmatively require insurers to indemnify for all attempted cures which are legally rendered.[35]

The Indiana case held that an insurer need not pay for care rendered by a podiatrist, but the court's view of the policy behind the law would seem to permit the insurer to exclude physicians who refused to cooperate with cost-containment measures so long as some range of choice was left to the insured. An insurer that wished to reduce the legal doubt still further might simply increase the copayment requirement for all care rendered by noncooperating doctors or hospitals. Such an arrangement might even overcome a more far-reaching requirement, such as Utah's apparently unique prescription that "the right of any person to exercise full freedom of choice in the selection of a duly licensed . . . [provider] shall not be restricted. . . ."[36] It would not appear that closed panel plans amount to "unfair discrimination" as prohibited in many States or that statutory provisions designed to expand the opportunities of nonphysician personnel, such as podiatrists, optometrists, and so forth, should be read to prohibit the exclusion of some physicians from participation in a closed panel. It would also seem acceptable for the closed-panel plan to impose qualitative controls such as govern admission to a hospital's medical staff. Another means of escaping restrictions in the insurance code may be through employer self-insurance. While the law of each State must be investigated with care, opportunities for productive innovation in cost containment do not seem to have been foreclosed.

Entry barriers facing HMO's are an important factor inhibiting the market's provision of cost-containment services. The Institute of Medicine's 1974 policy statement entitled *HMOs: Towards a Fair Market Test* documented the many legal and nonlegal problems which HMO's face and the failure of the Federal HMO Act of 1973 to address them constructively.[37] Under present conditions, the successful creation of an HMO is a triumph of managerial, legal, political, financial, marketing, and negotiating skill. Somehow one wishes it were not so difficult and that plan's medical capability were the decisive factor in its success or failure. The severe difficulties faced by HMO's, which Congress has done more to create than to alleviate, make all the more important the encourgement of other private-sector efforts.

Legitimate cost-containment efforts by HMO's and others are at least potentially curtailed by the law of medical malpractice[38] and by PSRO's.[39] Although cost-cutting could jeopardize the quality of care unduly, these two mechanisms for preventing overeconomizing draw their norms primarily from prevailing fee-for-service practice, which is precisely the source of the problem and the thing from which departures must be sought if benefits and costs are to be better equated at the margin. The costly distortions in insured-fee-for-service medicine brought about by automatic third-party payment and the "defensive medicine" which it facilitates could well be perpetuated by the courts and by PSRO's unless economic considerations are somehow introduced.

Even though there seem to be no insurmountable legal obstacles to private-sector provision of cost-containment services, there is little expertise available and considerable uncertainty about how to begin. More seriously, there is some doubt that the private health insurers, who are in the best position to develop the expertise and initiate the effort, have sufficient interest in doing so. Private insurers have made only limited moves to date and seem to be in general agreement about the limits of their powers.[40] Moreover, limiting coverage and controlling costs would only limit their premium income and the size of their reserves, making cost containment seem unattractive from the insurers' point of view. But this observation holds only for the industry as a whole, not for the individual firms, since any one firm could expect to increase its market share substantially if it could come up with an effective mechanism for providing essential coverage at low cost. Once the first olive was out of the bottle, competition would force the remaining firms to develop mechanisms of their own.

It still remains to inquire why insurers and others have done so little up to now. One cannot ignore the possibility that a tacit conspiracy exists among health insurers to adhere to traditional practices. If real competition in the design of insurance would ultimately reduce premium income, the industry members may feel that the transitory gains to them individually from getting a jump on their competitors would be offset by the ensuing uncertainty and the longrun prospect that all would share a smaller pie. In antitrust terms, "oligopolistic interdependence" or "conscious parallelism" may prevail, perhaps strengthened by regulation, by a traditional resistance to innovation and competition, and by frequent industry pronouncements that everything possible is being done and that governmental intervention, not competition, is the answer.[41] Conspiratorial explanations for the industry's inaction may seem inadequate, however, when it is recognized that insurers have in fact attempted some major innovations, primarily HMO development, and that other innovations, such as those suggested herein, would have produced a major confrontation with the medical profession. Even if it could hope to be successful in introducing a change over medical society objections, an insurer could anticipate incurring high costs that subsequent imitators would not incur. Under these circumstances, the better part of valor may be to do what health insurers have done—very little. This reflection leads me to conclude that the problem at the moment is not the health insurance industry, which may simply be behaving rationally given the climate for innovation, but is, instead, the medical profession, which has dictated that the climate for innovation is a stormy one indeed. For this reason, it seems to me that the ultimate key to stimulating competition in cost containment lies in reducing the power of organized medicine to resist initiatives that are not to doctors' liking.

COMBATING ORGANIZED RESISTANCE TO COST CONTAINMENT

The greatest obstacle to third-party cost containment is the willingness, even eagerness, of doctors to act collectively to halt, dilute, co-opt, or capture any cost-containment measure that they find objectionable or threatening. The question I wish to examine here is whether the antitrust laws can be employed to bring about an environment in which insurers and bulk purchasers of care can innovate freely in seeking cost containment.

As a result of their long enjoyment of substantial professional autonomy, physicians now respond almost reflexively to outside interference in "their" affairs by taking collective action through their local, State, and national professional associations. Indeed, professional societies are so accustomed to guarding their frontiers against intrusions—by other health professionals, by lay groups representing consumers' interests, or by government—that they will not take kindly to even the suggestion that some of their customary defensive practices may violate the antitrust laws. Yet, at least since the Supreme Court's 1975 decision in *Goldfarb v. Virginia State Bar,* [42] it has been clear that the so-called "learned professions" must obey the Sherman Act's prohibition against "every contract, combination . . ., or conspiracy in restraint of trade." As "combinations" of competitors, professional organizations must be prepared to defend themselves against the charge that their activities unreasonably restrict competition and deny consumers the benefits of a functioning market. Although professional groups may be allowed some leeway not allowed industrial trade associations, there are certain practices that, while common, are not likely to be permitted to continue.

The Law of Group Boycotts and Trade Associations

The legal doctrine most pertinent to improving the climate for private-sector cost-containment initiatives is that which outlaws concerted refusals to deal, or group boycotts, such as a medical society might engage in or stimulate as a means of enforcing its will against some outsider. A sense of the problem can perhaps be gained from the following purely hypothetical case taken from a recent examination in the Antitrust course at Duke Law School; the whimsical tone, introduced for the students' benefit, should not obscure the seriousness of the issue:

> *American Medical Views,* a weekly newspaper published by the American Medical Alliance (AMA), the leading national professional organization of physicians, has reported the following:
>
> "INSURER REQUIRING PRIOR APPROVAL OF ELECTIVE ADMISSIONS
>
> "Providential Insurance Co., affectionately known throughout the trade as 'the Pro,' is not likely to be thought of in affectionate terms by doctors or its insureds when its current practice of requiring prior approval of all elective hospital admissions becomes widely known. 'It is only an experiment,' says J. C. Commerce, president of the Pro. 'But we think a great deal can be saved by not accepting doctors' judgments automatically as proof that an expense incurred for hospitalization should be paid for under our policy. We also think, incidentally, that elective surgery,

and the fees for it, should be approved in advance, and we are investigating ways of doing it.'

"Doctors' are expressing strong views about the Pro's 'experiment.' 'It violates ethical insurance principles and threatens to deprive needy patients of hospitalization which their doctor believes is essential,' says Dr. George Good, president-elect of the AMA. 'I have heard doctors say that they are not admitting patients insured by the Pro simply because of the red tape involved. They are running a malpractice risk as a result, but life is too short for this paperwork on top of all that the government requires.'

. . . .

". . . [D]octors' organizations are considering . . . direct action. Next week's meeting of the Iowa Medical Society will probably adopt a resolution condemning the Pro's admission review program as 'unconscionable and unethical.' A special mailing by the Society to member and nonmember doctors recently spelled out the Pro's policy and cited instances of hardship created by its use. The Pro denounced the mailing as misleading and unfair.

"An entire morning session at last week's meeting of the Ohio Medical Society was devoted to the Pro's practices. Dr. Charles Fine, chairman of the Society's insurer relations committee, was the featured speaker and called on doctors to 'consult your consciences to see if you can cooperate with this wealthy company's systematic neglect of your patients' health needs in an effort to save itself a few dollars.'

"Speakers from the floor called for aggressive action against the Pro, including a refusal to have any direct dealings with it. They proposed, for example, that bills not be sent directly to the Pro but be sent to the patient instead, making him seek reimbursement from the insurer. Several speakers declared their intention to give up their 'piece of the Rock,' a reference to the Pro's slogan used in advertising its other lines of insurance.

"Many Ohio doctors are refusing to provide their patients in advance with the records they need to satisfy the Pro that the proposed hospital stay should be paid for. Others have refused altogether to see patients with Pro coverage, advising the patients by a standard form letter that they cannot fulfill their ethical obligations if a third party intervenes in this way.

"The Pro admits that its plan to save money at patients' expense may fail. 'We still think many hospital admissions are unnecessary,' says Mr. Commerce, 'but without a reasonable level of doctor cooperation we cannot make our review effort stick. It's too bad we are all alone in this effort and that the other insurers, especially Blue Cross, are so unwilling to challenge the doctors.'

"National Blue Cross spokesmen, privately critical of the Pro's plan, said that they encourage local plans to employ hospital-based review machinery, similar to that now accepted by HEW, to cut down on unnecessary admissions. Dr. Good of the AMA says that what Blue Cross does is what all 'ethical' insurers should do. He also said that the Pro 'would have our full cooperation in arranging a review program under medical society or hospital staff auspices. It is critical that patients' rights not be infringed, however. There is such a thing, after all, as the right to health care.'"

Just as the students were asked to do, I propose to discuss the antitrust questions raised. The principles involved are well developed in the case law of antitrust, and it is significant that my students, knowing nothing about health care, were able to make quite a lot of sense out of the problem. Thus, we are not theorizing in a vacuum but have the benefit of substantial experience with analogous situations and of insights into human behavior under comparable conditions developed over a long period of time.

To start with, although a medical society's call for a boycott of the insurer or its insureds would be clearly unlawful under a long line of cases,[43] we have nothing quite so blatant here. Nevertheless, an unlawful conspiracy to boycott can sometimes be inferred from collective actions likely to produce uniform behavior amounting to a boycott. For example, in a 1914 case in which some retail lumber dealers' associations published a list of wholesalers who also traded at retail in competition with the associations' members, the Supreme Court said,

> . . . when, in this case, by concerted action the names of wholesalers who were reported as having made sales to consumers were periodically reported to the other members of the associations, the conspiracy to accomplish that which was the natural consequence of such action [i.e., refusals to deal] may be readily inferred.[44]

Even if a conspiracy to boycott could not be inferred in a particular case,[45] the actions of a medical society are still actions taken by competitors in concert and must be analyzed under antitrust principles to see if they are unreasonable as themselves to be classed as restraints of trade. Thus, in our problem, the "Iowa" medical society resolution condemning the health insurer's ethics could well be said to restrain unduly the insurer's freedom to act in accordance with its own business judgment concerning consumers' desire for cost-containment services.

The problem is complicated, however, by the competing antitrust principle that, although true group boycotts are illegal *per se,* unilateral refusals to deal are normally not suspect.[46] Indeed, the freedom to do business with whomever one chooses is part of that same "freedom of traders"[47] that the rule against group boycotts is itself designed to vindicate. Arguably, the physicians in our problem might have their own personal reasons for refusing to cooperate with the hypothetical cost-containment program. Thus, not only might the paperwork burden be seen as excessive, but the individual doctor might be so outraged by the insurer's action that he is willing to give up some patients and some income to keep his conscience clear and to strike a small blow for patients' rights and professional independence. Although the "Ohio" facts in the problem demonstrate that physicians could well have been acting for reasons of their own and not with primary regard to what other doctors were doing, the fact remains that, through the use of code words and signals, the "Ohio" doctors invited an outpouring of sentiment designed and calculated to discipline and harass the insurer. The numerous individual refusals to deal were therefore, it seems clear, decided upon with some expectation that others would act in parallel fashion, and many such refusals would not have occurred without that expectation. Moreover, the medical society's role in whipping up enthusiasm is apparent. A court or jury could, I think on such facts infer the existence of a conspiratorial boycott[48] or, alternatively, could hold that the medical society's provision of meeting time and leadership on the issue unreasonably contributed to the ensuing trade-restraining activities of its members.

Despite the foregoing logic, one case suggests that the courts may not be quick to characterize as a boycott medical society activities of the sort found in the problem. In *United States v. Oregon State Medical Society,*[49] decided by the Supreme Court in 1952, the trial court had found insufficient evidence of a medical society boycott directed at certain private "hospital associations" engaged in objectionable cost containment. The Supreme Court commented on these findings as follows:

> The record contains a number of letters from doctors to private associations refusing to accept checks directly from them. Some base refusal on a policy of their local medical society, others are silent as to reasons. Some may be attributed to the writers' personal resistance to dealing directly with the private health associations, for it is clear that many doctors objected to filling out the company forms and supplying details required by the associations, and preferred to confine themselves to direct dealing with the patient and leaving the patient to deal with the associations. Some writers may have mistaken or misunderstood the policy of local associations. Others may have avoided disclosure of personal opposition by the handy and impersonal

> excuse of association "policy." The letters have some evidentiary value, but it is not compelling and, weighed against the other post-1941 evidence, does not satisfy us that the trial court's findings are "clearly erroneous."
>
> . . . .
>
> Appellees' evidence to disprove conspiracy is not conclusive, is necessarily largely negative, but is too persuasive for us to say it was clear error to accept it. In 1948, 1,210 of the 1,660 licensed physicians in Oregon were members of the Oregon State Medical Society, and between January 1, 1947, and June 30, 1948, 1,085 Oregon doctors billed and received payment directly from the Industrial Hospital Association, only one of the several private plans operating in the State. Surely there was no effective boycott, and ineffectiveness, in view of the power over its members which the Government attributes to the Society, strongly suggests the lack of an attempt to boycott these private associations. A parade of local medical society members from all parts of the State, apparently reputable, credible, and informed professional men, testified that their societies now have no policy of discrimination against private health associations, and that no attempts are made to prevent individual doctors from cooperating with them. Members of the governing councils of the State and Multonomah County Societies testified that since 1940 there have been no suggestions in their meetings of attempts to prevent individual doctors from serving private associations. The manager of Oregon Physicians' Service testified that at none of the many meetings and conferences of local societies attended by him did he hear any proposal to prevent doctors from cooperation with private plans.
>
> If the testimony of these many responsible witnesses is given credit, no finding of conspiracy to restrain or monopolize this business could be sustained. Certainly we cannot say that the trial court's refusal to find such a conspiracy was clearly erroneous.[50]

Despite the Court's explanations of the evidence, it certainly seems that messages were received even though none were obviously sent. Nothing could be more suggestive of the subtlety of intraprofessional communication and of the difficulty of curbing the profession's propensity to concerted action. Moreover, the Court's assertion that the boycott was ineffective reveals a judicial failure to recognize the total success of the doctors' campaign in bringing the hospital associations to heel and terminating their objectionable methods of cost containment.[51]

The *Oregon State Medical Society* case is important authority, to be sure, but it is quite possible that in the years since 1952 we have come to a greater sophistication about health-care costs and about the power exercised by the medical profession over the conditions and financing of medical practice. A recent review of the record in the *Oregon* case by Lawrence G. Goldberg and Warren Greenberg, two FTC economists, is most revealing of the methods and the success of the medical society in that instance and should help the courts to avoid repeating their mistake. As a sign of the difference in the times, it is notable that the trial judge's findings of fact, by which the Supreme Court felt bound, contained, as the Court observed, "irrelevant soliloquies on socialized medicine, socialized law, and the like, which . . . do not add strength or persuasiveness to his opinion. . . ."[52] It seems probable that somewhat greater alertness to the hazards arising from physician harassment of third parties would have produced a different result.

Today, it is possible to observe the considerable extent to which medical societies are in fact using their weight to shape the private financing system under which physicians operate. Recent studies by the Council on Wage and Price Stability of private-sector cost-control efforts revealed a number of instances of professional associations' resistance to health-care cost-control measures which employers and unions sought to introduce.[53] Another instance, a classic one in many ways, occurred a few years ago when the Aetna Life and Casualty Company instituted the practice of helping its insureds defend themselves in court against claims by physicians for fees which the insurer had determined were excessive; medical society response was vigorous, and the Aetna was forced to conform to professional demands.[54] At the present time, there are a number of ongoing struggles over attempts by health insurers to implement various kinds of second-opinion programs designed to curb unnecessary surgery. For example, in the Detroit area, three medical societies are negotiating the precise nature of these plans with the insurer.[55] Some of their demands are apparently non-negotiable, however, and a threat of boycott undoubtedly hangs over the proceedings.

While antitrust has still not visibly affected the tendency of local medical societies to make it their business to certify the propriety of insurer practices, there is some evidence that the AMA is beginning to resist its own anticompetitive impulses. *American Medical News* reported in December 1976—interestingly enough, just two days after my students confronted the examination question quoted above—that an AMA committee had, on the advice of antitrust counsel, withheld from the AMA's membership a report critical of health insurers' second-opinion plans, substituting a milder report in its place.[56] But, although the AMA's lawyers have recognized that antitrust principles require professional associations to take more neutral positions on developments in private health-care financing, the lesson has been hard to get across to the doctors themselves. For example, consider this news report of events at the AMA's 1977 Annual Convention:

> At the behest of antitrust counsel, the delegates reluctantly gagged themselves on several other issues, but rebellion finally broke out on the matter of mandatory second opinions, which some third parties are opting for as a means of cutting costs. The House was clearly eager to accept a resolution opposing mandatory consultation, but the cautious legal department wanted time to study the implications first.
>
> "This resolution is a clear statement of our views and we ought not to be afraid to adopt it," thundered Georgia's Frederick W. Dowda. "If we ran our offices the way the legal department wants us to run this House, we'd see one patient a week." The delegates cheered and adopted the resolution overwhelmingly.[57]

It would appear that a show of force by the antitrust agencies is called for.

Professionalism as a Defense

Even though the *Goldfarb* case indicated that the so-called "learned professions" are subject to the antitrust laws, that case, as well as common sense, also suggests that the concept of professionalism may permit certain collective activities by professional societies that would not be permitted if undertaken by industrial trade associations.[58] The broadest indication of this general principle appears in the *Oregon State Medical Society* case, precisely at the ellipsis in the lengthy quotation set forth above:

> Since no concerted refusal to deal with private health associations has been proved, we need not decide whether it would violate the antitrust laws. We might observe in passing, however, that there are ethical considerations where the historic direct relationship between patient and physican is involved which are quite different than the usual considerations prevailing in ordinary commercial matters. This Court has recognized that forms of competition usual in the business world may be demoralizing to the ethical standards of a profession. . . .[59]

This dictum, which the Court indicates was not necessary to the decision in the case, stands as a general expression of the special prerogatives which the medical profession may enjoy. The case law has still not defined the precise scope of those prerogatives.

There is no question that the foregoing quotation from the *Oregon* case, when read in the context of the boycott discussion, strongly implies that the medical profession might be allowed to engage in coercive boycotts, enforcing professional "ethics" against third-party insurance carriers and others.

We do not know for certain, of course, whether the Court would in fact tolerate such action. However, given its strongly expressed opposition in other contexts to "agreements . . . [which] cripple the freedom of traders and thereby restrain their ability to sell in accordance with their own judgment."[60] it would be surprising if the Court would permit the medical profession to enforce its preferences by such coercive means. Moreover, such a result would depart widely from the holding in the 1943 case of *American Medical Association v. United States,*[61] where the Supreme Court upheld the conviction of the AMA for criminal violations of the Sherman Act in its activities in opposition to Group Health Association, Inc., a Washington, D.C., prepaid group practice plan. Among the offenses charged in the *AMA* case were expulsions from membership of doctors who participated in the Group Health program, with the consequence that such doctors found it difficult or impossible to obtain access to hospital facilities. Denials of association membership and the like have never been as unfavorably regarded by antitrust courts as concerted refusals to enter into commercial relationships. Yet the court of appeals addressed the issue in strong terms:

> [A]ppellants were permitted to organize, to establish standards of professional conduct, to effect agreements for *self-discipline* and *control.* There is a very real difference between the use of such self-disciplines and an effort upon the part of such associations to destroy competing professional or business groups or organizations.
>
> . . . [A]ppellants have open to them always the safer and more kindly weapons of legitimate persuasion and reasoned argument, as a means of preserving professional esprit de corps, winning public sentiment to their point of view or securing legislation. . . . Neither the fact that the conspiracy may be intended to promote the public welfare, or that of the industry, nor the fact that it is designed to eliminate unfair, fraudulent and unlawful practices, is sufficient to avoid the penalities of the Sherman Act. Appellants are not law enforcement agencies. . . . [A]nd although persons who reason superficially concerning such matters may find justification for extra-legal action to secure what seems to them desirable ends, this is not the American way of life.[62]

This language seems more carefully weighed and more responsive to the true issues than the Supreme Court's dictum in the *Oregon* case. It would not seem that a meaningful distinction can be drawn between attempted destruction of a competitor, as in the *AMA* case, and destruction of the benefits of competition by dictating the terms on which dealing will occur.

The courts have still before them the considerable task of reconciling antitrust principles with the recognized self-regulatory responsibilities of the organized professions. To guide them, the antitrust enforcement agencies and the courts have their earlier experience in using antitrust policy to structure and direct industrial self-regulatory activities so as to curtail the potential for abuse while retaining the public benefits which flow from such activities. Perhaps the leading case is *Silver v. New York Stock Exchange,*[63] in which the Court used antitrust principles to impose upon the Stock Exchange an obligation to employ certain procedural safeguards to minimize the risk that self-regulatory powers would be used to injure competitors of Exchange members. It would be surprising if the implied self-regulatory powers of professional associations were any broader than the statutory powers exercised by the Stock Exchange or were entitled to any greater deference. The principles of the *Silver* case seem most relevant to the exercise of the disciplinary powers of such medical organizations as specialty societies and hospital medical staffs.

Looking beyond the profession's disciplinary powers over its own members, the medical societies appear to have a much weaker claim to a voice in the structuring and administration of third-party payment plans and other developments in the private financing and delivery of care. Their best legal argument would probably be based on an analogy to "seal-of-approval" and other standard-setting progams which have been tolerated, within limits, by the antitrust authorities in many industrial and other settings.[64] A medical society might, for example, invite insurers to apply for approval and, though administering its program in an open and seemingly reasonable way, nevertheless dictate conditions for approval that primarily served—in the name of ethics, the quality of care, and the doctor-patient relationship—to protect the profession's economic interests and to frustrate cost-containment efforts. While no official boycott might be imposed against plans denied or not submitted for approval, many providers, and indeed many consumers or consumer groups, would be influenced in their decisions to participate or to enroll. Obviously, the result could well be a perpetuation of the present situation unless the courts were prepared to recognize the danger that even a partially effective physician boycott could curtail important cost-containment initiatives. Of course, there would be no substantial problem if it were possible to arrange it so that the society's endorsement was conveyed only to consumers, who could make up their own minds, and not to the profession as a whole, many members of which might take it as a signal to cooperate with approved plans alone.

A "seal-of-approval" program does not usually present the hazard of stimulating a group boycott by members of the accrediting association since such members are not usually in the position of dealing individually with applicants. But, in one case where certain utilities allegedly refused to supply gas for use in a gas burner unapproved by an association of which they were members, the Court held that a violation had been pleaded even though a utility might have had good reasons of its own for unilaterally honoring the seal of approval program;[65] although an actual conspiracy to boycott was not clearly pleaded, the Court reacted to the hazard it perceived. In another case, an educational certification program was upheld despite somewhat arbitrary policies, but the evidence established that the schools constituting the accrediting organization freely adopted their own policies toward graduates of the unaccredited school, accepting many transfer students.[66] It would appear that a medical "seal-of-approval" program would be in great jeopardy if it was widely respected by the profession.

The social utility of "seal-of-approval" mechanisms is greatest in areas of great technical complexity, where consumers require special assistance and protection. It is not at all that third-party cost-containment initiatives present issues requiring scientific or technical expertise or that consumers and individual providers cannot protect themselves adequately against third-party abuses and make competent decisions without medical society assistance. In view of the differing balance between social benefits and social harm, specialty certification, supplying useful information to consumers, would have much stronger claim to recognition by an antitrust court than would a plan for certifying third-party payment mechanisms as acceptable to organized medicine.

Although many issues remain to be resolved in the process of harmonizing the long-standing tradition of professional autonomy under State law with Federal anti-trust principles newly applicable following *Goldfarb,* it seems probable that the medical profession's attempts to dictate to outsiders on issues on cost containment and financing mechanisms will not fall within the scope of legitimate professional activity, even under a tolerant application of antitrust doctrine. On such issues of economics, the profession cannot escape a severe conflict of interest which makes it an unreliable authority. Even though professing to speak for patients' interest—to the extent even, in our hypothetical exam question, of embracing the "right to health care"—the profession cannot competently represent patients' concern about costs. Use of the antitrust laws to confine professional societies' role seem very much in order.

Devising a Remedy

To recognize the perniciousness of medical-society orchestration of concerted professional resistance to private cost-containment initiatives is only to identify the problem, not to solve it. It is manifestly impossible to prevent altogether, or even to deny the legitimacy of, professional interchange concerning business developments such as we are discussing. I wish to examine here some of the problems of devising a remedy imposing on professional associations a requirement of neutrality toward cost-containment measures taken by private third parties. As frustrating and threatening as some of my suggestions will be to medical society activists, a fundamental premise of anti-trust is that private groups do not make and enforce laws and that freedom to innovate in the interest of consumers should not be curtailed by concerted action.

If meaningful competitive exploration of cost-containment strategies is to have any chance to begin, prompt clarification of medical societies' responsibilities under the antitrust laws is necessary. In order to avoid long drawn-out proceedings and the uncertainty attending case-by-case development, the FTC might consider the possibility of initiating a rulemaking proceeding to clarify in a "trade regulation rule" what is and what is not permissible in the way of medical society responses to private cost-containment initiatives.[67] I am not prepared to propose finally the content of such a rule, but it might go so far as to prohibit an association of competing physicians (other professions might be covered as well) from officially expressing (by way of resolution, official statement, editorial, or otherwise) either approval or disapproval of a particular third-party initiative or of a general method of cost containment. The rule would have to specify a number of things with particularity and might include some examples, perhaps drawn from the FTC's investigations, of the kinds of things prohibited or regarded as permissible. One advantage of using the rulemaking approach here would be that it would involve accusing no one directly of wrongdoing but would simply enunciate a clear rule to govern future conduct. I see no more painless way to effectuate the revolution in the status and governance of the professions than is implicit in the *Goldfarb* case.

Simply declaring that the medical society must remain neutral on private cost-containment ventures initiated without its advice would probably not be sufficient to create an environment conducive to effective private initiatives. It would probably be necessary to prohibit as well the approval (or disapproval) even of programs that were voluntarily submitted to the society by their proponents. Otherwise, a *de facto* "seal-of-approval" scheme would emerge, with the possible result that all plans lacking the society's imprimatur would be discriminated against by physicians acting in part in defense of the profession's collective welfare. The experience revealed in the record of the *Oregon State Medical Society* case demonstrates that, if the profession is allowed a chosen instrument as a financing vehicle (a Blue Shield plan in that case), it may succeed in setting the rules for all insurers even without explicitly calling for boycott.[68] Because application of the antitrust "rule of reason" in situations such as this allows a balancing of expected public benefits against expected harms, there is ample authority for the courts—or for the FTC in developing a trade regulation rule—to assess the probabilities and conclude that the public interest lies in the more extensive prohibition.

In developing rules for medical societies, particular problems could be anticipated in the presentation of "news" to the members through society-sponsored publications, and consideration should probably be given to prohibiting society-sponsored publicity tending to induce a boycott, such as reporting of explicit proposals for boycotts or of inflammatory opinion not balanced by opposing views. It is also not obvious just how a rule could effectively prevent a medical society from allowing its meetings to become forums for conspiracy-making; but the enforcement agencies and the antitrust courts have had experience with trade association meetings in other industries[69] and should be able to define potential abuses and thereby reduce the society's ability to inspire a sufficiently large number of physicians to act with primary regard for mutual self-interest. Finally, it is elementary that the medical society should avoid actions designed to penalize individual physicians who elect to cooperate with cost-containment efforts, including identification of such individuals by name so as to invite their colleagues to exert pressure upon them.[70]

Such restrictions on the medical society, its officers, and its newsletter, if they should be adopted, would undoubtedly be perceived as extreme measures, but anything less might be deemed inadequate to break the organized profession's grip on developments not within its legitimate domain. It is arguable, of course, that such a remedy is more appropriately imposed as a remedial measure in an FTC cease and desist order, following a finding of a specific violation, than in a trade regulation rule designed to clarify the substantive offense. Nevertheless, if investigation confirmed the existence of a real hazard of boycott and harassment due to the medical profession's receptivity to signals flashed in code from society headquarters, the mere sending of such signals could be barred as creating such a danger to the public and carrying so little public benefit that it can be classed as a restraint of trade or, under the Federal Trade Commission Act, as "unfair method of competition."

Antitrust enforcement has encountered in other contexts the same kinds of "free speech" objections that would inevitably be offered against prohibitions of the type suggested. The leading case involved a trade association of railroads accused by competing motor carriers of using the media in deceptive ways in a campaign to induce the enactment of legislation restricting the truckers' opportunities.[71] The Supreme Court refused to allow the antitrust laws to be used to restrict the railroads' use of the media to influence legislation, arguing, in effect, that the "marketplace of ideas" could take care of itself. A later case, however, upheld an antitrust complaint that charged a truckers' association with abusing their fundamental right of access to the administrative and judicial arms of government by systematically opposing before a State regulatory commission and the courts, without regard to the merits, all applications for new entry into the trucking business.[72] Despite the argument that the truckers were simply petitioning their Government, the case was held to fall within the so-called "sham" exception to the general principle that antitrust should not frustrate the exercise of political rights. It was held that, if the truckers acting in concert had in fact abused governmental processes for anticompetitive purposes, they would be guilty under the Sherman Act.

As shown in the cases cited, a trade association's free speech rights protect it only in petitioning the Government in good faith on behalf of its members. When a medical society involves itself in areas where it is not petitioning government and where it has no guard-governmental function of its own, it is subject to antitrust controls and to all the rigors of the antiboycott rule. Because its members' concerted political activity constitutes protected speech, a medical society could protest a Medicare policy that it found objectionable, even to the extent of prompting many doctors to refuse Medicare patients; indeed, it is not clear that the antitrust laws would prohibit an organized doctors' strike to obtain a change in the State Medicaid program, although the injury to innocent parties, the Medicaid beneficiaries, would sorely tempt the courts to find a remedy and to ignore the claim that the strike was political action.[73] On the other hand, developments in private financing mechanisms are, by definition, not political or governmental, and the rigorous antitrust rules against policing private economic behavior would apply. (Indeed, this distinction is one reason why some people regard the private sector as offering a better opportunity for ultimately breaking the medical profession's grip on the financing and delivery system.) Of course, the medical society might try to send its signals to the membership in the form of a complaint that "there ought to be a law" against whatever some third party was doing, but that attempt to disguise a call for a boycott as political speech would face a severe test under the so-called "sham" exception mentioned earlier, which the Supreme Court stated as follows:

> There may be situations in which a publicity campaign, ostensibly directed toward influencing governmental action, is a mere sham to cover what is actually nothing more than an attempt to interfere directly with the business relationships of a competitor . . . [in which case] the application of the Sherman Act would be justified.[74]

The overriding object of the FTC's confrontation with organized medicine should be to change medical societies from virtual arbiters of the private financing system's features into mere advocates whose point of view must compete with others in the marketplace of ideas and the political process. The medical societies will decry the potential abuses they see in free private-sector developments, and it is quite possible that reduction of their powers could allow some truly objectionable practices that might have been prevented. Nevertheless, the medical societies "are not law enforcement agencies"[75] nor are they suitable spokesmen for consumer interests. Moreover, other protections against abuse are available and wholly adequate. For these reasons, organized medicine should be confined to the use of persuasion directed either toward consumers or toward political bodies. In particular, the emerging health systems agencies (HSA's) seem to provide an excellent local forum for the medical society to advocate its view without simultaneously stirring up the profession to vigilante action. Indeed, the HSA's have a remarkable opportunity both to assist the antitrust enforcers in policing medical society behavior and to facilitate and encourage consumer-oriented initiatives in cost containment.

The Medical Society as Collective Bargainer

One implication of the foregoing legal analysis is that the medical societies are, or can readily be, prohibited from engaging in negotiations with health insurers, unions, employers, and other consumer groups over the nature and details of financing arrangements, even if those negotiations are initiated by others. The underlying reason why such negotiations have become customary, and the reason why they should be foreclosed, is the implicit threat of boycott facing any plan which departs from accepted practice without professional approval. Although private advice would be available from the medical society, there would no longer be any necessity for obtaining the society's agreement and therefore no necessity for negotiating the terms of cost-containment initiatives.

Removing the medical society from its accustomed role may seem counter-productive in view of certain socially beneficial changes that have been introduced as a direct result of insurer-provider negotiations in the past. Society-sponsored peer review mechanisms have been put in place in many communities to check excessive fees and utilization, and costs have seemingly been controlled by such developments as the so-called "foundations for medical care," which are second-generation Blue Shield plans controlled by the medical establishment but accepting some cost-containment responsibility. But these improvements seem minor compared to what would probably have been achieved in the absence of the boycott threat.[76] By the same token, removal of that threat should permit competition finally to stimulate insurers and others to develop more effective cost-containment measures.

Health-care providers' practice of combining for the purpose of bargaining with third-party payers has a venerable history, giving it an apparent legitimacy that argues for its continuation. The practice was obviously inherent in the original status of Blue Cross and Blue Shield plans as creatures of provider organizations; bargaining between plan and providers was inconsequential as long as the service plan was already charged with carrying out providers's collectively expressed wishes. But as the Blues came to be more independent, facing competition on the one hand and the demands of consumers and regulators on the other, the bargaining process became more intense. Nevertheless, given the gradualness of the evolution away from strict provider control, it probably never occurred to anyone at any point that providers should be negotiated with only individually and not collectively. In any event, there was usually no agreement on actual prices to be charged or paid, which varied with costs or circumstances and were handled either by a cost-related formula (in the case of hospitals) or by reference to usual and customary fees or charges. Thus, the most obvious antitrust concern—price—was not aroused, and it was possible to see other issues, such as cost-containment measures, merely as questions of ethics and administrative detail.

Bargaining between the Blues and organized providers has more than just historical acceptance behind it. The special relationship with providers is expressly recognized in many State laws. Moreover, under the Federal McCarran-Ferguson Act, the antitrust laws are expressly waived for the business of insurance as long as State regulation is in place. Further, the Blue plans were very large in many places, giving rise to a need on the part of providers to organize to protect themselves against potential exploitation once their direct control was weakened. Indeed, insurance commissioners in some States have leaned heavily on the Blues in an attempt to use their monopsony power in just this way, producing confrontations that are as much political as economic and therefore seem to make a collective industry response appropriate.[77] I would have to agree that it would be unfortunate if the antitrust laws were applied to deny self-help to providers confronted by a state-created and state-maintained monopsonist.

The problem faced by the FTC and the courts is to find ways of breaking down providers' united front toward third-party cost-containment measures wherever collective bargaining cannot be justified as a legitimate exercise of political or countervailing economic power. This is a complex undertaking. One possibility might be to recognize the Blues' special status in the community and their special relationship to providers by allowing collective bargaining with them while at the same time protecting the right of commercial insurers, unions, employers, and other consumer-operated plans to negotiate with providers individually. However, this approach runs the risk that the Blues will become (or remain) the providers' chosen instruments, with results similar to those in the *Oregon State Medical*

Society case. While the political environment might prevent this from occurring, it does not seem to have done so yet, since commercial insurers seem unable to go much beyond the Blues in cost-containment endeavors. The Blues' apparent status as models for insurer behavior, just as the Blue Shield plan was in the *Oregon* case, flows directly from collective bargaining, and the legitimacy accorded their mild efforts serves to make any more aggressive effort appear illegitimate because not professionally validated. For these reasons, it seems highly desirable to put the Blues on the same footing as everybody else, treating them more like private insurers and less like political instrumentalities. Even where some provider control remains under State law, that need not provide the warrant for actual face-to-face bargaining. Like other insurers, the Blues should negotiate with individual providers, not a cartel.

Although a Blue plan or a large buying group might wield monopsony power in some communities, that problem could be dealt with on an *ad hoc* basis where specific abuses appeared. Buyer coalitions should be controlled by antitrust principles, too; but in the present climate pragmatism suggests tolerance of consumer self-help measures taken against a background of past abuses by providers and the demonstrated stubbornness of the medical monopoly.[78]

SUMMARY AND CONCLUSION

This paper began by examining what the private sector, unrestrained and with normal incentives, might be expected to do to contain health-care costs. In such a market, the predicted tendency would be away from comprehensiveness in health insurance coverage and toward defining benefits with great precision so as to exclude from coverage care that is not likely to be worth to the patient its cost to the plan. Competition would drive health insurers and other plan organizers to seek the best combination of benefits (financial protection), exclusions (protection against moral hazard), administrative efficiency, and acceptability to both patients and individual providers. It is probable that various closed-panel arrangements would prove most satisfactory from all of these points of view, facilitating each plan's internal monitoring as well as its negotiation of charges with individual physicians, hospitals, pharmacists, and so forth.

That these speculations seem somewhat other-worldly is precisely the point and leads to an inquiry into the factors that have prevented the private sector from exploring the many avenues seemingly open to it. On the demand side of the market, one finds that the tax law's treatment of health insurance as an untaxable fringe benefit is the engine that, more than anything else, has driven the private sector off the track, distorting the demand for medical care. By making cost containment unrewarding—a dollar saved in premiums is worth only 60 to 70 cents to employees after taxes—the tax law undercuts the private sector's will to act and makes wholly unfounded both the frequent charge that the private sector is irresponsible and the frequent assertion that the market has failed. If government really wants to control health care costs, it has only to unleash the private sector by changing the tax law to make those citizens who do not require special subsidy pay for marginal health insurance coverage in after-tax dollars. Given the availability of this approach or some modification of it, it is simply wrong to say, as is so often said, that there is no alternative to trying to solve our problems by regulation. Moreover, government's special responsibilities toward those disadvantaged citizens who are now underinsured or dependent on the Medicare and Medicaid programs can be discharged in ways that rely upon and foster, rather than undercut, private-sector cost containment.[79] It is regrettable that we have shown so little imagination in our approach to assuring the accessibility of adequate medical care to all and that Congress, which largely created the cost-escalation problem, has shown no interest in solving it by withdrawing government from its dominant role and correcting the distortions it has introduced into the market for health insurance and health care.

While extremely important to any understanding of the private sector's performance, tax considerations do not explain the failure of the private sector to generate adequate cost containment even at the new margin—where the dollars at stake are worth just 60 to 70 cents. At this point, restraints on the supply side of the market are of great immediate importance. Legal restrictions, though significant and sometimes of uncertain scope, do not appear ultimately to stand in the way of many promising initiatives. The real crunch on the supply of cost-containment services comes when the medical profession's preference for blank-check spending authority is seriously challenged. Any suggestion that providers break ranks and participate in privately initiated cost-containment ventures is met with strong counterattacks having a powerful deterrent effect on innovative undertakings. Having identified this trade-restraining activity by organized medicine as the crucial issue, this paper advocates vigorous and immediate use of the antitrust laws to eliminate altogether the medical societies' dictation of or participation in the design of third-party financing schemes and alternative delivery systems.

It is a distinguishing feature of American society that the economic behavior of private interest groups, however powerful and elite, may be scrutinized by nonpartisan antitrust prosecutors and the judiciary, and many achievements of antitrust in controlling the exercise of private power could be cited.[80] Precisely because of its nonpolitical character, antitrust denies powerful interest groups their usual weapons and defenses and makes possible change that is both dramatic and effective, not just incremental or cosmetic, as legislative measures so often are. The new availability of antitrust, since 1975, for dealing with problems of the health sector is, for these reasons, an important development of unappreciated promise. This paper has attempted to identify as the crucial antitrust target the influence exercised by organized medicine over private financing mechanisms and their cost-containment initiatives. Because the FTC appears to have assumed the primary responsibility for implementing anti-trust policy in the complex health services industry, this paper suggests that an FTC trade regulation rule might be the appropriate weapon to employ to combat well-established professional practices and attitudes.[81]

Fortunately, activation of antitrust as an instrument of change in the health-care industry does not immediately depend on Congress or the Department of Health, Education, and Welfare to do anything at all. Of course, the Carter administration and Congress will eventually have to decide whether the United States should adopt an approach to national health insurance that undercuts, or one that builds upon, the private sector. I, for one, believe we should value the market mechanism highly and allow it a prominent part, not only because it, better than anything else, can contain costs and force the system to give value for money, but also because it preserves consumers' and providers' opportunity to express their other values and preferences on some highly personal and difficult matters.[82] It seems to me that bargaining in a relatively free environment between consumers, many of them organized in groups, and providers organized in competing closed panels can come substantially closer than government to finding the right balance among all the conflicting and competing values at stake in medical care. Moreover, it is at least possible that, before the final, fateful choice of a mechanism of social control is made for the health-care sector, we will have had a fairer test than ever before of what the private sector can in fact do. The essential prerequisite for such a test of the market's capability, it seems to me, is a prompt and authoritative clarification—and perhaps also a forceful demonstration—of what the antitrust laws require of organized medicine.

We have all had the experience of seeing a seemingly broken mechanical contrivance—a motor or a wrist watch, for example—start operating again without obvious explanation. Sometimes all that is needed is a kick or a shake. I think that the antitrust laws could be administered to provide just the kick or shake-up that could set the market for private health-care cost containment purring, or ticking, in a most surprising way. Even if it only sputters, the market would be of some value as a complement to public efforts and should not be displaced. Certainly government itself sputters a lot about health-care costs, but its machinery has yet to make much headway on its own.

NOTES

1. Schultze, "The Public Use of Private Interest," *Harper's,* May 1977, at 43.

2. *See* V. Fuchs, *Who Shall Live? Health, Economics and Social Choice* 60, 94-95 (1974).

3. *See* Havighurst & Blumstein, "Coping With Quality/Cost Trade-offs in Medical Care: The Role of PSROs," 70 *Northwestern University Law Review* 6 (1975).

4. *See* Havighurst, Blumstein & Bovbjerg, "Strategies in Underwriting the Costs of Catastrophic Disease," 40 *Law and Contemporary Problems* 122 (1976).

5. *See* Havighurst, "The Ethics of Cost Control in Medical Care," 60 *Soundings* 22 (1977).

6. *See, e.g.,* Council on Wage and Price Stability, "Employee Health Care Benefits: Labor and Management Sponsored Innovations in Controlling Costs," 41 *Federal Register* 40,298 (Sept. 17, 1976); Nash, Garfinkel, & Bryan [Research Triangle Institute], *Quality Assurance Methodologies Employed by Selected Third Party Carriers of Prepaid Dental Plans* (FR 24U-1007, Nov. 1976); Havighurst, "Controlling Health Care Costs; Strengthening the Private Sector's Hand," 1 *Journal of Health Politics, Policy and Law* 471, 472-74 (1977).

7. The most extensive application of the economizing-by-limiting-coverage principle is found in Martin Feldstein's concept of "major risk insurance," which entails copayments large enough and over a broad enough range to put consumers in the position of having to economize on most health expenditures while still having their maximum exposure limited to a fixed annual amount based on income. Feldstein, "The High Cost of Hospitals—and What to Do About It," 48 *Public Interest* 40 (1977).

8. *See generally* Feldstein, "The Welfare Loss of Excess Health Insurance," 81 *Journal of Political Economy* 251 (1973). For the most complete treatment of health insurance benefits, see A. Donabedian, *Benefits in Medical Care Programs* (1976), which nevertheless is quite vague on the issue of selectivity versus comprehensiveness and fails to identify the role of tax law (see text at notes 26-27 *infra*) in inducing comprehensive coverage.

9. Most studies of demand elasticity do not disaggregate demand beyond distinguishing between inpatient and outpatient services. This obscures the fact that the elasticity found is an average of many differing elasticities of demand for a wide variety of services. *See, e.g.,* Newhouse & Phelps, "New Estimates of Price and Income Elasticities of Medical Care Services," in *The Role of Health Insurance in the Health Services Sector* 261 (R. Rosett ed., 1976).

10. Demand curves reflect not only variations in preferences but also income differences, since some of the fall-off at higher prices may be said to reflect consumers' inability, not their unwillingness, to pay. The relevance of this observation for social policy is not clear. On the one hand, some observers would completely reject demand elasticity as a relevant consideration, endorsing proposals for comprehensive coverage and contending, in effect, that the "welfare-loss triangle" reflects inequality, not inefficiency. On the other hand, it can be argued that demand elasticities provide a good index of relative medical necessity despite income differences, which probably affect the slope of all demand curves to about the same degree.

11. Interest is being expressed currently in closely defining a minimum benefit package as the basic entitlement under a national health insurance program. *See* Rosenthal, "Setting the Floor: A Missing Ingredient in an Effective Health Policy," 1 *Journal of Health Politics, Policy and Law* 2 (1976). Similar selectivity in designing the benefit package would also be appropriate in private insurance schemes, which allow groups of people to choose their own "entitlement," but with the costs in view. The Government could help consumers in making informed choices about the optimal scope of private coverage by sponsoring research into particular procedures' cost effectiveness and demand elasticity.

12. Blue Shield Association recently announced an intention to exclude 28 medical procedures from coverage on the ground that they "are widely acknowledged as obsolete and inappropriate." *Boston Globe,* May 19, 1977, at 19, col. 1. Blue Shield was generally expressing the medical profession's idea that anything not bad medicine should be covered by insurance. The point here is that exclusions could be based on other grounds.

13. Medicare allows supplemental billing for physicians' services but not for other services. For example, the "maximum allowable cost" regulations covering drugs deny Federal beneficiaries the option of paying the difference in price between generic and brand-name products. 45 C.F.R. §19.1-19-6 (1976). Medicare will, however, pay for the more expensive product if the doctor certifies that it is "medically necessary." For variations on the use of cash indemnity payments, *see* Newhouse & Taylor, "How Shall We Pay for Hospital Care?," *Public Interest* 78 (1971). The latter source proposes also that insurance premiums reflect a choice of hospital so that those willing to use the community hospital rather than the university hospital will pay less.

14. *See* Havighurst & Blumstein, *supra* note 3.

15. *See* Havighurst, *supra* note 6 at 484.

16. The medical profession has found it convenient to define "unnecessary surgery" as equivalent to fraud, and many politicians have accepted this characterization. The correct conceptualization would have reference to the elasticity of demand and to the appropriateness of insurance coverage, not the surgery itself. For the medical view, implying an obligation on the part of third-party payers to pay for anything that is not fraudulent, *see* Paulshock, "Unnecessary Surgery: Who'll Have the Final Say?," *Medical Economics,* Mar. 7, 1977, at 75.

17. *See* Council on Wage and Price Stability, *supra* note 6, at 40303-07; Research Triangle Institute, *supra* note 6.

18. Some insurers have dropped the exclusion of cosmetic surgery, seemingly a rather straightforward and sensible one, because of difficulty in policing claims. Doctors apparently go quite far in casting their diagnoses to help patients obtain coverage.

19. It is notable that HMO's do not explicitly limit coverage but undertake to provide all needed care. Limitations are introduced indirectly, however, by various rationing mechanisms, including waiting time and limited resource availability. The lower hospital utilization rates in HMO's seem to flow from medical decisions but are comparable to what would happen under plans which would pay for hospitalization only under limited circumstances. It is possible that consumers and physicians are happier with this kind of cost containment, perhaps because it seems to leave decisions more completely in the treating doctor's hands, but there is the one drawback that, while some out-of-plan care is sought by HMO subscribers, the patient is not always free to purchase extra care if he should wish to do so.

20. Indiana Blue Cross and Blue Shield describes as follows its reasons for insisting on a "prime contractor" role in its relation with HMO's:

> This will allow the HMO to be an "Alternate Blue Cross and Blue Shield Program" and not a competitive alternative because Blue Cross and Blue Shield will continue to maintain the membership regardless of the option selected by the enrollees.
>
> Historically, Blue Cross and Blue Shield plans which assume only ancillary roles in ADS development and the operation gradually become dispensable in those roles and are eventually displaced by the growing capacity and capability of the ADS program.
>
> If the HMO enrollees are not Blue Cross and Blue Shield members, then Blue Cross and Blue Shield is merely merchandising its expertise of administrative capacity and doing nothing in the way of addressing its resources and leverage toward improving the delivery and financing of health care. The indications are clear that employer groups and consumers in

general are increasing their demand that Blue Cross and Blue Shield lead rather than follow and do more about cost containment in health care.

Thus, the Blue Cross and Blue Shield resources and leverage must become the tools with which effective change is brought about in health care.

Indiana Blue Cross and Blue Shield, Conditions for Partnership: Alternate Delivery Systems, Prepaid Group Practice 1 (no date). It requires some straining to read this as something other than a declaration of intent to monopolize.

21. *Cf. United States v. Pan American World Airways, Inc.*, 193 F. Supp. 18 (S.D.N.Y. 1961), *rev'd on other grounds,* 371 U.S. 296 (1963).

22. *See* test at notes 68 and 76 *infra.*

23. *See* Reynolds, "A New Scheme to Force You to Compete for Patients," *Medical Economics,* Mar. 21, 1977, at 23.

24. *See, e.g., Webster County Memorial Hospital, Inc., v. United Mine Workers of America Welfare and Retirement Fund,* 536 F.2nd 419 (1976) (upholding a union's bargaining with a hospital for fixed per diem charge).

25. *See, e.g.,* Washington Business Group on Health, *A Working Paper on a Private Sector Perspective on the Problems of Health Care Costs* (April 1977).

26. *See* Feldstein, "How Tax Laws Fuel Hospital Costs," *Prism,* Jan. 1976, at 15.

27. *See,* the somewhat fuller discussion of this proposal in Havighurst, *supra* note 6, at 475-78.

28. *See, e.g.,* Council on Wage and Price Stability, *supra* note 6.

29. *See* Hansen, "Laws Affecting Group Health Plans," 35 *Iowa Law Review* 209, 211-19 (1950); Laufer, "Ethical and Legal Restrictions on Contract and Corporate Practice of Medicine," 6 *Law and Contemporary Problems* 516, 522-27 (1939).

30. *Cf. Gibson v. Berryhill,* 411 U.S. 564 (1973); *North Dakota State Board of Pharmacy v. Snyder's Drug Stores, Inc.,* 414 U.S. 156 (1973).

31. *American Medical Ass'n v. Weinberger,* 522 F.2d 921 (7th Cir. 1975).

32. The court suggested that regulatory review "may have the effect of directly influencing a doctor's decision on what type of treatment will be provided, thus directly interfering with the practice of medicine." *But see Association of American Physicians and Surgeons v. Weinberger,* 395 F. Supp. 125 (N.D. Ill, 1975), *aff'd mem.,* 423 U.S. 975 (1976). The courts' confusion on these issues also appears in their assessments of the States's efforts to limit their exposure under Medicaid. Attempts to limit coverage of deferrable surgical procedures have been invalidated by reading Federal law to require coverage of all "customary" services. *Medical Society of the State of New York v. Toia,* CCH Medicare & Medicaid Guide. § 28364 (E.D.N.Y. 1977). But arbitrary limits on the length of hospitalization are permissible. *Virginia Hospital Association v. Kenley,* 427 F. Supp. 781 (E.D. Va. 1977). One might have thought that the latter type of restriction might cause greater hardship than the former (but for the hospitals' willingness to continue to provide services without payment).

33. The theory of the case is criticized in Havighurst & Blumstein, *supra* note 3, at 55-58, and in Havighurst, *supra* note 6, at 496-497, n.62.

34. *E.g., Arizona Rev. Stat.* §20-1403 (1975); *Indiana Code Ann.* §27-8-5-10(c) (Burns 1975).

35. *Insurance Commissioners v. Mutual Medical Insurance, Inc.,* 241 N.E.2d 56, 61 (Ind. Sup. Ct. 1968).

36. *Utah Code Ann.* §31-27-24(2) (1974).

37. *See also* Testimony of C. Havighurst, *Hearings on Competition in the Health Services Market Before the Subcommittee on Antitrust and Monopoly of the Senate Committee on the Judiciary,* 93d Congress, 2d Session, part 2, 1036, 1078-82 (1974).

38. *See* Bovbjerg, "The Medical Malpractice Standard of Care: HMOs and Customary Practice," 1975 *Duke Law Journal* 1375; Havighurst, "'Medical Adversity Insurance'—Has Its Time Come?," 1975 *Duke Law Journal* 1233, 1237-40.

39. *See* Havighurst & Bovbjerg, "Professional Standards Review Organizations and Health Maintenance Organizations: Are They Compatible?," 1975 *Utah Law Review* 381.

40. *E.g.*, Bailey, "Rising Health Care Costs—A Challenge to Insurers," 8 National Journal 608 (1976).

41. *See generally* Posner, "Oligopoly and the Antitrust Laws: A Suggested Approach," 21 *Stanford Law Review* 1562 (1969). I find the health insurance industry too actively engaged in conferring on what is and is not possible. The Health Insurance Association of America, in developing its political position, necessarily engages in evaluations of competitive strategies such as HCA's.

42. 421 U.S.773 (1975).

43. *E.g., Fashion Originators' Guild of America v. Federal Trade Commission,* 312 U.S. 457 (1941).

44. *See Eastern States Retail Lumber Dealers' Association v. United States,* 234 U.S. 600, 612 (1914).

45. An inference of conspiracy would not be compelled if the information circulated was otherwise difficult to obtain and had value to the members above and beyond its utility as a signal for concerted action. *Cement Manufacturers Protective Association v. United States,* 268 U.S. 588 (1925); *McCann v. New York Stock Exchange,* 107 F.2d 908 (2d Cir. 1939).

46. *E.g., United States v. Colgate & Co.,* 250 U.S. 300 (1919).

47. *Klor's, Inc. v. Broadway-Hale Stores, Inc.,* 359 U.S. 207, 212 (1959).

48. An inference of conspiracy from "conscious parallelism" is not compelled where the putative conspirators might have had reasons of their own for acting as they did. *Theatre Enterprises, Inc. v. Paramount Film Distributing Corp.,* 346 U.S. 537 (1954). But arguable reasons for independent actions should not preclude a fact-finder's inference of conspiracy where an element of interdependence remains. In the *Theatre Enterprises* case, the jury had found for the defendants, but it is unlikely that a finding for the plaintiff would have been overturned. See note 66 *infra.*

49. 343 U.S. 326 (1952).

50. *Id.* at 335-37.

51. *See* Goldberg & Greenberg, "The Effect of Physician-Controlled Health Insurance: *U.S. v. Oregon State Medical Society,*" 2 *Journal of Health Politics, Policy and Law* 48 (1977).

52. 343 U.S. at 331.

53. Council on Wage and Price Stability, *supra* note 6.

54. *See* Goldberg & Greenberg, *supra* note 51.

55. *See* "MDs Winning 'Second Opinion' Fight," *American Medical News,* April 18, 1977, at 1.

56. "Second Opinion Statement Weakened," *American Medical News,* December 13, 1976, at 12.

57. "Trade Restraint: Listening to Lawyers," *Medical World News,* July 25, 1977, at 17.

58. 421 U.S. at 787-88, n.17:

> The fact that a restraint operates upon a profession as distinguished from a business is, of course, relevant in determining whether that particular restraint violates the Sherman Act. It would be unrealistic to view the practice of professions as interchangeable with other business activities, and automatically to apply to the professions antitrust concepts which originated in

other areas. The public service aspect, and other features of the professions, may require that a particular practice, which could properly be viewed as a violation of the Sherman Act in another context, be treated differently. We intimate no view on any other situation than the one with which we are confronted today.

59. 343 U.S. at 336.

60. *Keifer-Stewart Co. v. Joseph E. Seagram & Sons, Inc.*, 340 U.S. 211, 213 (1951).

61. 317 U.S. 519 (1943).

62. 130 F.2d 233, 248-49 (D.C. Cir. 1942).

63. 373 U.S. 341 (1963).

64. *E.g., Structural Laminates, Inc. v. Douglas Fir Plywood Association,* 261 F. Supp. 154 (D.Ore. 1966), *aff'd per curiam,* 399 F.2d 155 (9th Cir. 1968), *cert. denied,* 393 U.S. 1024 (1969); *Rooffire Alarm Co. v. Royal Indem. Co.*, 202 F. Supp. 166 (E.D. Tenn. 1962), *aff'd,* 313 F.2d 635 (th Cir.), *cert. denied.* 383 U.S. 949 (1963) (insurers' testing organization lawfully refused to test plaintiff's fire alarm which failed to meet organization's threshold standards).

65. *See Radiant Burners, Inc. v. Peoples Gas, Light and Coke Co.*, 364 U.S. 656 (1961).

66. *Marjorie Webster Jr. College, Inc. v. Middle States Ass'n. of Colleges and Secondary Schools, Inc.*, 432 F.2d 650 (D.C. Cir.), *cert. denied,* 400 U.S. 965 (1970). For a case involving the medical profession, see, *Community Blood Bank of Kansas City Area, Inc.*, 70 F.T.C. 728 (1966), condemning a boycott of commercial blood banks despite evidence of possible individual motives for uniform action.

67. The FTC's jurisdiction over nonprofit associations, such as the medical societies, is unfortunately in some doubt, and the FTC has unsuccessfully sought legislation to broaden its powers. There is, on the other and, no doubt that the Antitrust Division of the Justice Department could bring suit against medical societies.

68. *See* Goldberg & Greenberg, *supra* note 51.

69. *E.g., American Column and Lumber Co. v. United States,* 257 U.S. 377 (1921).

70. *See id.* at 411, which speaks of a conspiracy relying "for maintenance of concerted action . . . upon what experience has shown to be the more potent and dependable restraints, of business honor and social penalties. . . ."

71. *Eastern Railroad Presidents Conference v. Noerr Motor Freight, Inc.*, 365 U.S. 127 (1961). For discussion of the application of these principles in the context of professional self-regulation, see *Feminist Women's Health Center, Inc. v. Mohammad,* 415 F. Supp. 1258 (N.D. Fla. 1976).

72. *California Motor Transport Co. v. Trucking Unlimited,* 404 U.S. 508 (1972).

73. For the view that such boycotts are illegal and a review of the litigation (so far inconclusive), see Weller, "Medicaid Boycotts and Other Maladies from Medical Monopolists: An Introduction to Antitrust Litigation and the Health Care Industry," 11 *Clearinghouse Review* 99 (1977).

74. 365 U.S. at 144.

75. *See* text at note 62 *supra.*

76. *See* Havighurst, "Health Maintenance Organizations and the Market for Health Services," 35 *Law and Contemporary Problems* 716, 767-77 (1970), for a discussion of society-sponsored foundations as combinations in restraint of trade because of their preemptive effect on competitive developments.

77. *See, e.g. Frankford Hospital v. Blue Cross of Greater Philadelphia,* 417 F. Supp. 1104 (E.D. Pa. 1976).

78. *See id.; Webster County Memorial Hospital, Inc. v. United Mine Workers of America Welfare and Retirement Fund,* 536 F.2d 419 (1976).

79. For some brief suggestions, see Havighurst, *supra* note 6, at 477-78.

80. The New York Stock Exchange's fixed commission rates, dating from the 18th century, were recently eliminated due to pressures from antitrust authorities.

81. *See* text at note 57 *supra.*

82. Government seems, by contrast, a poor vehicle for saying "no" to health services that people want or for distinguishing needs and weighing values. This thesis is developed at length in Havighurst & Blumstein, *supra* note 3, and Havighurst, Blumstein & Bovbjerg, *supra* note 4. *See also* Havighurst, *supra* note 6, at 490-92, nn.70, 86.

Comment*

John Pisarkiewicz, Jr.
Glassman-Oliver, Inc.
Economic Consultants
Washington, D.C.

Professor Havighurst views the lack of cost containment efforts in health care as a market failure, and he examines both the demand and supply sides of the market to understand and develop suggestions for correcting that failure. On the demand side, he sees the tax treatment of health insurance premiums as the primary culprit.[1] In taking this position, he is, of course, in the company of Martin Feldstein and the editors of the *Wall Street Journal* who recently advocated that appropriate changes be made. On the supply side, where Professor Havighurst focuses, he sees the key to the resistance of organized medicine to third party cost-reducing or cost-limiting initiatives that are not to the doctors' liking. To remedy this, he recommends vigorous antitrust activity including perhaps a trade regulation rule. This kind of activity should establish a climate which would allow normal market forces to operate and effectively dampen cost increases.

While neither of these two suggestions is new, they are ones with which I fully concur and ones which I think deserve much repetition. Consequently, Professor Havighurst's paper is of considerable value in this respect.

The FTC, in my view, embarked upon a program of trying to inject competitive forces into the market for health care services with the issuance of the complaint against the American Medical Association and others in December 1975. This program has as its root the idea that the country ought to give the invisible hand a chance to operate and show us what can be accomplished before considering the method of the visible hand and some form of national health insurance. To date, we have made some progress, but I am disappointed with the speed of that progress. What is also disappointing is the lack of recognition of our efforts by parties not directly involved in the cases and investigations. With the exception of A. F. Ehrbar,

---

*The views expressed herein are those of the author and not necessarily those of the Bureau of Economics or the Federal Trade Commission

the many recent articles I've seen on the problem of the rising cost of health care do not mention the role which the FTC is trying to play. Hopefully, this conference and Professor Havighurst's paper will remedy that situation.

In addition to the value of repetition, I also noted that Professor Havighurst's thoughts and observations are fine in theory but may be quite difficult to achieve in practice. He does not neglect this point, but it is one which I wish to emphasize. In doing so, I do not wish to appear hostile to the basic idea of relying on free market forces, but I think it is necessary to be realistic. If the market for health care services is ever permitted to function freely, we should allow it an extensive period of time to operate before judging the adequacy of its performance.

Professor Havighurst thinks that it will be difficult but not impossible to achieve adequate cost containment through the market mechanism. For example, he foresees health insurance companies devising plans which can distinguish between services for which demand is elastic and those for which demand is relatively inelastic. The companies could then tailor policies to cover service for which demand is relatively inelastic and thereby reduce what Professor Havighurst calls moral hazard. I think the transactions costs involved in devising such plans could be extraordinarily high. Dichotomizing a particular medical service or procedure into two different classes is a fairly easy task when viewing aggregate health statistics. For example, four professors from the Harvard School of Public Health recently indicated that in their judgment there were too many hysterectomies, tonsillectomies, and appendectomies, etc., and that surgery of this type is not needed in many cases in order to assure adequate care. In their opinion, cost-benefit analysis should play a vital role in making these kinds of decisions.[2] While I agree with this, it seems to me that examining aggregate health statistics is one thing and talking to an individual patient who is ill is quite another. It might be quite difficult to convince that patient that his proposed operation either does not square properly with national health statistics or that his own doctor's original plan to operate was not upheld by a second opinion.

Another difficulty I foresee involves the behavior of the health insurance companies themselves. Professor Havighurst feels that once an adequate climate is established by antitrust forces, it will simply be a matter of getting the first olive out of the bottle before numerous cost-cutting initiatives are developed. Frankly, it may not be such an easy process. Health insurance firms have been regulated indirectly by the medical profession or directly by the Government for a considerable period of time, and it may be that they have learned to prefer the quiet comfort of a regulated existence to the vagaries of a competitive situation.

Another indicator of the level of competition which might result if threats from organized medicine are removed is the level of competition existing in the life insurance industry. Here only State regulation is a factor and yet there appears to be some dissatisfaction with the performance of that market. This industry is currently being studied by the staff of the FTC and perhaps their efforts will result in insights into the nature of the problems and how they might be corrected.

Finally, one very positive note. Professor Havighurst sees a variety of cost containment proposals flowing directly from the actions of HMO's, IPA's, HCA's, and others, if these alternative delivery systems are allowed to flourish. He is concerned, however, that exisiting prohibitions on the practice of corporate medicine will prevent the proper development of these alternative delivery systems. I totally concur with the idea that these other systems can have a pro-competitive effect. But with regard to the prohibitions on the corporate practice of medicine, I note that those which flow from the AMA's Code of Ethics are a target of the suit against the AMA issued in December 1975.

NOTES

1. Strictly speaking, this should be characterized as a market distortion rather than as a market failure.

2. See *The Washington Post.*

REFERENCES

A. F. Ehrbar, "A Radical Prescription for Medical Care," *Fortune,* February 1977, 164.

Wall Street Journal, May 18, 1977, 22.

Washington Post, May 24, 1977, A-12.

Comment

Richard E. Shoemaker
Assistant Director, Department of Social Security, AFL-CIO

It is indeed difficult to discern any semblance of a market at all in the health industry. In this age of specialized disciplines, it is difficult not to interpret reality in terms of the concepts and assumptions of the discipline rather than, first, understanding in depth the object or focus of study and then modifying or, in fact, even rejecting the application of that discipline as an appropriate tool for interpretation, explanation, or prediction.

Too many economists, for example, apply demand and supply analysis to the health marketplace and assume, therefore, the consumer will or can make rational choices as to how he may allocate his or her financial resources. This view correctly interprets insurance against the risk of illness to have a distorting effect on the optimum pattern of delivering health care effectively and efficiently.

This type of analysis is fallacious because it is the physician and not the consumer-patient who not only supplies the services but creates the demand for health services. It is now a well accepted fact that about 80 percent of the demand for health care is induced by the physician. We do not have twice as much surgery in this country as in England or Sweden because Americans need or demand twice as much surgery as the British or the Swedes. We have twice as much surgery because we have twice as many surgeons.

The work of Victor Fuchs and Marcia Kramer has demonstrated the relationship that, in fact, supply determines the demand in the medical care marketplace. However, laymen such as you and I understand this without the necessity of "proof" for we all behave pretty much the same way. We go to a doctor when we don't feel well, or have pain or, in some instances, think it is time to have a "checkup." The doctor is unlikely to make a precise diagnosis without ordering some tests which he deems essential. This is his decision, not mine or yours. The patient does not have enough knowledge to contradict his doctor.

After the diagnosis is made—hopefully a correct one—the patient's regimen is established by the physician.

Consumers do not "shop" around for a "best buy" in doctors. Information about charges for doctor's office visits are rarely available. If a patient is in distress and has not yet established a "doctor-patient relationship," he is likely to go to a physician nearby, or consult the telephone directory, or ask his friends whom he should see.

Nor does the patient shop around for a hospital. He goes to the hospital where the doctor arranges for his admission, likely the only hospital with which the doctor has an affiliation.

The fact is that the medical marketplace is dominated by physicians and, therefore, the medical marketplace is a monopoly of the medical profession. This power extends into the hospital. Hospital administrators live in virtual fear of offending their customers who are the medical staff and not the patients. The loss of even the affiliation of one doctor can result in the loss of a quarter of a million dollars in revenue to the hospital.

Businessmen know where the power is, even if some economists do not. Pharmaceutical manufacturers devote almost their entire advertising budget to doctor "education" because they know it is the doctor who prescribes the medicines for which the patient has to pay.

Financial incentives placed on the consumer cannot be effective. Unless financial leverage is placed on the physician, unless he is given a financial incentive to use health resources appropriately, unless his monopoly power is broken, cost containment becomes just another academic discussion between interdisciplinary teams of the non-medical profession.

The insurance industry, which is composed of Blue Cross, Blue Shield, and commercial insurance, has yet to challenge the power of the medical establishment. It is true that in recent years Blue Cross made a substantial contribution in the direction of supporting the development of Prepaid Group Practice Plans. However, most of such programs remain under the control of Blue Cross. As a consumer, I have a question as to how far Blue Cross will, in reality, seriously compete with itself in its capacity as an underwriter of traditional forms of practice. In fact, Blue Cross and Blue Shield are very much a part of the medical power structure, and their activities with respect to supporting the development of alternate forms of medical care delivery have had overtones of restricting competition among different plans in Rochester, New York, and Washington, D.C. The same conflict-of-interest potential exists where alternate delivery systems are sponsored or promoted by the commercial insurance industry. This is an area which should be carefully monitored by the Federal Trade Commission.

Insurance itself, as it has been applied to health care, has, indeed, caused a massive distortion in the delivery of health services. The principles of casualty or risk insurance involve the payment of relatively small premiums for infrequently occurring risks that involve catastrophic costs to the insured. Thus, hospitalization, because it was the most expensive modality of treatment, was the first benefit to be insured; surgery followed, with routine medical care last.

If, however, the purpose of a health program is to prevent catastrophic illness, then the most important coverage is for routine medical care, but such coverage does not fit the definition or concepts of casualty insurance. The concept of insurance, therefore, reinforces and financially supports high-cost episodic care. Catastrophic insurance would further distort the delivery of health services to high-cost technological care that benefits very few to the detriment of routine health maintenance which helps many and prevents many from needing treatment for catastrophic illness.

The principles of casualty insurance are not compatible with providing health service in a cost effective manner and should be dropped. The principle of prepayment should be adopted in its place. This is the principle in which, for a periodic payment made in advance, the beneficiary receives whatever care he or she needs regardless of how little or how much. This principle works as the prepaid group practice plans have demonstrated for over 40 years. This principle even appears to work with fee-for-service reimbursement as some independent practice associations have demonstrated. It should be noted that prepayment places the provider at risk and for this reason the interest of the physician becomes that of keeping his patients well and out of the hospital.

I do agree that the antitrust laws can be very helpful in breaking the monopoly of the medical profession. Were it not for the lawsuits that charged the profession with a conspiracy to restrain trade and which were won, there would be no Group Health Association in Washington, D.C., no Kaiser Foundation Health Plans, nor other prepaid health plans. The use of antitrust law is a most important element in curbing the power of the medical societies, and I do agree that it is most important that the FTC adopt rules to govern the conduct of the medical profession. This would be most helpful.

REFERENCE

V. R. Fuchs and M. J. Kramer, *Determinants of Expenditures for Physicians' Services in the United States 1948-1968,* Washington 1972.

Comment

Jesse L. Steinfeld, M.D.
Dean, School of Medicine,
Medical College of Virginia, Virginia Commonwealth University

Before I begin, I should and will emphasize that I speak for no organization, not the Medical College of Virginia, nor the American Medical Association, nor the American College of Physicians, both of which latter groups I am a member; nor do I speak for any other professional organization. I should add that if I were speaking to physicians and hospital administrators, I would emphasize the need for constructive change within the health system rather than defense of the status quo; but since I'm speaking to economists, I will take a modified position.

As the second physician on this program, I will make general comments rather than restrict my remarks to a critique of Mr. Havighurst's paper.

First, in any conference or discussion, we must specify our goals. If our goal is improved health (in the World Health Organization sense of the word—good mental, physical, and emotional health); to repeat, if our goal is improved health for the American people, we will emphasize health education, exercise, good nutrition, avoidance of tobacco, alcohol, and other drugs, the use of preventive techniques, and allocate appropriate resources for biomedical research, all of which can be accomplished by establishing a rational, national health policy to develop an improved health system. Notice I did not say "health care system." As we have conquered the killers of the past, the infectious diseases—lifestyle and personal behavior patterns have become the germs of the 1960's and 1970's. If our goal is to decrease the income of physicians, that may or may not improve the health of the American people. If our goal is to increase competition among physicians and hospitals, that also may or may not improve the health of our people. As a matter of fact, we teach our students in medical school to *cooperate* for the patient's benefit with the appropriate other necessary specialists and other members of the health care team, including members of the patient's family.

There is a recent newspaper article indicating a severe outbreak of infectious disease in California by an infectious agent, for which we have an effective immunizing agent—which apparently is not being used adequately. This clearly emphasizes the need for preventive techniques and lends further emphasis to the fact that appropriate use of preventive and other techniques could lower the Nation's total health bill while improving health.

Secondly, with respect to those economists who advocate an unrestrained free market system in health, I would add that people who are not familiar with history are doomed to repeat it. In the United States in the last century and in the early part of this century, we had an unregulated system without effective licensure, and the havoc and misery created by those free market institutions led to the Flexner Report, the development of standards and accreditation for medical schools, tightened State licensing of physicians, specialty licensing, hospital accreditation, and the like. Our system is still evolving but it does represent medicine's response to society's demands. Certainly our current multisystem can be markedly improved: e.g., the numbers, kinds, and distribution of physicians, other health professionals, and physicial resources; we must also lower our citizens' unrealistic expectations from medical care. It seems every group and in this conference, especially economists, wants to make national health policy in isolation from the many complexities comprising "health and health care" in modern society.

The third point relates to the fact that health is a social good. While one can state that many physician-patient encounters are unnecessary, one can only determine that after the fact. While it is true that health care has been less important than public health measures in increasing the lifespan of the American citizens since the turn of the century, I should add that society has a vested interest in its citizens' health, just as in their education. The G.I. Bill after World War II contributed immensely, in my opinion, to a great deal of our intellectual and technical progress in the last three decades (although I'm sure the bill for higher education was expensive compared to both the cost and the educational opportunities available before World War II). Well, you say, we know all these obvious things, but health care costs are getting out of hand. Health care is consuming proportionately too much of the gross national product, so let's regulate to the nth degree and socialize medicine, or else deregulate entirely. Of course, it is true we can limit the production of the number of physicians or limit the number of hospital beds which consume the major portion of the health dollar, and thus we can restrict elective surgery and other elective hospital admissions. I should point out parenthetically my experience in the Soviet Union where there is one of the highest, if not the highest, physician-to-patient populations in the world, where physicians clearly are in a socialized medicine system and do not fare well economically. Yet the Deputy Minister of Health in the Soviet Union, Dr. Dmitri Venidiktov, informed me a few years ago that the pressure from

Soviet citizens to build more medical schools was so intense that they were building them and educating more and more physicians, even though there was no medical or other social need for additional physicians in the Soviet Union.

My fourth point (and I learned this during my sojurn in Washington) is that our society—perhaps for political reasons—wants simple answers to complex questions. I submit that we would be further ahead if we could articulate our goals into a national health policy and then examine how each of the many proposals facing the U.S. Congress and the regulatory and other Federal agencies fit into that overall policy. Otherwise, we'll have HMO's, PSRO's, and other O's proposed as solutions becoming problems instead, after the original legislation becomes a "Christmas Tree" during the legislative process.

This Nation does need a national, rational health policy and does not now have one. I hope this FTC meeting will move us along toward that goal. The development of such a policy is complex, as illustrated by the failure of the health group of the Commission on Critical Choices for Americans to develop such a policy after months and months of deliberation.

Fifth—and this relates to my third and fourth points—our society has moved increasingly to the concept that health care (or alternatively, some measure of health) is a right, not a potential purchase for the American citizen. Education is also considered a right—but up to a point—each child is not guaranteed a Ph.D. Similarly, I believe that in setting health policy and recognizing the value of health, we will have to set priorities—on personnel, facilities, programs, expenses, and the like.

Sixth, I was surprised to hear very little about systems. While it is true that the method of payment has organized our present system of health care, it is not required that we continue to use the present payment system to exert leverage to change what we now have. Really, we should have a more ambitious goal for the American people. There can be new health systems incorporating the schools, the communications media, the transportation system, cooperation amongst institutions, and personnel. What are the incentives to develop new systems? Are they all economic? I firmly believe that the next fifty years of biomedical research will be as productive as the past fifty years. But again, we need a policy and a plan. Using halfway technologies to treat end-stage kidney disease with little research on prevention and little use of resources on the available preventive techniques to avoid kidney disease, or even early detection and treatment of early kidney disease such as pyelonephritis, is not good national health policy—unless you are one of the unlucky ones who already have end-stage renal disease. In this same vein, preliminary data from family practice versus internal medicine training programs suggests that family practitioner trainees tend to treat diabetics as outpatients in a number of situations in which internal medicine residents admit the patient to the hospital. Do not misunderstand. I believe in specialization in medicine as well as family practice. These are not mutually exclusive; rather, what I'm saying is that we have done too few experiments in health care delivery—and practically none in large-scale citizen health education and experiments with citizens practicing preventive medicine in cooperation with their physicians.

The seventh point is that, while I agree that better educated citizens would be better patients, I don't believe it's practical to provide citizens with cost estimations as a sole criterion of choosing physicians or a hospital. Adding quality criteria (which we are currently unable to do) would improve the situation but I believe we must settle the major issues such as equity, priorities in national health policy and programs and proceed from there.

Eighth—I'd be remiss if I did not remind the audience that physicians' fees are not the major ingredients in health care costs. Hospitalization, malpractice insurance, physicians practicing defense medicine, and a host of other factors account for a large portion of our current increase in health care costs.

Ninth, do I believe in competition? Certainly. There is competition amongst students to get into medical, dental, nursing, pharmacy schools, and the like. There is competition among biomedical researchers to be the first to discover the causes of cancer, arteriolosclerosis, diabetes, and so forth. I even believe in economic competition in the health arena, but only as part of an overall health policy and health structure. I am familiar with the fact that Government agencies disagree, just as physicians and economists. It is less likely for programs to backfire if they are part of an overall whole. I believe this Nation is moving toward national health insurance, and I hope we can reach our goals cooperatively and without any social disruption.

Tenth, and finally, I would suggest that the new programs be phased in, with a realistic timetable. Health professionals and health facilities do not appear or become transformed in the periods usually visualized by politicians—namely, before the next election. So I would add patience to the complex equation I have spelled out earlier.

With these caveats—and though I do not speak for any segment of organized medicine and though I agree that costs are high, and that some physicians are less than honest and that there is an over-emphasis on technology, yet I do believe progress through cooperation as well as competition can be achieved. I also believe that the time is opportune for development of a national health policy, programs, and priorities. I believe an appropriate role for the Federal Trade Commission is to cooperate and participate in the development of that policy. I believe that costs can and will be contained as part of that overall policy. Just as I believe no one professional group should set national health policy, so I would advise the Federal Trade Commission not to attempt to set new national health policies in isolation, but to cooperate and participate with other concerned groups in the development and implementation of national health policy. The time now is ripe.

Regulation as a Second Best

Stuart H. Altman
Dean, Florence Heller Graduate School for Advanced Work in Social Welfare, Brandeis University
and
Sanford L. Weiner
Research Associate, Graduate School of Public Policy, University of California, Berkeley

In a recent article, Clark Havighurst (p. 578) argues that:

> The policy options in medical care no longer include (if they ever did) the possibility of not regulating the health sector at all or of placing primary reliance on market forces.

Yet, on the adjoining page, he also cautions that "as a remedy for problems of public policy, regulation is overprescribed. . . . [It] has often proved neither efficacious nor safe as a remedy for the ills of the body politic" (p. 577).

It is this dilemma—that policy trends in medical care make regulation necessary if not desirable—that we wish to explore. We first review the recent growth of the medical care sector, and the questionable benefits provided by these additional resources. Then we evaluate possible strategies for constraining the system. Since the erosion of market forces is unlikely to be reversed, public regulation becomes the inevitable "second best" alternative. But regulation is not all of a kind, so we need to examine the variables that influence its effectiveness.

This analysis therefore makes effectiveness of regulation the key policy issue. Traditional patterns of regulation often fail by attempting to constrain only the outputs of the system—leaving its underlying incentives untouched. We believe health-care regulation can only be effective when it is explicitly designed to change the incentives which motivate hospitals and physicians. The final section compares our view of effective regulation with the new Administration plan for hospital cost containment.

THE RISE IN MEDICAL CARE COSTS: INFLATION OR GROWTH?

Rising costs are the most prominent and probably the most significant policy issue concerning the medical care system today. Higher costs not only are an added burden on those who pay for care, they are a major deterrent to extending public involvement into other important and often neglected human service needs. Indeed, the capacity to generate just the additional revenue needed to maintain current benefits is of serious concern to Federal policymakers, and several States have been forced to reduce their Medicaid eligibility standards rather than see their budgets continue to soar.

There has been considerable discussion about whether these rising costs represent inflation—more resources needed to deliver the same output—or growth and change in the services delivered as well. It is of course not sufficient to note that the "cost per patient day" has risen steadily, since the average patient day can represent a changing mix of medical services. We must disaggregate the average into cost increases generated by overall inflationary pressures in the economy and those that result from the special character of the medical sector including more intense patient services.

When this is done, as in a recent study by Martin Feldstein and Amy Taylor, it becomes clear that the rising cost of hospital care does indeed represent more than just normal inflationary pressure. The authors, controlling for overall inflation, still find that the cost of a day in the hospital rose five times from 1950 to 1976 from $21.66 to $102.33 at 1967 prices (p. 8).

Analysts within the hospital industry have argued that an important share of these excess cost increases could be accounted for by the increased earnings of hospital workers, which have risen faster than the earnings of comparable workers in other industries. These were described as "catch up" increases because of the prior lag in hospital wages, and were partially due to increased unionization. However, Victor Fuchs (1976) has now documented that the catch up is over, earnings are now comparable, and that its impact was relatively slight:

> For the quarter century 1949-1974 the earnings of hospital workers improved about 37 percent compared with those of all private, nonagricultural workers. This relative wage gain however explains only a small part of the very rapid rise in the cost of a day of hospital care relative to other prices (p. 426).

According to the Feldstein/Taylor estimates, only about one-fourth of the increase of hospital prices in excess of the general inflationary levels is a result of these above-comparable earnings increase.

Hence, one has to look elsewhere—to the increased and enriched real resources that make the medical care system of today considerably different from that of 10 or 20 years ago. In 1955 there were about 2 full-time employees for every patient day of treatment; by 1975 the number of workers per patient day had grown by almost 75 percent to 3.39. The 1975 hospital worker is better educated and provides a more specialized service than his/her counterpart did in 1955. In addition, far more sophisticated and costly equipment backs up the average hospital bed today than a decade or two ago. In fact, despite their better paid, better trained labor, hospital payroll costs have dropped from 62 percent (1955) to 53 percent (1975) of their budgets because non-labor inputs—supplies and new technology—have grown even faster.

Only half the twenty-year cost growth can be attributed to changes in factor costs—the other half represents additional employees, new technology, and other changes in hospital activities. When one looks specifically at the rise in hospital per diem costs above the general levels of inflation, only 25 percent can be attributed to excess factor costs—the other 75 percent represents increased inputs of services. So we strongly concur with Feldstein and Taylor that "hospitals use more inputs to produce an increasingly sophisticated style of hospital care. It is this change in the character of the hospitals' service that accounts for the unusually rapid rise in hospital costs" (p. 29).

One policy option is to accept this system as it is now developing: i.e., to decide that decentralization, unconstrained access (for those with insurance), and quality (as defined by individual physicians) are the dominant objectives, whatever the cost. Many participants in the system implicitly advance this view. We prefer, however, to ask whether the patient and society are getting benefits commensurate with the billions of dollars in additional real resources pumped into the industry annually. If the answer is no, then the issues become: Why has this come about; should something be done to constrain the system; and if so, what is the most effective means to do it?

ARE WE GETTING OUR MONEY'S WORTH?

While the growth in medical resources has continued unabated, there have been growing doubts concerning both the efficiency and the efficacy of the system of care that absorbs these resources.

On the efficiency side, about 25 percent of the 931,000 non-Federal, short-term general beds remained empty on an average day in 1974. This occurred, despite greatly increased utilization, because the supply of beds has also expanded—from 1960 to 1974, it rose over 45 percent. This overexpansion of capacity is of greater concern today than in previous decades because of the growing costs of maintaining such redundancy;[1] the hospital day that cost $23 in 1955 or $48 in 1966 is about $150 today. We suspect that if national data were available, it would show a similar picture for the utilization of trained manpower. A pilot study by Edward Hughes *et al.*

(1972) found that surgeons at a suburban New York hospital were operating at about one-third their estimated capacity. Victor Fuchs (1974, p. 71) concluded that "there is no reason to believe that the findings from this study are atypical of the general situation."

In each case, prepaid groups financed on a capitation basis, which place greater constraints on the use of specialists, hospital beds, and marginal hospital care, have found it possible to provide acceptable care with far fewer resources. Edward Hughes and others' (1974) comparative study of surgery in a west coast prepaid group found surgeons doing triple the work per surgeon, and considerably more minor procedures on an outpatient basis. Milton Roemer and William Shonick have also found that prepaid groups tend to have fewer beds per capita and hospitalization rates 25-40 percent lower.

These questions about the efficiency of the system are paralleled by the even larger issues of its ultimate efficacy. There has been an increasing realization (Fuchs, 1974; Aaron Wildavsky, 1977) that the factors that most significantly affect health status today are not supplied by physicians. Instead, they are in the province of public health (vaccination, sanitation), personal lifestyle (diet, exercise, smoking), or broader social and environmental conditions (housing, poverty, factory carcinogens).

The reason acute care medicine is not included among these factors is that, as Lewis Thomas (p. 37) has noted, we do not yet have the underlying scientific understanding to control any of the major causes of mortality:

> We are left with approximately the same roster of common major diseases which confronted the country in 1950, and, although we have accumulated a formidable body of information about some of them in the intervening time, the accumulation is not yet sufficient to permit either the prevention or the outright cure of any of them.

This does not mean that medicine cannot play an important part in "supportive care, the amelioration of symptoms, and sometimes the extension of life." It's just that these elements are not the same thing as the prevention of deaths from heart disease, stroke, and cancer, which caused 70 percent of all the deaths in 1974.

In fact, it is precisely the attempt to ameliorate the symptoms of diseases we cannot control with the "half-way technologies" now available that drives up the services used and resources absorbed (Ivan Bennett). Indeed, the medical profession has carried this effort so far (for reasons described in the next section) that many technologies have gained widespread acceptance without ever having passed controlled trails of their effectiveness. H. G. Mather's studies in Britain, for example, have now raised serious doubts about our unquestioned use of coronary care units.[2] Even where the scientific evidence does exist, as with the negative aspects of tonsillectomies, physicians have been slow to change their accustomed biases.

The implication of the facts that many factors other than medicine impinge on health, and that in any case much medical treatment is of uncertain benefit, is that, at the margin, additional resources devoted to current technology will have negligible impact on health outcomes. So we must conclude with Lewis Thomas (p. 46) that:

> If our society wishes to be rid of the diseases, fatal and non-fatal, that plague us the most, there is really little prospect of doing so by mounting a still larger health-care system at still greater cost for delivering essentially today's kind of technology on a larger scale.

THE EROSION OF THE MARKET

Why then are we spending more than we should for medical care? We would support the thesis that one major cause of the rapid cost growth has been the parallel growth in health insurance coverage, which has completely undermined consumer incentives. Since hospital stays and other medical activities can be costly and often unanticipated events, there is a strong incentive to insure against them. As the cost rises, the incentive for obtaining insurance grows as well. In this country, private incentives have been supplemented by public insurance plans (Medicare and Medicaid) whose origins stem from the same rationale.

So the out-of-pocket costs for hospital care, which amounted to half the total in 1950 and a quarter as late as 1966, have declined rapidly. About 90 percent of all hospital costs are now paid through either private or public insurance. (Inpatient physician fees are also largely covered.) As a result, real hospital costs have more than tripled in twenty years while leaving out-of-pocket costs per day essentially unchanged (table 1). The consumer bears directly the costs of only a minor portion of the services he consumes. For outpatient physician services, insurance coverage is not quite as pervasive but still amounts to almost 60 percent of total charges.

However, providers of health care also have an independent interest in the nearly complete financial protection for most health services, and have taken at least equal advantage of it.[3] Even before the complete spread of hospital insurance, the medical professional had special influence, for the imbalance of knowledge between consumer and professional concerning the efficacy of service provided has always made this a highly unusual marketplace. This innate consumer uncertainty, as Kenneth Arrow (pp. 965, 966) describes it, leads to considerable delegation to the physicians, and a reciprocal obligation on their part not to compromise in the care provided:

> The patient must delegate to the physician much of his freedom of choice. He does not have the knowledge to make decisions on treatment, referral, or hospitalization. To justify this delegation, the physician finds himself somewhat limited, just as any agent would in similar circumstances. The safest course to take to avoid not being a true agent is to give the socially prescribed "best treatment" of the day. Compromise in quality, even for the purpose of saving the patient money, is to risk an imputation of failure to live up to the social bond.

The dominance of the third-party payment system has now transformed this negative professional injunction, to provide quality or fail the patient into a strong positive norm. Physicians, like other professionals, are trained to apply their skills up to the point where the marginal benefits approach zero. With most professionals, constraints on resources limit the services provided to far short of this level. But physicians are now essentially free to provide as much care, and the type of care, that they find appropriate. In fact, the norms in American medicine highly value new technology as a prime expression of the quality of the medical process. There is only minimal concern about the costs generated, and even the ultimate medical outcome is often a secondary consideration. As the system operates there are few external constraints on these professional desires. The usual tests of innovation in more traditional industries, that they must reduce costs or clearly improve quality, are absent.

A third important force in the push for more and "better" health care has been government, particularly the Federal Government. This has happened first through the indirect route of tax subsidies for health insurance premiums,[4] and then through direct subsidies—Hill-Burton Construction grants and loan guarantees, and the underwriting of a major expansion of the Nation's health professionals' training capacity. Between 1946 and 1971, about 30 percent of all hospital construction projects were assisted under the Hill-Burton program.[5] It has been a major force in the very sizable expansion (or over expansion) of the Nation's acute-care inpatient hospital capacity. To some this is a vivid example of Wildavsky's (1976) view that highly successful programs often create their own new problems.

Unfortunately, we do not seem to learn from past mistakes. Increasing numbers of analysts are now concerned that the heavy subsidization of the country's health professional training institutions by the Federal Government and the governmental pressure to expand their training capacity will generate large increases in future supply of health professionals and concomitant large increases in the spending for medical services. Since 1963 the Federal Government spent more than $5.0 billion for health manpower training with enrollment in schools of medicine and osteopathy almost

Table 1 Insurance and the Net Cost of Hospital Care (Short-term, Non-Federal, General Hospitals)

	1950	1955	1960	1966	1970	1972	1974	1975
Percentage of costs paid by:								
1. Private Insurance	29.3	44.7	52.5	51.4	45.6	45.4	45.4	43.6
2. Government	21.1	19.9	18.8	25.5	37.8	41.1	42.8	44.5
3. Direct Consumer Spending	49.6	35.2	28.7	23.1	16.6	13.5	11.8	11.9
Average cost per patient day	15.62	23.12	32.23	48.15	81.01	105.21	128.05	151.53
Net consumer cost per patient day	7.75	8.14	9.25	11.12	13.53	14.20	15.11	18.03
Average cost per patient day (1967 dollars)	21.66	28.83	36.34	49.54	69.66	83.97	86.70	94.00
Net consumer cost per patient day (1967) dollars)	10.75	10.15	10.43	11.44	11.63	11.34	10.23	11.18

Source: Martin Feldstein and Amy Taylor, tables 8 and 9

doubling. By 1990 this expansion will translate into a per population growth in the number of physicians of almost 50 percent. If, as many now believe, physicians can induce increases in demand for their services, the implications for increased health spending of this growth in supply of health providers is obvious and staggering. As Reinhardt suggests:

> Abstracting from the availability of physician services, it seems clear that the reduction in health-care expenditures (health-care income) to be had from a say 10 percent reduction in the stock of physicians would be manifold that to be had by reducing the net incomes of that stock of physicians by 10 percent. *The implications for cost containment policies are obvious* (Uwe Reinhardt, pp. 42). [Emphasis added.]

Wennberg's studies in Vermont and Maine have demonstrated the potential outcomes from this system. Neighboring towns with comparable populations and insurance coverage display per capita rates for surgery that vary up to 200 percent, and for specific procedures 300 percent or more, depending on the local mix of professional tastes and available resources. (These studies control for patient flows.) Even in medicine, similar rates of patient contact with physicians lead to widely varying hospital admission rates (tables 2 and 3). In these instances, physican discretion seems clearly dominant.

But if unconstrained professional choices supported by governmental spending are at the heart of the problem, what can be done? Most economists have come down in favor of strengthening the marketplace and in particular strengthening the role of the consumer. For example, Martin Feldstein's mechanism for bringing this about would be to impose very high deductibles, as much as 10 percent of family income up to a present limit, on any comprehensive insurance package. In this way families would again feel the direct costs of the great proportion of care provided. Other economists, including Thomas Schelling and Joseph Newhouse and Vincent Taylor, have proposed analogous plans whose central feature is also consumer choice.

However, these schemes fail on two grounds. First is the basic imperfection in the medical marketplace, as described by Arrow. While it is undoubtably true that at some level direct costs will deter utilization, this is a matter that involves not only consumer preferences, but also consumer income, and most important, physician advice. The level of out-of-pocket costs likely to deter physicians and their middle-class patients together, would probably prove over-severe for lower income groups. Moreover, the plan would also have to ban the strong middle-class disposition to insure privately against these direct costs, as has taken place with Medicare.[6]

Table 2 Variation in Number of Surgical Procedures Performed Per 10,000 Persons for the 13 Vermont Hospital Service Areas and Comparison Populations, Vermont, 1969. (Rates Adjusted to Vermont Age Composition.)

Surgical Procedure	**Lowest Two Areas**		**Entire State**	**Highest Two Areas**	
All Surgery	360	490	550	610	690
Tonsillectomy	13	32	43	85	151
Appendectomy	10	15	18	27	32
Hemorrhoidectomy	2	4	6	9	10
Males					
Hernioplasty	29	38	41	47	48
Prostatectomy	11	13	20	28	38
Females					
Cholecystectomy	17	19	27	46	57
Hysterectomy	20	22	30	34	60
Mastectomy	12	14	18	28	33
Dilation and currettage	30	42	55	108	141
Varicose veins	6	7	12	24	28

Source: J. Wennberg, "PSRO and the Relationships among Health Need, Elective Surgery and Health Status," *Perspectives on Health Policy,* Boston University Medical Center, 1975.

We realize that these arguments against relying on increased co-payments as the primary mechanism for limited health-care spending have left most economists unconvinced. However, we are unlikely to have the opportunity to test their proposals on a national scale, because such schemes also lack political feasibility. While small deductibles and co-payments can play an important role in inducing cost consciousness on the part of both consumers and providers, an enforced major reduction in current insurance levels runs exactly counter to the decade-long trend in public policy toward "more and better."

We see little evidence that reduction in first-dollar health coverage is at all likely. Unions continue to push for broad and comprehensive coverage for their members, with no co-insurance. Similarly, no major insurance company has seen fit to market actively a high deductible co-insurance plan. And when President Ford tried to increase the co-payment rate under Medicare by only 10 percent, and use the money for increased program services, his proposal received almost no congressional support on either side of the aisle.

No doubt one major reason why organized labor continues to press for ever larger health-care benefits paid for through the employer is because of

Table 3 Age-Adjusted Discharges from Hospital Per 1,000 population, Maine Comprehensive Health Planning Regions and Constituent Hospital Service Areas (1973)

	Southern Maine	Tri-County	Kennebec	Northeast	Aroostook
Region as a Whole	150	157	197	152	204
Hospital Service Areas Ranked within regions:					
Highest	212	192	235	249	309
Second Highest	193	158	234	230	283
Second Lowest	127	153	204	146	185
Lowest	117	134	157	127	172
Ratio of highest to lowest ranked hospital Service Areas	1.81	1.43	1.50	1.96	1.80
Coefficient of variation*	18%	15%	18%	21%	22%

* The coefficient of variation includes all HSA's within a planning region except those with populations less than 4,000.

Source: J. Wennberg, *et al.,* "Health Care Delivery in Maine II: Conditions Explaining Hospital Admission," *J. Maine Med. Assn.,* Oct. 1975, 255-261.

the large health insurance tax subsidies involved. Yet, when the House Ways and Means Committee was asked to consider eliminating these subsidies, such a change was overwhelmingly voted down.

We are also at a loss to find other countries which reversed the trend toward first-dollar coverage and introduced moderate or extensive amounts of co-payments in their standard health insurance policies.[7]

Thus, it seems that rationing by price is no longer considered acceptable in this area. If we see any changes in the public involvement in medical care, they almost certainly will provide greater insurance coverage, not less. For, as Theodore Marmor (p. 32) puts it, "if these plans were fully implemented, they would reintroduce the financial barriers to care that many national-health-insurance advocates see as the access problem in the first place."

It has been suggested that a network of health maintenance organizations (HMO's) offers a solution to this problem. We strongly believe that the pattern of constrained resources found in successful HMO's is to be encouraged. However, HMO "success" appears to be a delicate balance of management and untypical professional norms, mediated by bargaining. Where HMO's have not been able to constrain the supply of hospital beds, or recruit from the minority of physicians who believe ambulatory care is to be preferred, their performance has been less bright. Even among successful groups or across Kaiser regions, different bargaining outcomes have led to considerable variations in utilization. And for every Kaiser success in California there is a prepaid group in New York or Rhode Island that has foundered. For HMO's to substitute effectively for consumer choice, a substantial majority of practicing doctors and existing hospitals would have to be absorbed into them—a highly unlikely prospect.[8] Therefore, we cannot look to HMO's to play the central role in reorganizing the incentives of the existing system.

So the medical marketplace has two sources of imperfection. One stems from the nature of medical knowledge as a commodity; the other derives from the trend of public intervention in medical care. Wherever one might put the emphasis between them, together they undermine the hope and assumption that consumer incentives will ever be the driving force in the medical sector again.

THE IMPERFECT MARKET FOR HEALTH INSURANCE

Organized buyers often provide market discipline as a substitute for individual consumers. Wildavsky (1977, p. 109) is not the only one to have asked why we don't see this behavior in health "insurance companies. Why are they left out of almost all discussions of this sort? Why don't they play a cost-cutting role in medical care as they do in other industries?" In theory, insurance companies could either refuse to pay what they consider excessive amounts or control their payments by contracting with institutions in advance to provide the covered services for a negotiated rate.

In practice, we have seen no example of such an undertaking being tried, let alone successfully completed. The reasons lie in the incentives created by the structure of the health insurance market itself. Most private health insurance is obtained by individuals through their place of employment. Encouraged by Federal tax subsidies, and by insurance companies which find the work place an excellent screening device against individuals who are bad medical risks, most private health insurance is employment linked.

For most employers, health insurance is now an accepted and expected benefit that must be offered to attract a qualified labor force. However, employees of any one firm will often live scattered throughout a metropolitan area, going to many different physicians, who have privileges in several hospitals. Few employers wish to be seen as injecting themselves into the relationship between an employee and his/her physician. Hence, the idea of buying insurance coverage from a company with only a limited number of participating providers and hospitals is unattractive to most employers—even if such coverage were cheaper. This has been a major problem for prepaid group health plans. (Once implemented, the Dual Option provisions of the 1973 HMO Act will require that firms with over 25 employees make such plans, where they exist, available to their workers.)

Employers are similarly reluctant to take steps to control health costs that might be interpreted by their workers as a reduction in benefits. For example, few employers are willing to include a provision for the use of second opinions before surgery in their contract unless it is asked for or approved by the workers or the union.

For their part, most insurance companies are not in a market position to negotiate with major health service suppliers; they are simply price-takers. Those few who have sufficient market penetration are mostly Blue Cross plans, which do negotiate special contracts with hospitals. But these contracts for the most part maintain the practice of paying on a cost reimbursement basis. Whether because of their traditionally close ties with hospitals and the medical profession, or because of political pressures, few Blue Cross plans have attempted to exert their market power to limit what they consider to be excessive hospital cost increases. Most Blue Cross plans are regulated by State agencies, leaving their relationships with the hospitals open to political review. When they alone have attempted to push the hospitals too far (in the hospitals' view), they have faced strong criticism from elected State representatives. Hence, the preferred strategy of some Blue Cross plans has been to seek direct State action to regulate hospital cost. Other plans, opposed to State controls, have tried to develop enlarged private mechanisms to attack this problem.

Most Blue Cross plans and some commercial insurance companies have become active proponents, if not actual operators, of various types of health maintenance organizations. Most have supported the growth of the health planning movement and have encouraged States to introduce certificates-of-need legislation. But, the impact of these activities thus far has been very small, particularly when compared to the magnitude of the problem.

The recent major increases in health insurance premiums have persuaded several large employers to put increased pressure on their insurance companies to reduce the climb in health-care costs. These employers are also joining to sponsor educational efforts to explore the feasibility of new cost control efforts. In Michigan, the automobile firms were instrumental in blocking part of a Blue Cross rate increase request and in forcing the hsopitals to accept reduced rates of growth in their next year's expenses. But for the most part, employer concerns about rising health insurance premiums have been directed at marginal changes in the insurance companies' operations, through reductions in their overhead rate, rather than at the major problem of rising health-care costs. From a national perspective, the initiative of Blue Cross plans, commercial insurance companies, and employers can provide support and could be a critical element in the success of any governmental regulatory activity. But action from these groups alone cannot be expected to affect significantly the rate of growth of health-care spending.

We have now discussed the key private actors that influence the medical-care system. Consumers, health insurers, and employers all face peculiar market incentives that do not induce or permit any of them alone to control the cost of health care.

As in other sectors of the economy where market imperfections are substantial, we are forced to seek "second best" mechanisms for resource allocation. In the case of medical care, this inevitably will be some form of public regulation.

REGULATION AS AN ORGANIZATIONAL STRATEGY

Rather than repeat the litany of sins committed in the name of regulation, we think it more useful to discuss alternative forms of regulatory activity and their likely effectiveness.

Charles Schultze (p. 45) has recently noted that:

> Political action and economic theory treat the actual instruments of social intervention as a series of black boxes. One first identifies a market failure—environmental pollution or industrial accidents. . . . If the political system can generate a consensus that some form of social intervention is called for, the job is turned over to the black box.

Since we believe regulation is here to stay, it is increasingly important to get beyond black box descriptions of it and find out what's inside the boxes. Conventional planning and regulatory strategies often fail because they focus on constraining only the outputs of the medical-care system. They tend to assume simple motivations for the regulators and ready compliance by those regulated—ignoring the powerful and contrary incentives an open-ended reimbursement system may offer to both groups. In contrast, we believe that the effectiveness of regulation can be greatly enhanced by a strategy explicitly designed to change those incentives which influence hospitals, physicians, and local regulators.

Consider, first, the general approach of health planning advocates. To some observers the medical-care sector is characterized by decentralization, disorganization, unnecessary conflict, and suboptimality. The lack of a clear structure, including a central authority to decide what services should be offered and where, is very troublesome to them. They see planning agencies as the mechanism whereby information about the total health "needs" of the entire area can be used to coordinate and redirect this system, and thus bring rationality and efficiency to the medical sector. When these agencies fail to have serious impact on the system, their advocates see the need for the theory to be applied more forcefully. Typically, the agency is reorganized, with more formal authority, scope, and resources, but with the same mission in mind.

Economists have rightfully led the attack on these notions. No central agency will ever have the information, time, or wisdom to settle thousands of individual cases appropriately. Schultze (p. 56) cites the parallel example of the Environmental Protection Agency, which is mandated by law to calculate water pollution permits for each plant in the country. "To do this for 62,000 plant sources of pollution demands omniscience from EPA."

Nor would the wisdom necessarily be employed if it existed. Planning bodies made up of representatives from the major actors within the health sector often have far more incentive to protect the status quo than to constrain or restructure the industry. An important component of the new health planning structure is the requirement for an institution to obtain a certificate-of-need before acquiring new plant and equipment (over $150,000). But there is no constraint on the overall number of projects that can be approved, and hence little pressure to enforce relative priorities. Why should "our area" be denied expanded services when the reimbursement system will support them? There are even less pressures concerning spending for existing medical services and no ability to rechannel these resources to other areas.

Where planning agencies have tried to stand against the trend, they have rarely been successful. The incentives for the hospitals to invest in new technology, as we have seen, remain unchanged. They often have far more organizational resources and technical expertise than the planning agency, which can only react to their initiatives. As a result, the spread of expensive, exotic technology such as CAT scanners continues virtually unimpeded. Neither planning techniques nor regulation of new investment is strong enough alone to change professional behavior which is so fully encouraged and financed in other parts of the system.

However, the major alternative to health planning—economic regulation as a solution to market failure—often falls victim to the same ills. Traditionally, it has been believed that regulation is necessary where there are market structures, such as natural monopolies, where competition is likely to be inappropriate or ineffective. Here the injunction is to substitute a public utility regulatory approach for the imperfectly functioning market. The agency, in such a situation, usually defines its work as setting prices, quality standards, conditions of entry, etc.

But this approach is often insensitive, as well, to the pattern of incentives produced by the system and their impact on regulatory effectiveness. The early State prospective reimbursement experiments, for example, have probably suffered from their reliance on a public utility strategy. Given the clear problems of retrospective costs reimbursement, the logic of regulating hospital costs in advance is appealing.[9] Yet, the results in the practice of establishing prospectively set budgets have been mixed, at best.[10] The various schemes tried to date have concentrated too much on establishing rate ceilings rather than constraining the total budget of the institution. As a result, too little attention has been placed on explicitly incorporating into the control system incentives for behavior change within the hospitals. This is particularly true for those experiments which use the budget review or direct negotiation mechanisms. Only when these changes are the designed intent of mandatory programs can we expect to observe positive results. As long as the underlying incentives for growth remain unchallenged, it should not be surprising that the ceilings on outputs alone have little impact.

How, then, can we shift these underlying incentives? We believe the key to regulatory effectiveness is an explicit organizational strategy that concentrates on behavior within the hospitals. Then the objective for the regulatory agency becomes organizational change. While many of the same techniques are employed, they are used with different intentions and to different effect. Rate regulation becomes a means, not for setting prices per se, but of shifting the incentive structure for some of the professionals and administrators within the hospitals. This, in turn, can potentially shift the balance of power on the numerous detailed decisions made within the hospitals that aggregate to cost growth, and that no planning agency could ever process individually.

But shifting the balance of power within an organization could be the most difficult change to make. The experience of the Economic Stabilization Plan (ESP) from 1971-74 clearly highlights this phenomenon.[11] One of the implicit incentives created by these controls was a shift in power from the medical boards to the hospital administrators, who became the experts in what new services could fit within the regulations. Their increased importance for managing the external environment increased the administrators' influence within the organizations they served. This, surprisingly, was viewed with alarm both by the medical boards and the administrators.

The controlled index of hospital costs used in the final version of the ESP controls (Phase IV) was total expenditures per patient admission—much closer to an aggregate budget limit. The use of this measure rather than cost per patient day reversed the earlier incentive by rewarding shorter lengths of stay. The plan also attempted to deal with hospitals that would try to maximize revenues—and evade the controls—by increasing their total admissions. Significant increases in number of cases would be reimbursed at a declining cost per case.

The logic of the regulation was to allow for internal variation and flexibility, while demanding far more central control *within* the hospital over new services, technology, and costs, since these would come out of a constrained pool for the first time. The more the hospital sought to grow in a year, the more difficult its reimbursement position—thus reversing the inventives provided in a cost-based financing system. Hospital growth and change would not be frozen; rather, the external constraints were meant to create incentives for internal trade-offs and priority setting.

We cite the ESP experience, not to suggest that it produced final answers, but as a provocative illustration of a more effective approach to regulatory strategy. Even the Phase IV regulations left a number of issues unresolved. Most important was the lack of a regular mechanism (other than case-by-case appeal) for adjusting the limits for changes in a hospital's case mix. Both shifts between outpatient and inpatient departments, and more or less severely ill inpatients have significant service and cost implications. One potential perverse incentive, for example, would be to hospitalize a greater proportion of outpatients, generating numerous low-cost short stays to lower the hospital's average.[12]

While the key to the effectiveness of a health regulation system is its capacity to stimulate changes in the behavior of physicians and hospital personnel, we really know little about how to accomplish this end. To go with the extensive studies now in progress to chart the motivation for consumer behavior, we need profiles of the specific incentive structure within hospitals that motivates provider behavior. In parallel with the work on national health insurance financing, we need research on the regulatory mechanisms each NHI plan implies. Particularly useful would be more work on the structure of the regulatory agencies themselves, including the appropriate balance of State and Federal responsibilities.

Most important, we need to link our micro-theories of behavior and our macro-theories of regulation, to describe the specific impact of different regulatory schemes on internal incentives. Only in this way can we anticipate how regulation will actually change the pattern of hospital resource allocation, and thus the growth of the sector. For if we continue to ignore what's in the black box of regulation, we run the risk of creating a system much worse than second best.

THE ADMINISTRATION'S COST-CONTAINMENT STRATEGY

President Carter's new hospital cost-containment plan, presented to the Congress in April, displays both the potential and some of the unresolved difficulties of a regulatory strategy we discussed in the last section. It would control all inpatient revenues (not just public funds) received by a hospital, with some adjustment in the revenue limit for institutions with major changes (positive or negative) in the number of patients they treat. (New, chronic, and HMO-controlled hospitals would be exempt.)

The plan is the clear descendent of the Phase IV regulations, and thus designed with its potential impact on hospital behavior in mind. The proposal embodies several of the explicit incentives which we believe are critical for a regulatory strategy to be effective. Perhaps most important, it requires each institution to spend against a fixed and predetermined revenue limit. It anticipates that hospitals may attempt to evade this control through their capacity to influence the number of patients they treat. Indeed, the disincentives for increasing patient load are quite severe: For the first 2 percent increase in admissions (above the base year), no additional increase in the revenue limit is allowed; for increases from 2-15 percent, the allowable revenue limit is permitted to increase by only 50 percent of the average revenue per admission received by the institution during the base accounting year. When these negative incentives for treating new patients are combined with the positive incentives for treating fewer patients—admission can drop up to 6 percent before the revenue limit is reduced—the barrier may even be too strong.

The plan also provides for a national ceiling on certificate-of-need approvals. The Administration proposes to set this ceiling next year at $2.5 billion, about half of current spending for hospital capital investment. A formula would allocate this limited amount to each State. The logic is parallel to that for operating costs—a constrained pool for new projects is meant to encourage local tradeoffs. There is also a provision intended to begin the process of evening out geographical disparities. Areas heavily overbedded or where hospital beds are under-utilized will be subject to special controls requiring the removal of two old beds for each new one added. For the first time, these constraints put not only teeth but priorities into the planning system, which would be a notable gain.

By limiting the hospital budget controls to inpatient revenues only, the plan again consciously attempts to encourage a shift towards outpatient care. However, this is an area where inconsistent incentives may exist. In many hospitals, outpatient care has been subsidized by inpatient revenues. As inpatient funds contract, these institutions may seek to reduce "money-losing" services. In contrast, some hospitals have found that when overhead costs are appropriately weighed toward inpatients' services, the outpatient departments actually support themselves. But few hospitals will now be willing to reallocate costs and therefore potential revenues from the uncontrolled (outpatient) to the controlled (inpatient) segments of their budgets. So the intended simple incentive toward more outpatient care may not have its intended impact.

The Carter proposal also uses a highly questionable mechanism for responding to hospitals that attempt to avoid treating undesired patients, either those with limited insurance or those requiring expensive treatment. In these instances, other local hospitals are expected to complain to the local health planning agency which will then investigate and report its findings to the Secretary of Health, Education, and Welfare, who may impose certain punitive actions. Thus the basic design of the cost-containment program encourages hospitals to treat simple cases, and avoid complicated ones, and then attempts to stop such practices with an awkward and complicated "snitching system." This is the type of technique that we argued earlier is likely to be ineffective.

The proposal could ease future operational problems by taking one lesson from the ESP experience with other industries. There are numerous small firms, or hospitals, whose behavior even in the aggregate has little impact on a national program. The Price Commission eventually learned that these firms could be left to themselves without endangering national targets—leaving more resources to be elevated to the major actors. Similarly, exempting hospitals with under 50 beds from controls would reduce the number of hospitals regulated by 25 percent, while freeing from these controls perhaps 6 percent of the total beds. This does sacrifice formal symbolic equity for administrative simplicity—not always the best political tradeoff—but it has never been proposed, so its actual political feasibility remains untested.

On the other hand, the plan does include the perception of instability that plagued the early ESP. The bill was the product of a highly-constrained drafting process which required a plan that could be announced almost immediately, and implemented in time to be effective for the new budget year which begins in October. As a result, the plan carries the label "transitional"—meant even by its authors to be revised next year. But this conveys to the hospitals not a sense of flexibility but expectations of impermanence. That is not the climate most likely to inspire longrun changes in attitudes or behavior.

Yet, even so, when you compare the Carter plan to less comprehensive schemes, such as that introduced by Senator Talmadge, its virtues dominate its faults. The Talmadge bill offers a sophisticated idea for grouping hospitals, but its main focus remains the conventional strategy of per diem limits on routine hospital operating costs—not physician-controlled services. The constrained total budgets which we see as essential for shifting incentives, changing behavior, and producing effective regulation are found only in the Carter bill.

The Talmadge proposal is labeled "long term," in contrast to the "transitional" Administration plan. At least with respect to the limitations on total revenue, we would prefer the timing to be reversed. Forcing hospitals to save money by sharing their laundry services simply will not be enough.

NOTES

1. Apart from a slight rise after the start of Medicare and Medicaid, occupancy rates have been relatively stable. It is the growing costs of this extra capacity that is of concern.

2. See, also, A. L. Cochrane.

3. In few major industries is there such widespread use of nonnegotiated, cost-based reimbursement. For more than 50 percent of the dollars spent for hospital care, the hospital need only justify that it actually incurred a legitimate health-care expense and the money will be paid. For most of the remaining bills, an insurance company is required to pay whatever the hospital feels is an appropriate charge for its service. The market is such that insurance companies are forced to pay whatever the institutions selected by its policyholders (most likely selected by their physicians) charge for the services covered in the policy.

4. As fringe benefits, employer-paid health plans are a business expense to the firm, and free of income or payroll tax to the employee. Employee contributions are also partially deductible from income taxes.

5. Judith R. Lave and Lester B. Lave.

6. A recent RAND study by Emmett Keeler, Daniel Morrow, and Joseph Newhouse argues (p. 28) that "if there is no special tax benefit for supplemental health insurance premiums, demand for insurance that provides first-dollar coverage for out-of-hospital service is likely to be negligible." As we will note, longstanding political attitudes make this a big "if." The authors then say that "if present tax treatment of health insurance premiums is continued . . . supplementary insurance becomes considerably more attractive." But then, in a statement of faith, they conclude, "we would speculate that purchases [of supplemental coverage] would be small even with the tax subsidy." However, this analysis is for moderate deductibles applied to *ambulatory* care. They accept that "supplementary insurance that covers hospital expenditures only is more attractive." With Feldstein-level deductibles it would be more attractive yet.

7. We are aware of isolated groups within the U.S. and in other countries who have moved away from first-dollar coverage, but such reverses are a mere drop in an empty California rain bucket.

8. A full discussion of the organizational characteristics of HMO's properly deserves a paper rather than a paragraph, and we hope to deal with the subject elsewhere.

9. See William Dowling for an outline of the wide variety of schemes that might fit within this concept.

10. See Clifton Gaus and Fred Hellinger.

11. See Stuart Altman and Joseph Eichenholz, and Paul Ginsburg.

12. See Robert Derzon.

REFERENCES

S. Altman and J. Eichenholz, "Inflation in the Health Industry: Causes and Cures," in M. Zubkoff (ed.), *Health: A Victim or Cause of Inflation*, New York 1976.

K. Arrow, "Uncertanty and the Welfare Economics of Medical Care," *Amer. Econ. Rev.*, December 1963, 941-973.

I. Bennett, "Technology as a Shaping Force," *Daedalus*, Winter 1977, 125-133.

A. L. Cochrane, *Effectiveness and Efficiency*, London 1972.

R. Derzon, testimony in U.S. Senate, Committee on the Budget, Hearings on the First Concurrent Resolution on the Budget—Fiscal Year 1978, Volume III, *Rising Health Care Costs*, Washington, D.C., April 9, 1977.

W. Dowling, "Prospective Reimbursement of Hospitals," *Inquiry*, September 1974, 163-80.

M. S. Feldstein, "A New Approach to National Health Insurance," *The Public Interest*, Spring 1971, 93-105.

______ and A. Taylor, *The Rapid Rise of Hospital Costs*, Cambridge, Mass., January 1977.

V. Fuchs, *Who Shall Live?* New York 1974.

______, "The Earnings of Allied Health Personnel—Are Health Workers Underpaid?" *Explorations in Economic Research*, Summer 1976, 408-432.

C. Gaus and F. Hellinger, "Results of Hospital Prospective Reimbursement in the United States", presented at the International Conference on Cost Containment, Fogarty Center, Bethesda, Md., June 3, 1976.

P. Ginsburg, "Inflation and the Economic Stabilization Program" in M. Zubkoff (ed.), *Health: A Victim or Cause of Inflation?*, New York 1976.

C. Havighurst, "Federal Regulation of the Health Care Delivery System," *University of Toledo Law Review*, Spring 1975, 577-616.

E. Hughes *et al.*, "Surgical Work Loads in a Community Practice," *Surgery*, March 1972, 315-27.

______ *et al.*, "Utilization of Surgical Manpower in a Prepaid Group Practice," *New England J. Med.*, October 10, 1974, 759-63.

E. Keeler, D. P. Morrow, and J. Newhouse, "The Demand for Supplementary Health Insurance or Do Deductibles Matter?" RAND paper R 1958-HEW, Santa Monica, Calif., July 1976.

J. R. Lave and L. B. Lave, *The Hospital Construction Act: An Evaluation of the Hill-Burton Program 1948-1973*, Washington, D.C. 1974.

T. Marmor, "Politics of National Health Insurance," *Policy Analysis*, Winter 1977, 25-48.

H. G. Mather *et al.*, "Acute Myocardial Infarction: Home and Hospital Treatment," *British Med. J.*, 1971, 334-38.

J. Newhouse and V. Taylor, "How Shall We Pay for Hospital Care," in C. M. Lindsay (ed.), *New Directions in Public Health Care*, San Francisco 1976.

C. Phelps and J. Newhouse, "Coinsurance and the Demand for Medical Services," RAND paper R-964-1-OEO, Santa Monica, Calif. October 1974.

U. E. Reinhardt, "Health Manpower Policy in the United States: Issues for Inquiry in the Next Decade," unpublished paper presented to the Bicentennial Conference on Health Policy, University of Pennsylvania, November 1976.

M. Roemer and W. Shonick, "HMO Performance: The Recent Evidence," *Health and Society*, Summer 1973, 271-317.

C. Schultze, "The Public Use of the Private Interest: Excerpts from the Godkin Lectures," *Harpers*, May 1977, 43-50.

T. Schelling, "Government and Health," in C. M. Lindsay (ed.), *New Directions in Public Health Care*, San Francisco 1976.

L. Thomas, "On the Science and Technology of Medicine," *Daedalus*, Winter 1977, 35-46.

J. Wennberg, "PSRO and the Relationships among Health Need, Elective Surgery and Health Status," *Perspectives on Health Policy*, Boston University Medical Center, 1975.

______ *et al.*, "Health Care Delivery in Main II: Conditions explaining Hospital Admission," *J. Maine Med. Assn.*, October 1975, 255-261.

A. Wildavsky, "Policy As Its Own Cause," unpublished working papers, Graduate School of Public Policy, University of California, Berkeley, December 1976.

______ "Doing Better and Feeling Worse: The Political Pathology of Health Policy," *Daedalus*, Winter 1977, 105-123.

Comment

Harold A. Cohen
Director, Health Services Cost Review Commission, State of Maryland

My comments are divided into two parts. In the first part, I comment on the statements that lead Stuart Altman and Sanford Weiner to conclude that regulation is coming. Next, I discuss implications for hospital regulation to be drawn from other regulated industries and apply those thoughts, as the authors did, to the administration's Cost Containment Bill.

First, I would like to give an example of the practical use of second best theory in hospital regulation since several people in the audience might not understand it. Assume a planning agency drew up a hospital bed capacity plan which calls for 300 less beds in the north central part of an area and 300 more beds in the northwestern part of the area. This is the "first best" hospital delivery system. Assume the planners have no authority to close 300 north central beds. Now there is an application to open a 300 bed hospital in the northwest. Second best theory says that even though approval would move the system closer to the "first best" design, having all 600 beds might be worse than just keeping the "wrong" 300 beds.

I agree with the authors' comments that increases in cost per day don't simply represent inflation and that a principal factor further increasing costs is additional intensity. Further, I agree that much of what we choose to consume is not worth the money—but it doesn't follow that we spend too much.

The authors cite the literature which suggests that the "wage rate catch up" does not explain a great deal of the accelerated rate of hospital costs. The policy conclusions they seem to support do not follow even if the conclusion is correct.

Altman and Weiner review some of the reasons why the competitive model will not work in the medical sector. These areas, consumer ignorance, provider generated demand, insurance—especially first dollar coverage—have been evaluated in other papers and I won't discuss them. The authors discard, I think correctly, a voluntary shift to an HMO-dominated delivery system, but it should be given a chance without having to compete with a subsidized fee-for-service system. The authors then state that this will inevitably lead to some form of public regulation (due in part to the misconceived rate of inflation). Note that this is a political conclusion. There is no finding that regulation is a second best. Indeed, given the way physicians totally dominate all Government established regulatory methods directed at them, one might postulate that regulation is a "first worst."

I wondered why the authors didn't spend more time analyzing the other alternatives for second best (such as *laissez faire* with and without buttressing by the antitrust laws, Government ownership (i.e., socialized medicine), etc.). Mark Pauly's opening paper suggests why. There is no a priori way to demonstrate which of these alternatives is the second best.

By the way, the insurance problems could be handled in at least one interesting way under more Government ownership. The Government could provide everyone with indemnity insurance sufficient to pay for the least expensive level of service which can satisfactorily treat each illness. No supplementary insurance would be allowed. This would make everyone 100 percent self-pay on the margin and eliminate the access problems associated with large co-insurance and deductibles. I don't throw this out as politically possible, but to point out that it is at least possible that the major problem with much health insurance may not be the first dollar coverage but rather the last dollar coverage. You might want to consider this as a variant of a voucher system.

I cannot debate the authors on their political prognostication that more regulation is coming whether it's good or bad. I appreciate the feeling of job security it gives me. But I can discuss some of the suggestions the "litany of sins committed in the name of regulation" suggests for analyzing the Administration bill.

First, I agree that "the effectiveness of regulation can be greatly enhanced by a strategy designed to change those incentives which influence hospitals, physicians and local regulators." Indeed, I would argue that the principal function of regulators is to set parameters which the market would otherwise set and a climate for the providers to compete within those parameters.

For example, one outcome expected in a competitive market is for the marginal products of capital and labor to be proportional to their prices. Traditional rate-of-return oriented regulation leads to a higher capital/labor ratio. Will we reach the "ideal" in the "non-profit" hospital sector? Not with a system which allows wage rate pass throughs and limits capital to $2,500,000,000 nationally. We will have a reverse Averch-Johnson effect of magnificent proportions—especially since Commission data show hospital wages are already above market rates for identical job classifications in many parts of the country.

The Administration bill seems to assume that hospital capital and labor are never substitutable. That is very wrong. Indeed, proprietary hospitals have been shown to have higher capital/labor rates (and less of each) than non-profit hospitals.

I agree with the authors that the incentives should tend to lessen the quantity of ancillary tests and prospective revenue per admission (or per day) would provide that incentive; but the incentive in the bill is to lease out ancillary departments. Further, the variable cost volume adjustments should provide at least neutrality regarding the number of admissions.

The authors cite regulators' concern for quality, but don't discuss any meaningful way of using it.

One complaint about regulation involves the capture theory. The regulated firms are always presenting information to the regulator. In the hospital sector there are payers which might well become involved in hearings before the regulator; the most obvious example is Blue Cross and the Health Insurance Association of America. As Mark Pauly argued in his paper presented to the conference, it may well not pay an individual commercial insurance carrier or an individual Blue Cross carrier to seek to reduce hospital costs through this process. This is because cost savings would be shared with their competitors. The concerted participation by such payers should be viewed as a legitimate trade association activity by the Federal Trade Commission. Further, it should be noted that the Administration's proposal does not allow for such input by payers. A hospital may request an exception to the cap on payment per admission. If granted, that exception is binding upon Blue Cross and commercial insurance companies. If the Secretary denies the hospital's request, the hospital may appeal. Symmetry and fairness require that payers should have the right to appeal if the Secretary approves the hospital's request and payers should have an opportunity to provide input to the Secretary while he is making his decision. Regulators must be as responsible to the paying public when they say "yes" as they are responsible to the providers when they say "no."

The idea of opportunity cost is central to almost all important microeconomic ideas. Health planners traditionally do not recognize opportunity costs. Title II of the Administration's program as supported by Altman and Weiner would, in part, make planners recognize opportunity costs within the health sector. The Secretary, in determining the total amount of capital for health care construction on the national level, would have considered opportunity costs outside of the health sector. Title II does not require planners to consider the operating costs implications associated with capital projects. Capital is treated as a complement to labor, never as a substitute. Planners should not be indifferent between two capital projects one of which will save considerable labor costs while the other will cause considerable additional labor costs.

In summary, the authors do not present a case to show that regulation is a second best and argue for a form of regulation which, while sound in general terms, can be improved upon substantially.

REFERENCE

H. Averch and L. L. Johnson, "Behavior of the Firm under Regulatory Constraint," ***Amer. Econ. Rev.,*** **Dec. 1962, 1052-69.**

Guilds and the Form of Competition in the Health Care Sector*

Lee Benham
Associate Professor, Economics and Preventive Medicine,
Division of Health Care Research, Washington University

For many, the term competition is virtually synonymous with market competition. This notion is unfortunate because it often carries the implication that non-market solutions are not competitive and thus avoid undesirable consequences associated with (market) competition. It is clear that manifestations of competition differ depending on the nature of property rights and the mechanisms of social control, but whether these alternative forms of competition are less intense or more desirable cannot be determined a priori. In this paper, some implications of alternative forms of market intervention in the medical sector are explored by examining first the consequences of earlier interventions and then some parallels with modern reforms.

The alleged market failures in the medical sector are several. Perhaps the most common argument for market intervention is that because of the nature of medical care individuals cannot be wise consumers. The differential in knowledge between experts and consumers is allegedly great. Without severe restraints on market competition, patients would be exploited to their financial and physical detriment.

The externalities generated by the consumption of medical services are another concern. Communicable disease creates a conventional externality. In addition, even if consumer ignorance is not alleged to be a major problem, individuals may prefer a society in which others are constrained in their choice of medical services. Choice is often constrained through taxes (e.g., cigarettes and liquor) or through provision in kind (e.g., housing, food stamps, schools). In similar fashion, individuals may view the consumption of medical care by others in certain forms as undesirable. From one

---

* Many of the ideas in this paper reflect Reuben Kessel's influence. See in particular his article, "The A.M.A. and the Supply of Physicians," *Law and Contemporary Problems*, Spring 1970, 267-283.

perspective, constraining individuals to one choice of medical care is egalitarian, even if the care is not very good.

An institutional form of long standing has been available to deal with many such problems of quality control, consumer ignorance, and the unsavory commercial aspects of market competition: the guild. For centuries guilds have provided a widely accepted method of social control. Common types of problems which the guilds have sought sufficient authority to control are illustrated in a petition by the London Clockmakers in 1622.

"First, . . . [the clockmakers'] art is not only by the bad workmanship of strangers disgraced, but [the clockmakers are] disenabled to make sale of their commodities at such rates as they may reasonably live by.

"Secondly, for that divers strangers inhabiting in and about London do usually go to gentlemen's and noblemen's chambers and other places to offer their works to sale, which (for the most part) being not serviceable (the parties buying the same for the outward show only, which commonly is beautiful), are much deceived in the true value, which rests in the inwork only, and cannot be amended or by the Buyers perceived.

"Thirdly, . . . through the buyer's unskillfulness and the fugitiveness of the sellers, divers persons of worth have been utterly deceived of their money by strangers under colour of fair words and promises.

"Fourthly, . . . said strangers . . . grow so bold to intrude upon the privileges of this kingdom, that is not only to take apprentices with money for few years, but also to keep open shop, and those apprentices never being able to be made good workmen by them, the said strangers . . . leave those apprentices to make most unserviceable work, whereby the said art is not only disgraced but the buyers much abused and deceived."[1]

Similar themes run across the centuries. Many abuses decried by the clockmakers were alleged to exist in the practice of medicine in the United States at the turn of the century. There existed little professional or governmental control over medical education or medical practice at that time. Many medical schools were proprietary. Entry into medical school was relatively easy and the number of physicians per capita was large and growing. Wide variation existed in the type of medicine practiced, and consumers were alleged to be frequent victims of incompetents and quacks. Physicians were not doing well financially.

An assessment of the existing state of affairs and some suggested remedies were provided by the Flexner Report in 1910. To anyone with knowledge of guilds, the themes of this report sound familiar. Flexner argued that "quality" variation in medicine was unacceptable and that quality control could be maintained by requiring a specific production function in medical education with Johns Hopkins as the model. The report proposed that certified schools incorporate the Johns Hopkins model of medical education and that graduates of uncertified schools be prohibited from taking State licensing examinations. The recommendations were quickly adopted by the State medical boards.

The consequences of these changes were several. Medical education became longer, more expensive, and much more uniform. The number of medical schools and medical students declined. The shift in control over education and entry to the profession dramatically altered the basis on which individuals competed to enter medical school. For example, the shift from proprietary to nonproprietary medical schools and the increased curriculum and laboratory requirements resulted in a growing gap between costs and tuition revenue. This reduced the incentive of schools to offer medical training and to cater either to the demands of prospective students or to consumers of medical services. Tastes and preferences of key decisionmakers in medical societies and among medical school faculties became more important. The number of black medical schools fell from seven to two and the number of women in medical schools did not reach pre-Flexner levels in absolute numbers until after 1940.

Changes in the number and composition of individuals training to become physicians were surely not the result of radical change in preferences of consumers, prospective students, or even the decisionmakers in the medical sector. Reduction in the number of new graduates was a *sine qua non* of the Flexner reforms, and it should not surprise us that the successful members of the subsequent queue looked remarkably similar to those making the admissions decisions. Those excluded—women, blacks, and immigrants—were generally less troublesome to exclude, since they were less well connected. To modern eyes, the list of inequities is long.

The Flexner reforms brought about other unfortunate changes. Among these was a reduction in the incentive and opportunity for innovation in medical education. Most organizations introduce major innovations only where there is strong impetus to do so; it usually requires the prospect of a large gain to the relevant decisionmakers or the prospect of bankruptcy. Subsequent to the Flexner Report, the more prestigious medical schools could innovate without fear of sanction from the licensing authorities, but had little incentive to do so. Those organizations which would normally have the greater incentives to innovate, new schools or less prestigious schools attempting to move up, were severely limited in what they could do. Deviation from the officially sanctioned curriculum was risky for these schools, both directly, since they were vulnerable to decertification, and indirectly, because their graduates had to pass the official examinations, which in turn were based on the standard curriculum.

For many decades subsequent to the report there was little innovation in the character of medical education. This lack of innovation did not reflect a body of evidence that the Flexner model produced the most effective physicians. Indeed, comparisions between respected (or at least licensed) members of the association were discouraged, especially if such comparisons were to be made public. The notion of comparing the effectiveness of physicians trained in different schools violates the guild or professional notion that a uniformly high standard of service is always provided.

Thus, even if successful innovation were undertaken, it is unlikely the evidence documenting the success would be collected. Even if evidence were available showing a program to be superior, the evidence could well remain private information. Finally, even if the effectiveness of a new program were clearly demonstrated and widely disseminated, little incentive existed for relevant decisionmakers to respond. Had fundamentally different modes of training and practice been permitted, the incentives to generate and disseminate information about the effectiveness would have been greater, since survival of a particular mode would depend in part upon demonstrated success. It is difficult to imagine having less information about the efficacy of different modes of practice.

Lest I be misunderstood, I am not saying that the changes associated with the Flexner Report were without benefit. These changes did provide strong incentives for certain types of biomedical and clinical innovation. Heavy emphasis was placed on biomedical and clinical evidence concerning the efficacy of surgical and pharmaceutical intervention. The competition to provide new innovations in this area has been intense, and great strides have been made. Those responsible can take satisfaction from the progress in this area. However, the competition to translate the biomedical breakthroughs into effective medical practice has been considerably less intense. Even less attention has been given to problems of patient compliance and to improving patient knowledge as a mode of therapy. Practicing physicians' knowledge of nutrition has been notoriously limited as has been understanding of and interest in ways to improve patients' knowledge. The very definition of success reflects the underlying nature of competition. The issues are not merely technical—how do we perform better surgical procedures for problem X—but they reflect our priorities, our concerns about likely social and medical complications, the costs, the likelihood of compliance, the patient's preferences, and so forth.

The form of competition was fundamentally altered by the Flexner changes. In my view we have paid a heavy, although largely undocumented, price for that reform. Medical education and medical practice were cast in a particularly narrow mode by that reform and only in recent years have some schools become moderately innovative. The effects of the Flexner Report were not limited to the character of medical education. The controls over entry established in this and other similar cases appear to have altered dramatically the terms on which additional controls were introduced. The initial licensing process can be viewed as a technological innovation which reduces the cost to the profession of obtaining additional controls. At the same time, the incentives to introduce additional controls are increased; thus other controls are almost inevitable once control over entry is established. Establishment of jurisdictional lines becomes essential, for of what benefit is licensing if the non-licensed can practice? At the same time there is pressure to expand jurisdictions and to limit sharply encroachment by others.

Technological innovation presents another threat. Any guild will be alert to that type of innovation which is likely to have an impact on the demand for its services and will develop mechanisms to respond to undesired changes. While distinctions are not precise, innovations which improve the "quality" of service are more likely to be encouraged. These innovations are almost always consistent with and supportive of the overall objectives of the guild or profession. Indeed, a useful professional definition of an improvement in quality is that type of innovation encouraged by the profession. For example, innovations requiring more highly specialized and longer training are usually acceptable, as are innovations which are more expensive. Clear-cut pharmaceutical improvements like penicillin are certainly not resisted. There are, however, a wide range of innovations which are resisted. Innovation in the organization of the practice of medicine would be viewed with great suspicion for several reasons. Organizational innovation could lead to an increased division of labor, greater emphasis on cost effectiveness, increased competition among providers, and increased catering to the demands of patients. Organizational innovation could also reduce demand for providers' services and increase competition among providers—all undesirable from the viewpoint of providers collectively.

It is in this connection that the role of the entrepreneur becomes a matter of concern. The entrepreneur who has claim to residual profits has incentives to encourage specialization and organizational innovation, both of which are likely to reduce the role of and demand for professional or guild services. Maintenance of jurisdictional lines and guild or professional control is greatly facilitated if the role of the entrepreneur is sharply limited. This applies particularly to entrepreneurs outside the association, but also to those potential entrepreneurs who are licensed members of the profession. In this regard many professional regulations explicitly define the type of contract under which members can be employed and also limit the number and types of their employees. The arguments in defense of this are the same as those used originally to limit entry and to permit professional or guild control; namely, that competition among providers should be kept at a minimum and the expert provider should judge the extent of specialization. Thus, organizational innovations which move the locus of control away from the professional society and the individual licenses practitioner are likely to be resisted. The resistance by medical associations to prepaid group practice may have reflected some of these concerns.

Among the most important consequences of these guild-like controls are the altered incentives to produce and disseminate information. Guild systems are defended largely on grounds that consumers are ignorant and cannot make wise decisions. Yet, these organizations themselves go to considerable lengths to limit consumers' knowledge. As an example, the code of ethics of the American Dental Association states:

> It is unethical for a dentist to give lectures or demonstrations before lay groups on a particular technique (such as hypnosis) that he employs in his office.
>
> It is unethical for specialists to furnish so-called patient education pamphlets to general practitioners for distribution to patients where pamphlets, in effect, stress unduly the superiority of the procedures used by specialists. Publication of such so-called patient education material has the effect of soliciting patients.[2]

As another illustration of the importance placed on information constraints, consider the example of an occupation which has worked hard and successfully at following the pattern set by physicians: the optometrists. Excerpts here are taken from the 1969 rules and regulations of the Michigan Optometric Association:

> Eligibility for membership in the Michigan Optometric Association is based upon a point system. Initially, 65 points will be the minimum required for membership application.
>
> Members entering the association with fewer than 85 points must improve their point count standing a minimum of five (5) points *each* calendar year until at least 85 points are achieved. Thereafter, a minimum of 85 points must be achieved yearly to maintain membership.[3]

The point evaluation plan of this association, in condensed form, is as follows:[4]

	Total points possible for
Not advertising (refers to media advertising, telephone book listings, and window displays)	30
Location in a professional or office building as opposed to "an establishment whose primary public image is one of reduced prices and discount optical outlet"	25
Limiting office identification sign to approved size and content	15
Educational activities (professional meetings and activities)	14

Physical facilities (rooms and laboratory)	8
Functional facilities (equipment)	8
	100

Note that information constraints account for 70 out of the 100 possible points.

Providers benefit from such restrictions in that competition is reduced, but at the same time benefits from introducing certain cost-reducing efficiencies are also reduced. Where economies of scale exist in provision of a given service, it is necessary to attract a large clientele to take advantage of these scale economies. Without advertising to inform consumers of the cost savings, such innovation is often precluded. There is limited information on the magnitude of these effects, but Alexandra Benham and I estimated the effects of limits on information in the eyeglass market by comparing States with more and less strict controls on information. The prices were on the order of 25 percent or more higher in States with stricter controls.[5]

There are, of course, aspects to the information question other than advertising. Meaningful information about the quality of individual providers and the efficacy of alternative forms of therapy is difficult to obtain. Some information can be obtained from friends, personal experience, or trade names—for example, the Mayo Clinic. But for most people, most of the time, meaningful information is scarce. In this regard perhaps one of the most important inequities is the differential in knowledge which individuals have concerning their sources of medical care.

Ironically, the dearth of information about the efficiency of alternative methods and providers is itself partly a reflection of the desire to have uniformly good medical care. If a uniformly high quality of service is promised, and promised partly as a benefit of reducing competition among providers, then we can hardly expect to be given information about the differential abilities of the providers or comparative studies on institutional performance. Quite the contrary. Great effort will be expended to see that such information is not collected, and if collected not made public. The system has been around a long time and the rationale is widely accepted. It reflects a rather curious notion that as long as individuals remain uninformed about actual (or potential) alternatives, a sense of equity will prevail. The situation reminds me somewhat of the communist countries' method of dealing with unemployment. By definition there is no unemployment, so no unemployment statistics are collected.

Here I am not discussing the conventional question of whether individuals have access to a physician and how often that physician is seen. I am rather concerned about the difficulties a knowledgeable and sophisticated consumer has in determining the correct course of action in obtaining medical service. Many uncertainties cannot be reduced by more information, but the incentives in the system currently operate against providing accurate information about the uncertainties which do exist, or the information necessary to diminish those uncertainties which can be reduced, or information necessary to reward the good provider and penalize the bad.

Two examples will illustrate the point: First, guild members are generally encouraged not to criticize the services of another member publicly. Members are encouraged to deal with problems of other providers quietly and professionally. Consider a typical example of a professional code of ethics which states under the heading "unjust criticism":

"The dentist has the obligation of not referring disparagingly, orally or in writing, to the services of another dentist to a member of the public. A lack of knowledge of conditions under which the services were offered may lead to unjust criticism and to a lessening of the public's confidence in the dental profession. If there is indisputable evidence of faulty treatment, the welfare of the patient demands that corrective treatment be instituted at once and in such a way as to avoid reflection on the previous dentist or on the dental profession."[6]

A second example of the problems individuals have in obtaining information about medical practice is illustrated in a study by Nancy Ordway. She went to considerable effort to locate some of the most incompetent physicians in the United States. Some of the cases were notorious. She then attempted to find out what she could do about these physicians through normal channels, including the Illinois State Licensing Board, the Illinois State Medical Society, and the American Medical Association. Neither the Illinois State Medical Society nor the State Licensing Board would release information.

Inquiries to the American Medical Association's Department of Physician Information brought forth no derogatory information about the practice of medicine even in the case of physicians who had had their licenses revoked. Information on tax evasion and fraud was freely given. On reflection, it was probably unreasonable to expect a professional association to provide meaningful information about differences in quality of association members. But where can an individual obtain such information?

The guild method of social control exacerbates other problems it is supposed to cure. Our perception of what is the problem and what is an equitable solution largely determines the character of competition we favor in the medical sector. One way to characterize alternative forms of social control is by the problems that tend to be emphasized. Some problems emphasized by the guild approach have already been discussed. Extreme cases of failure or exploitation by non-licensed practitioners receive prompt and well-publicized attention. Contrast this with the attention given to a comparable failure by some respected (or at least licensed) member of the profession. Thus, by amplifying some issues and remaining quiet on others, the professions are in a strong position to influence the questions asked and the problems perceived. In particular, if the professional definition of the term "quality" is accepted, many of the restraints we observe imposed on competition are a foregone conclusion.

Let me illustrate an example of how information is selectively used. Alexandra Benham and I have done some analysis of the eyeglass field. One of the most frequently heard criticisms of our suggestion that advertising be permitted in this market is that quality of service will fall, that consumers will be exploited by bait-and-switch tactics, and that professional standards will be weakened. Spectacular examples are presented to buttress the case. Among my favorites is the story about the poor man in New York who, upon seeing glasses advertised for $15, went to the store. He ended up buying three pairs with gold-plated frames and a gold watch for a total of $1,500.

The introduction of advertising and more market competition into a market is alleged by the professional groups involved to have many undesirable consequences. The question is, how would we know? One method is to accept a professional assessment, but the problem here is obvious. Many professional standards are violated with increased market competition, and, consequently, by these standards "quality" must be lower. Some objective measures of performance could perhaps be developed and applied, but, again, the tests developed are very much a function of which standard is applied. Another approach is to look at the number and character of consumer complaints. This method is not without its flaws because of the way in which complaints are collected by the State regulatory boards. The likelihood that an individual with a particular problem will file a formal complaint depends in part on the encouragement that the individual receives from other sources of care.

The system of complaints is thus open to some indirect manipulation. It is with reservations that I accept the number of complaints filed with the State boards as an unbiased indicator of the true number of complaints. Nevertheless, it is of interest to examine what happened when price advertising was begun in Florida last year. Complaints registered at the State board went up. Keeping in mind the caveats listed above, quality declined by this standard.

Recently, however, an alternative standard was applied to this question. A study undertaken by Douglas B. Campbell and Thomas Borzilleri for the National Retired Teachers' Association and the American Association of Retired Persons examined the response of a sample of 2,564 retired persons in Florida to the law change permitting price advertising of eye glasses.[7] Only 1 percent of those surveyed did not wear glasses. Fifty percent of the membership strongly approved of the practice of price advertising by opticians and an additional 30 percent approved. Only 4 percent disapproved. Members of these groups obviously feld they benefited from this information.[8]

To get at the quality issue, Borzilleri and Campbell devised a simple but clever test by asking the respondents, "All things considered, the next time you buy eyeglasses or contact lenses, would you return to the same place where you bought your last pair?" Their responses were then matched to another question which asked if the place of last purchase advertised prices. The issue "Are consumers more dissatisfied with opticians which advertise?" was thus answered. "The results show that while 58 percent of the customers of non-advertising opticians indicated a willingness to give the seller repeat business, 86 percent of the advertisers' customers indicated they would return . . . only 8 percent of the customers of advertising opticians said that they 'probably' or 'definitely' would *not* go back. *A full 25 percent of the customers of non-advertising opticians gave the same answer."*

"In brief, if there is a quality problem it is not with advertising opticians. Rather it would appear that it lies with those who refuse to advertise their prices." [9]

These results are noteworthy in themselves; and also because they run counter to the officially maintained complaint record.[10] These results do indicate the need for a certain wariness toward professionally chosen indicators of quality.

A second striking feature about this study is that it is one of the very few times consumers have been given an opportunity both to experience a change in regulations and to say how they like the change. Such experiments are remarkable for their absence. In a more sensibly organized medical sector, experiments could be undertaken regularly with a subsequent sampling of consumer responses. I am uncomfortable with the notion that these collective decisions would form the basis of policy, but if quality standards are to be used as a basis for giving consumers "all or nothing" choices, then I think such experiments are needed.

While some of the most undesirable features of the guild system in the medical sector have been modified, the guild philosophy is still accepted in our attitude toward the role of competition, production and dissemination of information, and consumer choice. Furthermore, the incentive structure of the government regulatory agencies is in many ways similar to that of the guilds. For example, the definition of quality used to frame policy is often similar to, if not identical with, that used by the professionals involved. How often does a government agency resist a new regulation which will improve "quality"? How often are associated costs considered? How often are the competitive implications considered?

Pressures to expand regulatory authority at the expense of the market are considerable. It also appears to be the case, as with licensing, that once initial regulatory authority is set up, the imposition of certain types of additional control is greatly facilitated.

What can be done to improve the situation? Surely the comparative advantage of the Federal Government in this area is in providing information about the consequences of policies. A ridiculously small amount of useful information is available concerning the performance of individuals and institutions in the medical sector. I believe that any proposed rule change should be accompanied by some estimates concerning the price increases, the number of individuals likely to be adversely affected, and the number likely to benefit. I would also recommend that these estimated cost increases be attached to each licensing board or government bureau so that we know, not only how much tax money they are spending, but also how much their actions are costing. These costs could be compared with the benefits. The process is open to the usual perversions, but such changes would help shift the emphasis, if only slightly, to cost-reducing rather than cost-increasing innovations.

My own view is that we will probably have increasingly inefficient forms of competition, some combination of guild and bureaucratic competition, with the spoils going to those groups who can most effectively mobilize political support. If appropriate evidence were collected concerning the costs and distribution effects of these evolving forms of competition, I believe that most people, including those not ideologically committed to market solutions, would have reduced enthusiasm for these forms of social control. I am thus both an optimist and a pessimist. An optimist because I believe that the conflict of views concerning appropriate policy would be greatly reduced if the differences in outcome were more carefully documented. A pessimist because there is little incentive for the principal parties involved to undertake this analysis and a strong interest in continuing and expanding current policies.

NOTES

1. Joan Thirsk and J. P. Cooper, pp. 718, 719.
2. American Dental Association, p. 229
3. Michigan Optometric Association (1969)
4. Michigan Optometric Association (1969)
5. See Lee Benham and Alexandra Benham; and Lee Benham.
6. American Dental Association, p. 227.
7. Statement of the National Retired Teachers' Association and the American Association of Retired Persons, pp. 2, 3.
8. Statement of the National Retired Teachers' Association and the American Association of Retired Persons, pp. 3, 4.
9. Statement of the National Retired Teachers' Association and the American Association of Retired Persons, pp. 3, 4.

10. There is, of course, the question of what problems get filtered in and out of the formal complaint process by informal persuasion of various parties involved. That determination will require further study.

REFERENCES

L. Benham, "The Effects of Advertising on the Price of Eyeglasses," *J. Law Econ.*, Oct. 1972, 337-52.

______ and A. Benham, "Regulating Through The Profession: A Perspective on Information Control," *J. Law Econ.*, Oct. 1975, 421-47.

D. B. Campbell, "Attitudes of WRTA-AARP Florida Members Toward Eyeglass Purchase and Advertising," Planning and Research Department, National Retired Teachers' Association, American Association of Retired Persons, May 1977.

N. Ordway, "Does the Consumer Know, 'What's Up With His Doc'," Course Paper, Graduate School of Business, University of Chicago, 1974.

J. Thirsk and J. P. Cooper, ed. "The Clockmakers' Protest Against the Aliens, 1622" in *Seventeenth Century Economic Documents,* Oxford 1970, 718-719.

American Dental Association, "Principles of Ethics with Official Advisory Opinions, as revised November 1972", in Jane Clapp, ed., *Professional Ethics and Insignia,* Metuchen, N.J., 1974, 229.

Michigan Optometric Association, *Membership Point Plan Rules and Provisions,* 1-2, revised January 1, 1969.

Michigan Optometric Association, *Point Evaluation Plan,* (n.d.)

National Retired Teachers' Association of the American Association of Retired Persons on the Economics of the Eyeglass Industry before the Monopoly Subcommittee of the Senate Small Business Committee, U.S. Senate, May 24, 1977.

Comment

Anne R. Somers
Professor,
Department of Community Medicine and Department of Family Medicine,
College of Medicine and Dentistry of New Jersey-Rutgers Medical School;
Research Associate,
Industrial Relations Section,
Princeton University

Competition is generally the most desirable method of quality control, price-setting, and resource allocation. In theory, at least, the consumer has the final say, while producers or providers compete for his favor in terms of quality as well as price, thus maximizing the incentive to efficiency. Interference by Government or any other third party in the consumer-provider relationship is non-existent or minimal.

Even in the health care economy, with all its idiosyncracies, my philosophical bias is in the same direction. For years, I have urged greater attention to consumer choice and the prerequisite of intelligent choice, a well-informed and responsible consumer. As early as 1971, I spoke of the "uninformed consumer" as a "threat to any health care system," and listed "a national program of consumer health education" as Priority No. 1 in the reformulation of national health policy (A.R. Somers, 1971, pp. 80 ff.). In a new study that Herman Somers and I (p. 398) have just completed, we say that

> Responsibility for personal health rests primarily with the individual; not with government, not with physicians or hospitals, not with any third-party financing program. Meaningful national health policies must be directed to increasing, rather than eroding, the individual's sense of responsibility for his own health and his ability to understand and cope with health problems.

"Consumer sovereignty," in the economic sense, is clearly one important attribute of such an informed and responsible health consumer.

Second, I strongly agree with those economists who insist that quality and efficiency, as provider attributes, are not antithetical but complementary. I do not accept the claim, on the part of some physicians, hospitals, and other providers, that competitive pricing necessarily leads to poor quality. On the contrary, I believe that lack of concern with efficiency and price leads, more often than not, to lack of concern with quality, especially that essential ingredient of quality—appropriateness.

Third, I agree with those who criticize the performance of government as regulator of price and quality in the health care field. I oppose any tendency to jump blindly from the existing frying pay to the fire of doubtful public controls (A. R. Somers, 1977a, p. 138). The record indicates that government at all levels—Federal, State, and local—does not know how to regulate—or even how to "unregulate"—health care. Some agencies have the grace to admit they do not know. For example, I assume this conference is an admission of such ignorance on the part of the Federal Trade Commission!

Unfortunately for theory, however, there are all those special characteristics of the health care economy that vitiate the assumptions of a competitive market. Many have already been noted at this meeting. Two deserve special emphasis and are essential to my conclusions.

SOME SPECIAL CHARACTERISTICS OF THE HEALTH CARE ECONOMY

1. The peculiarities of the doctor-patient-hospital relationship mean that, for most of the health care economy, there is no such thing as a "sovereign consumer." Once the vertical consumer has become a horizontal patient, especially in the case of serious illness or disability, he ceases to be a consumer in the classical economic sense. The prevalence of third-party payment at this level of care is, of course, an important factor. But this statement would be generally true even in the absence of third-party payment. The typical patient, involved in tertiary or even secondary care, is usually in no position to engage in any financial bargaining. He has little or no ability to judge the quality or price of his care. His physician makes all the significant purchasing decisions: what diagnostic tests are needed, what therapeutic measures will be utilized, whether hospital admission is required and for how long, and what hospital will be used.

The doctor's role is particularly significant in relation to hospital care. No patient can be admitted to hospital on his own decision. The physician must certify to the need; he will determine what procedures will be performed, whether intensive care is needed, and when the patient can be discharged. Little wonder, then, that in the eyes of the hospital it is the physician who is the real "consumer." It is he who generates the hospital's revenues.

Although usually there are, in such situations, four identifiable participants—the doctor, the hospital, the patient, and the payer (usually an insurance carrier or Government)—the doctor makes the essential decisions for all of them. At least 75 percent of personal health care expenditures, and the purchasing decisions that determine these expenditures, are made by physicians, not patients. This includes not only expenditures for physicians services per se, but most hospital costs, a substantial portion of drugs and appliances, nursing home care, and other personal health care expenses. In such circumstances, to impose deterrent cost-sharing on patients, and to expect them to exercise informed and critical choice among various treatment modalities, is both unrealistic and unfair.

This is less true of primary care, however. Consumers can and do exercise some choice as to their primary care physicians, when and how often to see them, whether to join an HMO or not (if one is available), when and how often to request periodic health exams and other preventive procedures, what kind of eyeglasses to wear, whether and what over-the-counter drugs and vitamins to use and where to buy them. (Even in the area of long-term care, the patient and/or his family usually have more to say than in the case of acute-care hospitalization.)

Thus, in determining the feasibility of competition in the health care economy, it is essential to distinguish between two overlapping but distinguishable health care markets: (a) the market for primary care, and (b) the market for secondary and especially tertiary care. I will return to this distinction below.

2. The Government is already inextricably involved in virtually every aspect of decisionmaking. This involvement will inevitably increase as the implications of resource limitations become more obvious.

No matter how desirable it may be, theoretically, to keep decisionmaking entirely in the private sector, it is literally impossible to do so. I say this not only because of the historic need for some form of public safety controls, e.g., professional and institutional licensing; not only because of the historic need for some form of Government financing to assure universal access; but even more starkly today because we now know that the demand for health care in our type of society is virtually limitless, while resources—vast as they are in this multibillion dollar industry—must and do have some limits. Of the three major factors contributing to this demand—(a) the "technological imperative" inherent in modern biomedical science, (b) the three-way separation of decisionmaking, use, and payment, and (c) the blankcheck provider reimbursement principles sanctified in the Medicare "reasonable costs" and "reasonable charges" provisions—probably only the third is correctable. As a result, some form of rationing is inevitable.

To repeal the access programs we have already put in place is both morally and politically impossible—at least at the present time. There is no alternative but to use our democratic political institutions to try to develop as equitable and effective a rationing system as we can. It will not be easy; in fact, it may not be possible in a country that has become so permeated with the philosophy of limitless resources.

To recapitulate my theme thus far: Although an optimum economic model would keep Government out of the health care picture and rely on informed consumer choice to control price and quality, this is unrealistic in a situation where decisions determining the expenditure of three-fourths or more of the national health care dollar are made not by consumer-patients but by providers or third parties acting ostensibly on their behalf, and in a context of limited resources where it will be increasingly difficult to assure equitable access on the part of all Americans.

In such a situation, the intellectual debate over competition vs. regulation is essentially arid. I doubt if there is anyone in this room who would not prefer to minimize the role of Government and strengthen responsible private enterprise in the health care economy. The question is how to do so. The answer, or, rather, answers, cannot be ideological but will have to be highly pragmatic and will differ greatly among different sectors of the economy.

Let me hazard three broad propositions and follow each with a few specific suggestions.

THREE PROPOSITIONS

1. Competition can be meaningful, should be encouraged and, where necessary, protected, in one market—roughly one-fourth of the health care economy that has come to be known as primary care.

In this area, the vertical consumer-patient can generally make decisions for himself and exercise some meaningful choice. Policies that would help to maximize "consumer sovereignty" in this area include:

a. New emphasis on consumer health education respecting problems of personal health and illness and intelligent use of the delivery system. (The role of the Federal Trade Commission in discouraging "false and misleading advertising" in the cigarette industry could be of crucial importance in reducing the enormous toll of preventable disease resulting from smoking. This is also an area where economists might concentrate their ingenuity in the effort to develop financial disincentives to smoking.)

b. Resource-allocation and reimbursement policies assuring adequate attention to primary care, including prevention and long-term care. This calls for a substantial reordering of existing priorities, embodied in the benefit, as well as reimbursement, provisions of the pattern-setting Medicare program and most existing private health insurance.

c. Within the primary and long-term care fields, assurance of some consumer options as between various types of delivery systems; e.g., HMO's vs. fee-for-service, in-home services vs. nursing homes. In his area,

Government monitoring for attempts at "restraint of trade" will probably continue to be necessary.

d. Some cost-sharing at this level is probably acceptable. This should probably include some selectively heavy cost-sharing or deliberate non-coverage, on the one hand, balanced by cost-subsidies, on the other hand, of certain goods and services in accordance with basic health goals, e.g., *dis*couragement of promiscuous use of drugs and *en*couragement of selective cost-effective screening and counseling procedures.[1]

2. Competition can never be meaningful in that much larger health care market represented by secondary and tertiary care. Hence, a considerable degree of public regulation is unavoidable.

Given the fact that the hospital absorbs the largest portion of the health care dollar and that the physician is both the principal provider and the principal purchaser of hospital services, the regulatory effort has to be directed primarily at him and at the hospital. The main thrust of such regulation, however, should be to supplement and reinforce, *not* undermine, the highest ethical and professional commitments of the health professions and the hospital industry.

This means a large delegation of authority to the private instrumentalities to implement public goals and standards. It also means some acceptance of professional restrictions including restrictions on hospital privileges, in the interest of patient safety. However, this delegation and these quality restrictions must be within a context of clearly understood and clearly accepted public accountability. This concept, widely and loosely used today, is difficult and complex for both the public and private bodies involved. Speaking on the subject to a recent meeting of the American Psychiatric Association, I said (A. R. Somers, 1977b p. 959):

> The concept of "public accountability" involves, in my view, two essential ingredients: (1) genuine participation by private-sector professions and institutions in the formulation of public goals, and (2) a commitment to work toward such goals in a fiduciary or stewardship role, including an ongoing "accounting" to the public for this stewardship.
>
> Stated a little differently, the concept not only presupposes continued existence of the private sector, but a large degree of professional and institutional independence. The opposite side of the coin is that the professions and the institutions may expect to retain their private status only so long as they act as if they were public.
>
> This may seem a meaningless distinction but, to me, it seems very important. If we, in America, can achieve a combination of public goal-setting and private-sector implementation, avoiding

the evils of over-centralization and over-bureaucratization implicit in too much direct government control, we will have made a major contribution to the development of democratic self-government.

Public accountability might be likened to the "categorical imperative" propounded some 200 years ago by Immanuel Kant. At a time when philosophers were hotly debating the existence of God and the relevance of competing ethical principles, Kant concluded that, while this existence could not be proved, it behooved the prudent individual to conduct himself "als ob" or "as if" the universe were ordered in accordance with universally binding moral law.

The concept is particularly relevant and useful in the health field. Considerations of professional responsibility and public trust are deeply imbedded in the health professions and in hospital history. They are implicit in the Oath of Hippocrates and explicit in the state licensing laws. It is obvious that the government cannot take over and run the nation's health care system or even a single hospital without the cooperation of the majority of professionals involved. It is equally obvious, in this day of multi-billion dollar health care costs, that the private professions and institutions cannot function effectively without government participation and without implied acceptance of publicly-defined goals.

Pragmatically, we are already beginning to move in this direction with respect to resource allocation, quality, and utilization controls:

a. Resource allocation. Thus far, none of the Federal planning laws of the past decade has resulted in significant restraints on health care capital expansion. The industry is now over-capitalized and over-expanded. Restraints are urgently needed. But it is unrealistic to look to individual HSA's or State planning bodies to apply such restraints in the absence of a clear Federal mandate. The Carter administration's proposal for a $2.5 billion ceiling is one way of approaching this problem, although I would prefer to see the specific figure the product of negotiation rather than Federal fiat. And I doubt that there is any serious justification for the $2.5 billion. In the present context, we should start with an initial presumption of zero for any additional secondary or tertiary facilities or equipment.

Even more important is the mechanism for allocation and distribution of whatever figure is designated. For this purpose, I see no validity in the "provider" vs. "consumer" quotas currently mandated for the planning bodies. The meaningful adversarial relationship today is between primary and long-term care on the one hand and secondary and tertiary care on the other and between individual institutions within these categories. Obviously, all four modalities are needed but existing imbalances need correcting and the adversaries are incorrectly designated. Uninformed and unsophisticated consumers are not particularly helpful. The public interest would be better served by encouraging input from independent and knowledgeable individuals with a real stake in cost containment, regardless of provider or consumer background; e.g., board members of Blue Cross plans or HMO's, who are currently pretty much disqualified.

b. Quality. Despite some obvious shortcomings, which can and should be corrected, I believe that PSRO is essentially on the right track. The related malpractice controversy has also had some positive results which could be carried considerably further through joint public-private efforts.[2]

New initiatives are now needed with respect to certification and re-certification, licensure and relicensure, standards for and accreditation of educational programs for the health professions, including hospital residencies—the gateway to future specialization.

In all these areas, I believe the public interest will be better served by building on the strengths of existing organizations, such as the Joint Commission of Accreditation of Hospitals, the Coordinating Committee for Medical Education, the American Board of Medical Specialties, and the National Board of Medicare Examiners, rather than trying to discredit and undermine such bodies, some of which represent decades of dedicated efforts. To paraphrase Voltaire, if such organizations did not exist, they would have to be invented.

I do not claim that they are all disinterested or that they have done all that they should have done to protect the public interest. Obviously they have not. (Who of us has?) But I do say that the fault lies as much with the public sector as with the private: failure to define adequately public goals, failure to define adequately the mutual obligations of the two sectors, failure to implement public rewards and penalties in accordance with existing goals, failure to correct obvious inconsistencies and contradictions in public laws and regulations. What is needed is the development of clear, unambiguous codes or chargers of professional responsibility and public accountability governing the composition and conduct of these essential semi-public, semi-private bodies.

c. Patient cost-sharing, within practical limits, at the secondary and tertiary levels can have no significant deterrent effects and, I feel sure, will prove to be generally unacceptable. In so far as patients are subjected to unnecessary or inappropriate procedures or overlong hospital stays, according to PSRO and utilization review criteria, this form of malpractice can best be handled by denial of reimbursement.

3. A new approach to price-setting in the health care industry is needed. Competition does not and cannot work for the largest part of the industry. Unilateral rate-determination by the providers under the "reasonable costs" and "reasonable charges" formulas has brought us the intolerable inflation

of the past decade. Unilateral public rate-setting, imposed by Government on a single recalcitrant industry, is probably unworkable politically and possibly unconstitutional. Rate-setting by States, along the traditional public utility model, might produce some small deceleration in the recent rates of hospital cost inflation but such minimal gains do not appear to justify the considerable effort and expense involved, especially in view of the eventual federalization of Medicaid or its absorption into some form of NHI. The utility approach does not even address the issue of physician fees.

The ingredients most urgently needed to break the current impasse over cost controls are political acceptability to both parties and machinery for effective implementation. The instrument that seems most likely to meet these requirements is a set of *negotiated* rate and fee schedules, to be firm and binding on all purchasers for a fixed period of time (e.g., two years), arrived at through bilateral or multilateral negotiations between the principal representatives of the relevant provider groups and the major third-party purchasers of care, both public and private.[3] The numerous difficult technical questions involved in such bargaining, in a country of this size and in an industry of such complexity, would also be the product of negotiations. For example, the purchasers of care would probably find relative value scales necessary for the construction of equitable professional fee schedules as would the providers.

If ceilings or caps on the amount of annual increases in operating costs and in resource development are found to be necessary, these should also be the product of negotiations. In other words, both parties would be in on the take-off as well as the landing. Both would have tremendous stakes in the outcome of the negotiations, which is not now the situation under any current or proposed form of rate control. Some sort of quasi-judicial National Board of Review would be necessary as stand-by authority against a negotiating impasse and to assure due process on both sides.

I do not suggest that these three propositions offer an easy way out of our difficulties. I do suggest that they are not uncongenial to the thinking of some influential leaders of the health professions and therefore offer some promise of political viability.

The question before the American people today is not competition vs. regulation in the health care industry. The question is how to assure universal access to needed health services of good quality at a feasible price. We will never find the answer through ideology. We can only find it through a large-scale cooperative public-private effort, based on mutual respect, self-restraint, and a great deal of hard work on the part of all concerned. All of us—not just doctors, but economists, lawyers, administrators, whoever we are—should take to heart the Hippocratic injunction, "First, do no harm!" This means, among other things, do not play games with the lives of the American people.

NOTES

1. Lester Breslow and Anne R. Somers.
2. See Herman M. Somers.
3. See A. R. and H. M. Somers, 460-65.

REFERENCES

L. Breslow and A. R. Somers, "The Lifetime Health-Monitoring Program: A Practical Approach to Preventive Medicine," *New England J. Med.*, March 17, 1977, 601-608.

A. R. Somers, *Health Care in Transition*, Chicago, 1971.

———, (1977a) "Individual Comment," in American Hospital Association, *Hospital Regulation: Report of the Special Committee on the Regulatory Process*, Chicago, 1977, 138.

———, (1977b) "Accountability, Public Policy, and Psychiatry," *Amer. J. Psychiatry*, Sept. 1977, 959-965.

——— and H. H. Somers, *Health and Health Care: Policies in Perspective*, Germantown, Md., 1977.

H. M. Somers, "The Malpractice Insurance Controversy and Patient Care," *Health and Society/Milbank Memorial Fund Quarterly*, Spring 1977, 193-232.

Index

A

C

F

G

N

O

Q

W

Y

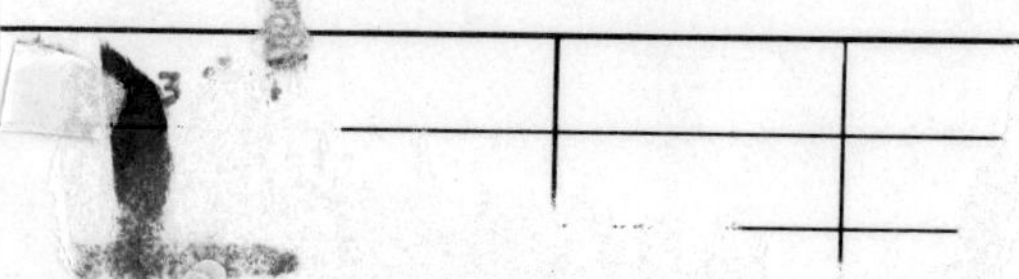